A Research Agenda for Biomedicine and Society

Elgar Research Agendas outline the future of research in a given area. Leading scholars are given the space to explore their subject in provocative ways, and map out the potential directions of travel. They are relevant but also visionary.

Forward-looking and innovative, Elgar Research Agendas are an essential resource for PhD students, scholars and anybody who wants to be at the forefront of research.

For a full list of Edward Elgar published titles, including the titles in this series, visit our website at www.e-elgar.com.

A Research Agenda for Biomedicine and Society

Edited by

ALEX FAULKNER

Emeritus Professor of Sociology, School of Global Studies, University of Sussex, UK

Elgar Research Agendas

Edward Elgar PUBLISHING

Cheltenham, UK · Northampton, MA, USA

Published by

Edward Elgar Publishing Limited
The Lypiatts
15 Lansdown Road
Cheltenham
Glos GL50 2JA
UK

Edward Elgar Publishing, Inc.
William Pratt House
9 Dewey Court
Northampton
Massachusetts 01060
USA

Authorised representative in the EU for GPSR queries only: Easy Access System Europe – Mustamäe tee 50, 10621 Tallinn, Estonia, gpsr.requests@easproject.com

A catalogue record for this book is available from the British Library

Library of Congress Control Number: 2025948516

This book is available electronically in the Elgaronline
Sociology, Social Policy and Education subject collection
https://doi.org/10.4337/9781035325511

Printed on elemental chlorine free (ECF)
recycled paper containing 30% Post-Consumer Waste

ISBN 978 1 0353 2550 4 (cased)
ISBN 978 1 0353 2551 1 (eBook)
ISBN 978 1 0353 8956 8 (ePub)

Printed and bound in the USA

Dedicated to researchers who care about our future

Contents

List of contributors

Erik Aarden is Assistant Professor at the Department of Society, Knowledge and Politics at the University of Klagenfurt, Austria. He has previously worked in Austria, Germany, the Netherlands, and the United States. He has done research on governance, resource distribution, and access in the context of medical research and technology in Europe, Asia, and the United States. His PhD dissertation focused on the integration of genetics in public health care delivery in three European countries. Much of his subsequent work has focused on the governance and operation of biobanks as medical research infrastructures.

Madeleine Akrich is Director of Research at Mines Paris – PSL (CSI-i3), France. She has devoted a significant part of her career to the development of a socio-anthropology of technology, with particular attention to the role of users. In a second phase, her interest has focused on the contribution of patients and people with health problems to the production of knowledge and expertise, whether through their participation in email groups or social networks, or in an organised setting within patient associations.

Andrew Bartlett is Research Associate in iHuman at the University of Sheffield, UK. His research is on the sociology of science, having worked on projects on the alcohol industry and on 'fringe' science, though he has been most prolific in studies of the contemporary life sciences. These have included work on the Human Genome Project, bioinformatics, psychiatric genetics, and advanced therapies. Themes common across these projects include questions of boundary work, interdisciplinary and extra-scientific collaboration, and the normative structure of different domains.

Edison Bicudo is Lecturer in the Department of Society and Politics at Aston University, UK. He is interested in the regulation, governance, digitalisation, and financialisation of health technology development. With a background in sociology, political economy, and geography, he also studies the ideological and cognitive underpinnings of health technology governance. His PhD focused on the cultural and economic impacts of international clinical trials. His book *Sociology, Cognition, and Linguistics* (2026) proposes a theoretical framework combining sociological interpretation and concepts from cognitive linguistics.

Stuart Blume is Emeritus Professor of Science and Technology Studies at the University of Amsterdam, the Netherlands. Educated at Oxford, he has worked at the University of Sussex, LSE, the OECD, and in the UK government, including in the Cabinet Office and as Research Secretary of the Black Committee on Social Inequalities in Health. He has been an adviser on bioethics to the World Federation of the Deaf, a 'Professor 2' at the University of Oslo, and a 'Prometeo' Fellow at the University of Cuenca (Ecuador). Key publications include *Insight and Industry* (1992), *The Artificial Ear* (2010), *Immunization: How Vaccines Became Controversial* (2017/2021), and *Immunization and States* (2021, co-edited). He writes regularly for *Psychology Today*.

Pascale Bourret is a former Professor at Aix-Marseille Université (SESSTIM), France. Her work focuses on the transformation of biomedical practices in connection to the development of genomic tools. She has published articles on bio-clinical collectives in the domain of BRCA testing, on regulation issues linked to new genomics tools, and on the emergence of genomic-driven clinical trials. Her recent work investigates the organisational and epistemic transformations surrounding the development of targeted therapies in the context of the development and implementation of precision oncology.

Alberto Cambrosio is Professor Emeritus of Social Studies of Medicine at McGill University, Montreal, Canada. His area of expertise centres on the sociology of biomedical innovation, with a focus on the application of genomics to the diagnosis and therapy of cancer. His publications include the following books co-authored with Peter Keating: *Biomedical Platforms. Realigning the Normal and the Pathological in Late-Twentieth-Century Medicine* (MIT Press, 2003; 2005 Ludwik Fleck Prize by the Society for Social Studies of Science) and *Cancer on Trial: Oncology as a New Style of Practice* (The University of Chicago Press, 2012).

Jorge Crespo Suarez is a PhD candidate at the Centre for Biomedicine, Self and Society at the University of Edinburgh, UK. He holds degrees in Psychology from the University of Havana and Public Health from the University of Melbourne. He works at the intersection of medical sociology and global health. His research explores how psychologists navigate the challenges of expanding care in Chile's public primary healthcare system. He brings extensive experience as a primary care psychologist in public healthcare settings, grounding his research on the sociology of psychology in everyday clinical realities.

Trang Do completed her PhD in Medical Anthropology at Monash University and currently works as a Senior Research Officer at Murdoch Children's Research Institute in Melbourne, Australia. Her work spans the disciplines of medical anthropology, global health, implementation science, health services research, and gender studies. Her research investigates how social and structural factors influence the way ill health is experienced among diverse population groups, particularly those in resource-constrained settings in low- and middle-income countries.

Alex Faulkner is Emeritus Professor of Sociology, School of Global Studies, at the University of Sussex, UK. His research has theorised the regulation, valuation, and uptake of technologies such as cell and tissue therapies, biomedical devices, PSA testing for prostate cancer, bioinformatics, and 3D bioprinting, variously in the UK, the EU, and India. His book *Medical Technology into Healthcare and Society: A Sociology of Devices, Innovation and Governance* was published in 2009 (Palgrave Macmillan).

He has recently investigated bio-therapies in elite sport and collaborated with a patient organisation to analyse Lyme disease policy in the UK. His current primary interest is in fiction-writing.

Amelia Fiske is Senior Researcher at the Institute for History and Ethics of Medicine at the Technical University of Munich, Germany. She holds a PhD in cultural anthropology from the University of North Carolina at Chapel Hill, US, and has been working in interdisciplinary bioethics contexts in Germany since 2017. Her work is situated at the intersection of cultural anthropology, science and technology studies, bioethics, and environmental justice.

Matt Hayler is Associate Professor in Contemporary Literature and Digital Cultures at the University of Birmingham, UK. Alongside Dr Danielle Sands and Prof Christine Daigle, he edits the Bloomsbury Academic series *Posthumanism in Practice*. He co-leads a scoping project on psychedelics and regulatory decision-making with Muireann Quigley and is also a UKCP trainee psychotherapist interested in the effects and potentials of new technologies for contributing to contemporary experiences of mental health.

Paul Martin is Professor of the Sociology of Science and Technology at the University of Sheffield, UK, and Co-Director of its flagship multidisciplinary research centre, the Institute for the Study of the Human (iHuman). His work sits at the interface of STS and medical sociology, and he is currently working on a major five-year project on high-priced 'orphan' drugs for rare diseases funded by the Wellcome Trust. In July 2024 he co-organised an international workshop on a Mixed Economy of Pharmaceutical Innovation which discussed many of the ideas in his chapter in this book.

Mianna Meskus is Professor of Sociology at Tampere University, Finland. She is also Director of the Tampere Centre for Science, Technology and Innovation Studies (TaSTI). Her research is situated at the intersection of sociology and feminist science and technology studies, with a specific focus on biopolitics, knowledge production, embodiment, and materiality. Current projects examine: biomedical shaping of reproduction and ageing; the processuality of 'sex' in biomedicine; animal experimentation and alternative research methods; and populations, ecological sustainability, and speculative futures.

Ingrid Metzler is Assistant Professor at the Division of Biomedical Ethics and Public Health Ethics at the Karl Landsteiner University of Health Sciences, Austria. She has been trained in Political Science and Science and Technology Studies. In her research, she engages with the ethical, social, and regulatory issues of emerging biotechnologies. Combining the framework of co-production with pragmatist lenses, she examines the situated moralities that shape uses of such technologies.

Maurizia Mezza is a PhD candidate in Anthropology at the University of Amsterdam, the Netherlands, and a Fellow at the Amsterdam Institute for Global Health and Development. Her research examines how vaccine safety evidence is produced post-commercialisation, with a focus on HPV and COVID-19 vaccines, gender, and intersectionality. She is affiliated with the Centre for Medicine, Information and Power at the Universidad Nacional de Colombia. In the non-governmental sector, she works on climate and health, particularly dengue and diarrhoea. Her interests include co-creative and transdisciplinary research methods.

James Mittra is Professor of Science, Technology and Innovation Studies in the School of Social and Political Science at the University of Edinburgh, UK. His research focuses on innovation and regulation of the health-related bioeconomy, with recent work on regenerative medicine exploring how advanced cell therapies navigate the difficult journey from bench to bedside. His work also critically engages with the concept of value (economic and non-economic) as it applies to public and commercial innovation processes.

Alan Petersen is Professor of Sociology, School of Social Sciences, at Monash University, Australia. He has expertise in the sociology of health and medicine, science and technology studies, and the sociology of emotions. His current projects include: a sociology of loneliness and digital technologies (funded by the Australian Research Council); a sociological study of safeguarding posthumous digital data (funded by ARC); and genomic governance (funded by the Medical Research Future Fund). His recent publications include: *Emotions Online: Feelings and Affordances of Digital Media* (Routledge, 2023), *The Handbook of the Sociology of Health and Medicine* (Edward Elgar, 2023), and *Pandemic Societies: A Critical Public Health Perspective* (Bristol University Press, 2024).

Martyn Pickersgill FAcSS is Chair of the Sociology of Science and Medicine at the University of Edinburgh, UK. He co-directs the Centre for Biomedicine, Self & Society, alongside the Wellcome Trust's 'One Health Models of Disease: Science, Ethics and Society' PhD Programme. His research explores the social, legal, and ethical dimensions of biomedicine. He is a member of the ESRC Strategic Advisory Network and the Scottish Science Advisory Council, and a recipient of the RSE Henry Duncan Medal.

Kiran Pienaar is Senior Lecturer in Sociology at Deakin University, Australia, with expertise in gender, sexuality and health. She is also Adjunct Senior Research Fellow at the Australian Research Centre in Sex, Health and Society (ARCSHS), La Trobe University, and an honorary Research Associate at Rhodes University, South Africa. She has published on topics related to gender, drugs, 'addiction', biopolitics and HIV. Her publications include a monograph titled *Politics in the Making of HIV/AIDS in South Africa* (2016) and an edited collection titled *Narcofeminisms: Revisioning Drug Use* (2023).

Barbara Prainsack is Professor at the Department of Political Science at the University of Vienna, Austria, where she works on the social, ethical, and regulatory dimensions of data-driven practices in biomedicine and the biosciences, as well as practices and institutions of solidarity in medicine and beyond. Barbara is also involved in policy-related work, for example, as Chair of the European Group on Ethics in Science and New Technologies, which advises the European Commission.

Muireann Quigley is Professor of Law, Medicine, and Technology at the University of Birmingham, UK, and Principal Investigator on the Wellcome Trust-funded Everyday Cyborgs 2.0 project. She has an interdisciplinary background that crosses medicine, ethics, and law. She leads a research project addressing the legal and philosophical challenges arising from the joining of persons and bodies with attached and implanted medical devices. She also co-leads a scoping project on psychedelics and regulatory decision-making with Matt Hatler. She is the author of *Self-ownership, Property Rights, and the Human Body: A Legal and Philosophical Analysis*, published by Cambridge University Press in 2018.

Vololona Rabeharisoa is Professor of Sociology at Mines Paris – PSL (CSI-i3), France. Her area of expertise intersects STS and health movement studies. She has explored the role of patient organisations in the production of knowledge and in the shaping of new forms of activism, notably around rare genetic diseases. Her recent work is on the involvement of patient groups in debates on pharmaceutical innovation and the pricing of advanced biotherapies like gene and cell therapies. She has extensively published on these topics.

Isabella M. Radhuber is Fellow of the transdisciplinary Academy (td-A), Research Fellow of the City of Vienna ('Wissenschaftsstipendium der Stadt Wien'), and Guest Research Scholar at the Equity and Justice Research Group (EQU), Population and Just Societies Program (POPJUS), International Institute for Applied Systems Analysis (IIASA), Austria. Her research interests include global inequalities, decolonisation, and resource distribution in the field of environmental and health politics, with a particular interest in the area of climate and health.

Margaret Sleeboom-Faulkner is Professor of Social and Medical Anthropology at the Department of Anthropology, University of Sussex, UK. For many decades, she has conducted anthropological research on social, economic, and regulatory aspects of the life sciences in East Asia and beyond. She has published profusely in the fields of academic nationalism and the social studies of reproductive technologies and regenerative medicine in China and Japan. Her latest book, *Regulatory Violence: The Global Dynamics of Regulatory Experimentation in Biomedicine and Health*, appeared in 2025 (Cambridge University Press).

Andrea Whittaker PhD, FASSA is Professor of Anthropology at the School of Social Sciences, Monash University, Melbourne, Australia. She is a medical anthropologist and Lead Researcher with the Centre to Impact AMR. Her work includes research on reproductive health and biotechnologies as well as social aspects of AMR. Her major publications include *Intimate Knowledge: Women and their Health in Northeast Thailand* (2000), *Women's Health in Mainland South-east Asia* ed. (2002), *Abortion, Sin and the State in Thailand* (2004), *Abortion in Asia: Local Dilemmas, Global Politics* ed. (2010), *Thai in Vitro: Gender, Culture and Assisted Reproduction* (2015), and *International Surrogacy as Disruptive Industry in South-east Asia* (2019).

Acknowledgements

First, I thank all the contributors to this book for their work on it – it has been a pleasure to take the project forward together.

I thank these colleagues for valuable reviews of drafts of chapters for the book: Madeleine Akrich; Edison Bicudo; Stuart Blume; Kathrin Braun; Tamara Hervey; Wen-Hua Kuo; Benjamin Marent; Paul Martin; Arima Mishra; James Mittra; Alan Petersen; Barbara Prainsack; Andrea Whittaker.

I thank Edward Elgar, especially Daniel Mather, for their support and helpful relationship during this project.

Finally, I thank my family, Margaret, Martha, and Ruth, for their support, good humour and tolerance.

Introduction: Navigating biomedical worlds

Alex Faulkner

The continuing incursion of biomedicine into healthcare and everyday life is fuelled by advances in scientific and bioengineering understandings of molecular, cellular, genomic and related biological processes. A myriad of new medical techniques and technologies are evolving through the biological sciences, the so-called 'life sciences' and software engineering. General scientific and technological trends propel these developments, including advances in informatics, digital data and AI. Biomedical technologies have been climbing up governments' policy agendas globally over the last 30 years, becoming part of political strategies to bring the 'bioeconomy' into being, for economic regeneration, industrial expansion and the advancement of human health.

These developments challenge deeply-embedded healthcare practices and organisational forms, clinical knowledge, definitions of diseases, standards of evidence for innovation adoption, professional and medical product regulation and people's experience of health and health services. Indeed, some technologies are seen to challenge the very definition of what it is to be human. At the same time, biomedical innovation has to grapple with societal and ethical concerns on issues such as health inequalities and disparities, institutional biases in access to care, 'global health', data sharing and privacy, citizen participation and citizen science, biosecurity and pandemic preparedness.

Societies worldwide are being exposed to a seemingly endless array of shocks to communities and healthcare systems, more or less long-lasting and with crucial consequences for biomedical and social science understandings. The SARS-CoV-2 (COVID-19; coronavirus) pandemic, atmospheric and water pollution and increasingly violent climate events are only the most obvious examples. Against this background, biomedical technologies have penetrated ever-deeper into our lives, everyday experiences and images of ourselves, both individually and in collective association. With the advance of genomics, and the associated proliferation of knowledge of biomarkers for disease presence or susceptibility, as the precision of testing increases, biomedical 'risk' never ceases to infiltrate our lives.

Whole new fields of biomedical endeavour, policymaking, research and commercial enterprise associated with these developments have been framed by interested stakeholders, including as 'Personalised medicine', 'Precision medicine', 'Regenerative medicine' and, possibly, 'Algorithmic medicine' (Marent et al., forthcoming 2026). The traditional fields of pharmaceuticals and medical devices adapt and incorporate innovations, for example in cell-based medicines, biosensors and AI/software-enabled medical devices, stretching the conventional boundaries of these industrial sectors and the corresponding regulatory regimes (Faulkner, 2012a). New classes of technology, such as 'Point-of-care' technologies and the European Union's 'Advanced Therapy Medicinal Products', become recognised.

Meanwhile and relatedly, there has been an increasingly obvious de-socialisation of social science scholarship. Not only has the human-made material world become seen as having agency or, at least, 'affordances' for action (Hutchby, 2001), but the perceived crisis of the natural environment and its human mediation are entering further and deeper into the theoretical repertoire, with the increasing salience of concepts of ecology, inter-species, relationality, flows, loops, process, entanglement and the like.

This book consists of invited contributions from a wide range of scholars from these fields with the aim of identifying approaches and societal aspects of biomedicine where the need for innovative, important and impactful research is evident. Social science and STS scholars are rising to meet the challenges posed by these innovations and must continue to do so. In the social sciences, scholarship around biomedicine is notable for the eclectic involvement of a range of cognate disciplines and fields of study, especially medical sociology, science & technology studies (STS), political science, social/medical anthropology, socio-linguistics and academic law.

Overall, the contributions here reflect the different contemporary approaches and perspectives noted above. Some chapters are relatively wide-ranging, focused on generic cross-cutting social/societal themes and concerns, while others are more focused on particular fields, though with broader application and theoretical implications. The chapters encompass a wide range of substantive health-related and biomedical fields, including pandemic vaccines; tissue and cell therapies; gene editing (CRISPR); pharmaceuticals; mental health app-based devices; diagnostics and biomarker tests, including reproductive genetic testing; bioprinting; climate change; cancer genomics; psychedelic therapy; and antimicrobial resistance (AMR) alternative therapy.

Below, I offer a selective view of key themes and highlights from the chapters, arranged in terms of three cross-cutting themes. Needless to say, the contributions do not fit easily into such pigeon-holes and readers are directed to the chapters themselves for their extensive detail and theoretical conceptualisation. Each chapter offers a range of issues, concepts and models that scholars in 'Biomedicine and Society' should build upon and take forward to better navigate, understand – and shape – the biomedicalised worlds that we unavoidably inhabit.

1 Multiplying and extending biosocial configurations

First, some of the chapters here testify to an extension and complexification of the biomedical world and societal responses to these developments. Emerging configurations are becoming wider, both spatially and socially, and longer elastically, ranging from prions and proteins to gene variants and epidemics and biospheres, connecting with and constituting novel societal, industrial and governmental organisational formations.

Radhuber et al. (Chapter 2) use the example of emergency flooding to illustrate the need for policies to support interdisciplinary research into the manifold health effects of climate change. There are clear impacts, such as on children's health that paediatrics must face; a 'climatological neuroepidemiology would probably bridge multiple fields and scales of analysis. It would merge insights from neurology, neurochemistry, environmental science, cognitive neuroscience and behavioural economics' (Gregory, 2023). Such study would also require the insights of sociology, STS, social anthropology and politics. The authors urge us to study especially the 'tertiary effects' of climate change, those that are modified by economic, political and social dynamics, such as poverty, resource scarcity and governance action itself. Scholars in biomedical STS should 'follow the climate', to adapt a well-known phrase, in all its ramifications.

The climate crisis is also affecting people's reproductive decision-making. As Meskus notes (Chapter 1), however, policymakers (in Norway, for example) might actively resist any discursive association between the climate crisis and a declining population. Meskus deals explicitly with an extensive scope ranging from molecular materiality to population-level dynamics, with the mediation and action of person-embodied processes and 'affective intensities'. Her material-feminist analysis shows 'life processes' being the object of scientific knowledge-derived governance that nevertheless encounters 'push-back' (my term) in the form of action 'encompassed and conditioned by … nonhuman but thoroughly social actors', such as IVF-related drugs.

Focusing on the pharmaceutical industry, Bartlett and Martin show how new actors are extending the social organisation of this arena, creating innovative production and business models. A 'new mixed economy' of pharma innovation and 'social pharma innovation' is emerging, involving patient groups, clinicians and third sector actors. A crucial aspect of this account is the extent to which 'unmet need' in public health, neglected by mainstream pharma, is being addressed in developments that hold some potential, at least, to do so. The authors provide a range of examples of new, promising configurations, and demonstrate the dimensions of an analysis that can be brought to bear on them. They call for a role for sociological research in supporting these seeds of re-formation.

A further form of bio-societal multiplication and extension can be seen in the realm of mental health, with the growing extension of psychiatry into the digital domain (Pickersgill and Crespa Suarez, Chapter 5). Drawing on sociologies of expectations, value and novelty, the authors trace the opinion-leading discourse that is propelling telepsychiatry towards digital device applications, showing both clinical resistance and promissory expectations around potential new psychiatric insights arising from digital deployment: 'psychotechnical novelty'. A range of issues, in tension, present themselves in shaping the promise of these developments: the presentation of psychiatric therapy online; 'clinical accuracy'; data privacy; monetisation; alternative psychopathological ontologies such as neurobiology vs. psychosocial models; empowerment vs. clinical responsibility; and the relative dominance or marginalisation of different key actors in the field.

2 Biopolitics of regulation and moralities

Biomedical innovation takes place in the context of an array of national and international laws, regulations and guidelines that try to anticipate innovations but are often seen to be playing catch-up. Regulation applies to many aspects of innovation, including experimental laboratories, clinical trials, data protection and 'post-market surveillance' of bio-products introduced to the market and healthcare systems.

Mezza and Blume in this volume shine light on the neglected field of pharmacovigilance, the collection of observational data on the performance of authorised, marketed products once in clinical application. They detail the poorly understood complexities of organisational and data systems set up by national and cross-national regulators. The field has been highlighted by controversies over the performance of novel vaccines for the SARS-CoV-2 virus pandemic. Side-effect data can typically be reported by healthcare professionals, but also by citizens/patients – ourselves. In the case of COVID-19, patient-reported issues, for example with menstruation, initially met with resistance from regulatory authorities. Mezza and Blume raise a plethora of research questions to better understand these issues: how do collections of reports trigger an 'adverse incident' warning to manufacturers and healthcare providers? How might public trust in pharmacovigilance systems be bolstered, and can vaccine hesitancy be reduced through this? Here, surely, is a prime case for a better 'public understanding of science'.

It is not easy to produce a novel, empirically based conceptual contribution in the overpopulated space of social science study of regulation in biomedicine, but Sleeboom-Faulkner does so in her critical, anthropological chapter here. Focusing on regenerative medicine trials in Asia and beyond, she shows how nation-states act strategically in international science collaborations, exploiting differences in national regulatory standards for clinical trials, leading to 'regulatory violence', where public health priorities are distorted by states' techno-economic ambitions, regulations are violated even within their own jurisdictions and actual harm to patients is foreseeably produced. Importantly, she shows how 'collaborations' typically hide a range of power imbalances, conflicting aims of scientists and clinicians, and ethical challenges for participant scientists, which warrant more public health-focused policy intervention.

Psychedelic substances have been enjoying a revival in attention as potential therapeutic interventions in the 2020s. Quigley and Hayler here provide an account of recent developments in regulatory assessments of trials and instances of some national authorities moving to adopt therapeutic models for psychiatric mental health, most notably Australia. The authors outline a series of challenges that the advocates of psychedelics face, ranging from the 'drug laws' of many jurisdictions and the dubious design and conduct of some crucial clinical trials (in the FDA, for example) to the simple availability of substances due to import/export rules. Psychedelics would typically be deployed in psychotherapy encounters, making for complicated issues for trialling, psychotherapy not being seen as straightforwardly falling within a pharmaceutical or device regulatory regime. Hence, the authors point to various problems of legitimacy that the psychedelic movement faces. Given that PTSD is associated with climate and other catastrophes, one might wonder if there will sometime be a role for therapeutic psychedelics here.

Moralities are often difficult to discern in regulatory and governance regimes and may be conspicuous by their absence rather than clearly stated (Faulkner, 2012b). In their chapter, Metzler and Aarden start to dig beneath the surface of governance regimes in the case of reproductive genetic technologies to unearth the seams of morality underlying them. Noting 'polycentric' regulation, they highlight the role of the private sector in carrying what they call 'biomoralities' into the health sphere. Biomoralities are often essentially competing with each other in shaping the direction of innovation and societal adoption of biotechnologies. The authors challenge us to consider how such direction might or might not 'do justice' to human nature expressed in societal values. Given Western democratic contexts, are communitarian and liberal moralities best serving the public health and the public good? What role can and should third sector actors play in the moral grounding of biomedical innovations?

3 Healthcare readiness, patienthood, bio-identities

The stabilisation of emerging, often controversial biotechnologies, both technically and institutionally, remains an enduring theme in social science scholarship of the biomedical domain. 'Technology identity' (Ulucanlar et al., 2013) has many dimensions shaping potential healthcare adoption and usership, as does the 'readiness' of healthcare organisations (Webster and Gardner, 2019). Likewise, the appearance of new bio-objects and bio-therapies can enable the formation of new social groupings, roles and identities – in the healthcare workplace, in research laboratory settings and among health-affected citizens.

The cancer immunotherapy, CAR-T, is analysed here by Mittra. Advocating the utility of concepts of 'process ontology' and 'craftwork' to understand this fragile technology, he examines the social and organisational conditions that might be needed – 'readiness' – for it to become established in healthcare practice. Interestingly, in analysing the very detailed biological-material-social logistics involved, Mittra shows how 'miscellaneous care' comprising relatively invisible, tacit 'ephemeral' working practices is essential to the adoption of this technology in a complex interweaving of multiple biosocial elements. Questions of valuation, patient selection and equitable access around this autologous therapy are also importantly raised.

A further example of a contested technology is analysed by Bicudo, deploying an innovative combination of sociological and linguistic analysis. How do metaphors and (less known) metonyms figure in the social organisation and political projects around a technology such as bioprinting (creation of bioactive therapeutic devices with live human cells by 3D printing), with its high degree of digital inscription? Bicudo shows how two alternate institutional modes of bioprinting are constituted through alternate linguistic strategies and hence world-views: an open-source model of communal innovation, largely, though not entirely, opposed by a business-oriented corporate model. Bicudo argues that ingrained alternate modes of embodied thought are mediated through these differentiated linguistic devices, provoking questions such as how not only linguistic but also visual metaphors and metonyms in mass media might be implicated in alternately constituted innovation pathways. Such an approach offers clear opportunities for application in other biomedical fields, as Bicudo outlines.

Echoing the 'extending configurations' noted above, multiplying socialities are also to be seen in the evolution of patient organisations: Akrich et al., with examples from France, discuss the emergence of new patient organisations and advocacy groups based around rare diseases, especially cancer-related genetic variations – 'oncogene-driven groups'. The authors' careful analysis suggests that such groups are not primarily identity-building but that novel biomedical entities are enacted as 'translational operators' to achieve medico-political goals of 'therapeutic actionability' that might alleviate suffering. Mobilising concepts of 'singularization' and 'mutualization' they show how such individualised, narrowly-focused associations are being developed and are brought into alliance with broader groups, seeking legitimacy in different ways. Not only are 'new kinds of partnership networks' produced, but even, provocatively, 'new kinds of people'.

What it means to be a patient, therefore, or indeed a citizen, is ever-evolving. Petersen and Pienaar's contribution here focuses on the relentless proliferation of new medical tests and biomarkers, which challenge these identities. In their overview, recognising that the social science study of testing is not new, they point to areas that require continuing and renewed attention. Adopting a broadly Foucauldian perspective on biopower, they raise the question of whether there is 'too much testing'. Genetic susceptibility, they note, is not related to diagnosis per se, and many diagnostic or 'screening' tests founder on the lack of corresponding treatments. Pointing to cases, among others, of ADHD, dementia and the discursive rhetoric of 'the obesity gene', and highlighting the competing actions of different – and differently powerful – stakeholders, the authors argue that such trends, boosted by the COVID-19 pandemic, are bringing the citizen experience of risk of, and actual, disease into closer proximity. So our citizenship and patienthood are embroiled in increasingly liminal sociobiomedical spaces. Should society find more ways of containing or shaping these proliferating trends?

Antimicrobial resistance (AMR) has become a very difficult phenomenon for healthcare policy worldwide and for patients who suffer its effects. Do and Whittaker here examine one therapeutic route taken by patients whose needs are not satisfied by routine care (in Australia). They show the individualised nature of help-seeking by patients suffering the multiple, often under-the-radar conditions associated with AMR, and focus on the 'medical travel' some patients undertake in search of alternative potential treatment, in this case phage therapy. Phage therapy is a controversial treatment among most clinicians (associated especially with a centre in Tbilisi, Georgia) but can in some jurisdictions be prescribed as an unlicensed medicine under compassionate use regulations. The authors point to the lack of any AMR patient group identity, given the wide variety of medical conditions that can be involved, and propose a need for support networks for the 'AMR survivor community'. As Will (2018) has suggested, the tension between health professionals trying to pursue careful 'antibiotic stewardship' and suffering patients might be ameliorated by better qualitative understanding of the meaning, causes and effects of different bacterial infections among patients themselves.

4 Forward-looking: Stretching concepts, magnifying focus

The scholarship in this book is testimony to the painstaking research and theorising efforts of the authors. The chapters contain multiple demonstrations and proposals for research that should be carried forward. They point to a number of trends for future research in the relations of biomedicine and societies worldwide.

In particular, we see efforts to acknowledge and understand the ever-increasing interrelatedness and interpenetration of the multitude of actors – human, biomedical and environmental – involved in human and planetary health. We see perspectives linking the cellular and the molecular with human population trends and with the continual social organising of healthcare, patients and citizens, and the reconfiguring of their relations. We see also, again in line with increasing interconnectedness and permeability of conventional boundaries, a move towards theorisation that grapples with the processual nature of biomedical entities and the 'work' (both metaphorical and literal) that social actors perform to understand, support but also stabilise and classify those fragile processes, to render them workable given the obduracy of their apparent affordances. Further, we see, and surely should support in judicious ways, the increasing involvement of citizens themselves in biomedical developments – as more or less responsibilised patients, but also as data-providers, actors shaping technology design, cell/tissue donors, charitable funders, advocacy collectives, DIY medical testers and more.

These developments imply some potentially radical re-thinking of various social and institutional boundaries. For example, does it still really make sense for social science scholars to speak simplistically of 'the pharmaceutical industry' with all its cultural and political semiotic baggage, if its organisational models are becoming so extensively multiplied (Bartlett and Martin, Chapter 4)? Is it justifiable, further, to conceptualise certain healthcare therapies as essentially 'medical', when so much of their delivery depends on 'invisible' ephemeral care-related practices (Mittra, Chapter 10)? Does it make sense, even, to draw a line around an arena of '*public* health' when it's clear that the climate-driven environment is equally enmeshed in the enterprise of shaping human and multi-species health (Radhuber et al., Chapter 2)? Should there be, and can there be, for example, planned provision of mental health trauma services in specific geographical 'hotspots' where severe climate emergencies can be foreseen? What role can infrastructures and devices of digital mental health play in severe mental distress as well as more routine mental health care (Pickersgill and Crespo Suarez, Chapter 5)?

Further, how might publics gain trust in regimes of biomedical product regulation when cross-national regulatory practices 'game' and essentially circumvent safety standards between different places (Sleeboom-Faulkner, Chapter 8), are unable satisfactorily to assess and act on quantified experiences of individual drug and vaccine-related patient side-effects (Mezza and Blume, Chapter 3) or have to deal with clinical 'evidence' that is easily challenged on methodological and other grounds (Quigley and Hayler, Chapter 13)? Can regulatory regimes be aligned more closely towards values and moralities accentuating the public good and avoiding regulatory capture (Metzler and Aarden, Chapter 6)? Relatedly, it is important to bring more consideration, pressure and innovation in human rights into the frame here (e.g., Ienca and Andorno, 2017).

What are the limits to the bio-entity-enabled formation of novel patient groupings (Akrich et al., Chapter 7)? What are the prospects for a critical mass of patient activism around AMR and similar widely fragmented medical conditions (Do and Whittaker, Chapter 12)? Equally, what are, or should be, the limits to the risk-shaping proliferation of biomedical testing for susceptibility to non-predictable diseases (Petersen and Pienaar, Chapter 9)? Can new sensitivities to embodied linguistic expression help steer biomedical infrastructures in more open, collaborative and equitable directions (Bicudo, Chapter 11)? How can 'speculative research' methods, as advocated by Meskus (Chapter 1), help societies (re)shape new biomedical innovations in favour of ourselves as citizens and patients?

We hope, collectively as authors of this book, that many of the topics, approaches and questions raised and discussed here will stimulate scholars to pick up the threads and develop them further, and to take them in new, valuable directions, to the eventual betterment of health and society broadly.

References

Faulkner, A. (2012a). Commensuration and proliferation: Similarity and divergence in law's shaping of medical technology. *Law, Innovation and Technology*, 4(2), pp. 165–184.

Faulkner, A. (2012b). Law's performativities: Shaping the emergence of regenerative medicine through European Union legislation. *Social Studies of Science*, 42(5), pp. 753–774.

Gregory, A. (2023). Children at 'existential risk' from climate crisis, UK's top paediatrician says. *The Guardian*. Available at: https://www.theguardian.com/society/2023/oct/21/children-at-existential-risk-from-climate-crisis-uks-top-paediatrician-says (accessed 24 March 2025).

Hutchby, I. (2001). Technologies, texts and affordances. *Sociology*, *35*(2), pp. 441–456.

Ienca, M. and Andorno, R. (2017). Towards new human rights in the age of neuroscience and neurotechnology. *Life Sciences, Society and Policy*, *13*(5). https://doi.org/10.1186/s40504-017-0050-1

Marent, B., Henwood, F., Petersen, A. and Neves, B.B. (2026, forthcoming). *Sociology of Health & Illness: Special Issue: Algorithms in Health and Medicine: Sociological Inquiries into Current Disruptions and Future Imaginaries*. USA: Wiley.

Ulucanlar, S., Faulkner, A., Peirce, S. and Elwyn, G. (2013). Technology identity: The role of sociotechnical representations in the adoption of medical devices. *Social Science & Medicine*, *98*, pp. 95–105.

Webster, A. and Gardner, J. (2019). Aligning technology and institutional readiness: The adoption of innovation. *Technology Analysis & Strategic Management*, *31*(10), pp. 1229–1241.

Will, C.M. (2018). Editorial: Beyond behavior? Institutions, interactions and inequalities in the response to antimicrobial resistance. *Sociology of Health & Illness*, *40*(3).

1 Populations, biologies, and futures: Research on the scientific governing of life

Mianna Meskus

1.1 Introduction

This chapter discusses social studies that explore biomedical knowledge production as a focal practice that modifies biological processes and, through that, shapes people's lives. Such studies contribute to a thematic and research agenda that I propose to term the scientific governing of life. My own and others' studies within this research agenda are interested in investigating and theorizing ways in which life processes are known, modified, and governed from the molecular level to the level of populations through modern, high-tech biomedical knowledge and technologies. Pervasive in contemporary societies, biomedicine provides a constant analytical challenge for social research. Biomedical practices such as reproductive medicine, biogerontology, epidemiology, and environmental and public health are looking glasses into how modern humans attempt to make sense of and intervene in life processes to prosper, live healthy and happy lives, and push against the embodied limitations, disturbances, and inequalities that life itself in its many forms gives rise to.

While biomedical knowledge targets life processes, it does not arise from a void, nor is scientific knowledge free from societal values and power relations. The aim of this chapter is to show that biomedical practice and social worlds co-constitute each other in many ways. The co-constitution of biomedicine and society is not a matter of unidirectional objectification and management of humans' and other living beings' vitality, morbidity, and mortality through knowledge. By this I mean that governing does not work only from knowledge production towards life processes. Rather, life as the object of governing is recalcitrant, volatile, and, as such, a persistent challenge to governing. Therefore, social research on biomedicine and society pays attention also to how and when various biological processes and peoples' experiences of them 'kick back' (Barad, 2007, p. 215). When this happens, the premises of scientific and policy practices are often problematized and reshaped. Thus, research within this area is interested in how peoples' bodies and experiences of health and illness are shaped through scientific knowledge but also in how resistance to governing emerges and shapes the premises of knowing.

Building on my own and others' research on, for instance, genetics, stem cell science, epidemiology, embryology, and related biotechnologies, I explore the scientific governing of life through three subareas of study: populations, biologies, and *futures*. Each of these areas addresses the shifting conditions under which biomedical practice shapes the life course. I introduce example studies within each theme that focus on biomedicine as a scientific practice concerned with the vitality of humans but also that of the more-than-humans involved.

Throughout the sections, I discuss the theoretical-methodological ambition that, I propose, is characteristic of many studies on the scientific governing of life: the aspiration to link together and move between *Foucauldian analytics of power* and *new materialist analyses* of the biopolitical and biomedical body. This conceptual development brings new aspects to (social) constructionist studies of science – to the constructed and mediated characters of entities involved in knowledge production (Latour, 2003). The combination of analytics of power and new materialist approaches gives rise to research on knowledge production at multiple sites and by a multitude of actors, some of whom are not human. Furthermore, I bring in a third discussion that involves the development of *speculative approaches* in the study of bioscience, biotechnology, and sociotechnical futures. To investigate uncertain futures shaped by emerging biotechnological solutions and experimental biomedicine, some scholars have turned towards methodological orientations that foreground the experiential production of knowledge and explore the value of 'not-knowing' or uncertainties in biomedical knowledge. Finally, in the 'Conclusion', I draw together the main points of the chapter and offer some suggestions on how research in this area could be developed further.

1.2 Populations

For Michel Foucault (2007), the notion of population refers to an idea that became important in the formation of social and political thought in Western societies. For instance, public health policies have been and are enacted in the name of the populations that are seen to make up nation-states. Foucault's historical analyses of the idea of population have helped scholars to see how it came to refer to a vital reality affected and governed in the form of a multiplicity of individuals. Foucault (2003) argued that through populations, *biopolitical* mechanisms and techniques focus on 'man as a living being'. Biopolitics refers to 'the endeavor, begun in the eighteenth century, to rationalize the problems presented to governmental practice by the phenomena characteristic of a group of living human beings constituted as a population: health, sanitation, birthrate, longevity, race …' (Foucault, 1997, 2008). Biomedicine, then, is one area of scientific governing where groups of people have been identified, counted, controlled, and cared for as 'a population'. Taking up this idea of biopolitical governing of populations, scholars continuing Foucault's work have shown that European social thought strongly builds on the importance of scientific and political governing of populations (Dean, 1999; Rose, 1999; Osborne and Rose, 2008; Lemke, 2010).

In line with the focus of this Elgar Research Agendas book, Foucauldian analytics of government has offered conceptual tools to study various forms of biomedical governing of populations (e.g., Bunton and Petersen, 1997; Rabinow and Rose, 2006; Rose, 2007). Some have explored genomic science and its effects in constructing race-based populations (e.g., Hinterberger, 2012; M'charek et al., 2014; Oikkonen, 2020), looking at, for instance, the intersections of forensics, DNA testing, and the governing of populations in the context of migration (e.g., Helén, 2014; M'charek and Wade, 2020). In recent scholarship, attention has also been turned to the deeply gendered constitution of population 'crises' (e.g., Schultz, 2015; Murphy, 2018; Sasser, 2018; Schuller, 2018; Wahlberg, 2018; Andersson et al., 2021). These crises have historically centered on women's reproductive capacities and behavior. Concerns about population have given legitimacy to a range of policy measures across past decades, from eugenic sterilizations and abortions to family planning and contraception campaigns to current debates on fertility decline and young people's reluctance to have children. These studies have also shown that population policies and programs across the world have been and continue to be constitutive of and entangled with gendered, colonial, and racist practice.

Research drawing from Foucauldian analytics of government has made a strong case for the complex relationship between population and environmental policies. That is, in the analytics of government, the way 'human populations' figure in scientific discussions on environmental degradation and species loss has gained new pertinence. For instance, Michelle Murphy (2017) and Jade Sasser (2018) argue that in the atmospheres of looming crises, population numbers legitimate demands for policy action. Scientific governing of life is conducted through projects and policies that focus on female lives, bodies, and reproductive choices, now in connection to environmental degradation and climate change (see Radhuber et al., 2026, chapter 2). This means that population issues such as 'overpopulation' in the face of climate crisis generate gendered and racialized forms of government of life (Ojeda et al., 2019;Dow and Lamoreaux, 2020). Furthermore, the population question and policymaking around it have become re-politicized in the name of reducing humanity's impact on nature and saving 'ourselves' from ecological catastrophe (Lappé et al., 2019). The global trends of fertility decline, increased longevity, and environmental degradation place knowledge production on populations at the center of biopolitical aspirations in novel ways.

Feminist discussion on population has proposed the abandoning of population as a conceptual framework, to distance social research from the longstanding natalist, gendered politics of reproduction (e.g., Clarke and Haraway, 2018). To counter pronatalist policies and the naturalist idea of biological kin-making, some scholars such as Donna Haraway (2016, 2018) have proposed that feminist studies should focus on and explore other concepts than population and, in relation to this, create alternative ways to theorize kin-relations (see also, Clarke, 2018; Murphy, 2018). Others view, however, that abandoning the framework of populations might even exacerbate racial, ethnic, classed, and gendered inequalities that are rooted in histories of stratified reproduction (Lewis, 2017; TallBear, 2018).

Viewing this debate from the perspective of the history of the Nordic welfare society, and as a researcher of scientific governing of life within a welfare system such as that of Finland, abandoning the concept of population as an analytical tool does not seem feasible. The concept and practice of population are elemental in past and current welfare society governance. Comprehensive population register data, for instance, are not only historical tools to know and enact the Finnish population but also the basis for authorities to decide on the eligibility of individuals for health and social rights, services, and benefits (Alastalo and Homanen, 2018).

The notion of population is informative also in investigating biopolitical imaginaries of Nordic welfare futures regarding demographic change. Together with Riikka Homanen, we have looked at how population policy discussions have invited and harnessed emotional orientation towards certain collective reproductive futures, while being disclosive of others (Homanen and Meskus, 2024). Building on Anderson's (2012) observation that biopower works on and through affect, we have traced the genealogy of 'affective biopolitics' of populations in Finland. We argue that the affective stakes of Nordic biopolitics are centered on persistent concerns about depopulation through ultra-low fertility. Analyzing population policy materials produced by the Family Federation of Finland from the mid-twentieth century until the present, we show that population anxieties have shifted from a focus on population quantity and quality, with a state-mandated pronatalism enmeshed with racial hygienics, to a more individualistic and encompassing demographic work where the numbers that 'matter' for population dynamics include numbers of births, pensioners, and migrants. In this research example, the scientific governing of life involves exerting a 'feeling for' the future welfare state. This conduct of affective orientation is based on the declining total fertility rate as a key concern in viewing the population and in problematizing its reproductive patterns. Biomedical practice, including reproductive biomedicine, has been expected to help in countering the fertility crisis through offering technological solutions to infertility.

In discussion with international feminist research on population, Homanen and I have also looked at how Nordic population anxieties face the climate crisis while being centered around the fertility issue. In the so-called developing countries, demographic and ecological futures are often seen as mutually constitutive (Sasser, 2018). However, the connection is not perceived as relevant to the Finnish welfare state (Homanen and Meskus, 2024). Indeed, our study shows there is an evident resistance to connecting population policy concerns with the climate crisis in the Nordic context. This is so despite a growing urgency to rethink what it means to be a citizen of the Nordic welfare state under conditions of environmental degradation and global warming.

To sum up, studies inspired by Foucault's thinking are informative in understanding the interconnections of bioscience, technology, and society. Scientific governing of life is conducted through populations in various ways. This is a historical and persistent rationale. Biomedicine plays a role here, particularly through the attention given to reproduction and fertility. Notwithstanding the increasing emphasis on individual choices and rights to services and care in current societies, research shows that interventions into human reproduction continue to find their legitimacy in the benefit of society – on the level of populations. This governing extends even to the cellular and embryonal level, as I show in the next section.

1.3 Biologies

The second theme to consider in the study of scientific governing of life involves biomedical science as it is conducted both in experimental science laboratories and in clinical settings of diagnosis and treatment. In this section, I turn to research on knowledge production at the level of complex, microscopic biological processes and mechanisms. Some scientists study, for instance, disease modeling that bioscientists conduct in laboratories with the help of cellular technologies and test animals. Others focus on patients' embodied experiences when they encounter biomedical knowledge and incorporate it into everyday practices. The general motivation for this area of study is to investigate the changes in the opportunities of shaping and managing processes of life and the political and personal expectations, fears, and hopes that accompany the biomedical governing of life.

Biomedicine and biotechnologies attempt to intervene in life processes and push against life's limitations. This is both a philosophical and a societal question. Studies have shown that human biology has become a promissory arena for capitalist appropriation of life, as biomedical care and biotechnology-based industrialization and marketing converge (Cooper and Waldby, 2014; Helosvuori and Homanen, 2022). More specifically, gene, cell, and tissue-based technologies provide a view into the development of the 'bioeconomy', or the economic aim to valuate, commodify, and marketize biological materials and biology-derived therapies more effectively than ever before (e.g., Waldby, 2002; Sunder Rajan, 2007; Mittra, 2016; Birch, 2017). Furthermore, turning biology into technology that is then scaled up and marketized as medical products and devices indicates a process of 'bioindustrialization' (Franklin, 2013) characteristic of current practices of governing life through biomedical knowledge. In other words, the sciences of life have become involved in the upscaling and standardization of the use of human biological material, at an industrial scale, in the prevention and treatment of disease. This bioindustrialization has vast implications for the ontology of human tissue (how it is sourced, used, and remolded), normative policy and ethical oversight, and clinical and consumer use (Webster et al., 2011; Koichi and Stephens, 2016; Stephens et al., 2021).

I wish to focus here on studies on biomedicine and society that emerge from the intellectual space that combines Foucauldian analytics of power and posthumanist feminist approaches, also called feminist new materialism. The relevant research acknowledges the embodied and material features in knowledge production that tend to go unnoticed. Here, the focus is turned onto how the production of knowledge and governing through bioscience depends on everyday embodied labor and material devices, apparatuses, and objects of scientific practice.

Recent developments in social and political theory involve a renewed theoretical interest in matter and materiality. Feminist posthumanist thinking has been focal in steering attention towards how human agents are continuously constituted by and in relation to the material world/s they live with (Pyyhtinen and Meskus, 2025). New materialist studies foreground more-than-human entities as shaping human action without becoming first-instance determining features of social relations or background explanations in the form of material structures. In the context of bioscience and biomedicine, studies have illustrated that human action responds to and is the effect of active biological entities from cells and bacteria (Hird, 2009a) to various research animals (Holmberg, 2011; Friese, 2013; Suzuki, 2015).

As it comes to Foucault's work, it is seen to offer important insight into the study of knowledge, power, and the biological body. Yet, it is also regarded as unsatisfactory in its anthropocentric orientation, restricting agency to human subjects without taking into consideration the agential properties of non-human forces (Lemke, 2015). For instance, Karen Barad (2007) argues that while Foucault indeed underscores that power is exercised through various apparatuses, his theorization on power-knowledge does not articulate the precise character and agency of material phenomena in power relations. To counter this, agents other than humans have gained attention, be they called, for instance, nonhumans (Latour, 2004), more-than-humans (Whatmore, 2006), critters (Haraway, 2016), vibrant matter (Bennett, 2010), or lively entities (van Dooren et al., 2016).

To empirically operationalize the premise of being attentive to humans and nonhumans alike, Bruno Latour has famously proposed the dubiously simple method of 'following actors around' (Latour, 1987) or 'following the trails myopically' (Latour, 2005), naming the approach 'slowciology' (Latour, 2005). In any empirical study, such an approach leads to the challenge of selecting which human and nonhuman elements should be considered when analyzing, describing, and explaining a phenomenon or a practice (Lehtonen, 2009). Studies on human-matter relationality tend to deploy a 'descriptivist' methodology, or 'descriptive empiricism' (Krarup and Blok, 2011). This invokes the issue of which actors to follow and what kind of materiality to sensitize to, given that research settings and empirical field work cannot extend to all possible directions.

The theoretical shift from Foucauldian analytics of power to new materialist studies is, I propose, closely connected to the methodological transformation where studying policy documents and other textual, archival materials has given way to or been accompanied by ethnographically-oriented research that involves participatory observation and engagement with study participants. I do not mean that research on knowledge practices and power relations with the Foucauldian approach has ceased. Rather, many scholars have attempted to renew the conceptual basis of their theorization on knowledge practices. This has brought in the constitutive relations between humans and more-than-humans as one unit of analysis, foregrounding the methodological issue of studying materialities as part of social practice.

The sciences of life are often studied in laboratory surroundings through ethnographic field work and in-depth interviews, to trace how biological entities, processes, and mechanisms are studied and modified in the everyday laboratory practices in the name of improved health and vitality. This can imply studying challenges in transforming scientific craftwork in laboratories into standardized and scaled-up production of biological research material (e.g., Jent, 2017; Meskus, 2018). Furthermore, laboratory ethnographies have traced how living biological material such as stem cell lines are collected and stored in national and supranational biobanks to pursue economic and science and health policy aims. The creation and maintenance of collections of tissue, cells, and other biological materials of human origin has become a much emphasized and politically-backed solution to the problem of moving biomedicine from 'the bench' to 'the bedside' (e.g., Stephens et al., 2008; Merleau-Ponty et al., 2018).

The materiality of the human body is at the center of attention here. In a key anthology on new feminist materialism, Stacy Alaimo and Susan Hekman (2008) argue that research needs to pay more attention to the materiality of the body itself as an active, sometimes recalcitrant, force (see also Barad, 2007; Hird, 2009b; Åsberg et al., 2011; Dolphijn and van der Tuin, 2012; Braidotti, 2013). Bodies have pain as well as pleasure, and diseases are subject to medical interventions that may or may not cure those bodies. Alaimo and Hekman state that 'we need a way to talk about these bodies and the materiality they inhabit' (2008, p. 4). For different strands of feminist new materialism, a uniting theoretical feature is the contestation of the notion of nature, or biology, as merely the inert scenery against which the humanist adventures of society and culture are played out (MacLure, 2013). For many scholars, the methodological point is to find ways of exploring the relationship of humans to nature without postulating that biological processes are 'pre-scriptive' to social action (Birke, 1986; Kirby, 2008). Thus, the point is not to identify, name, or use specific biological laws or regularities in arguing for causal explanations of people's experiences and social action. In the words of Deboleena Roy (2018), biology and biological processes need not be taken as essentializing or deterministic. Furthermore, according to Roy, a focus on empirical practices of working with and doing materiality prevents accepting scientific knowledge at face value.

In my own research, I have applied feminist new materialist thinking to the study of assisted reproductive technologies. Presenting a paradigmatic case for feminist new materialism that also draws from Foucauldian power analysis, in vitro fertilization (IVF) treatment is a socio-technical practice that contributes to making up families around the globe. IVF is an increasingly prevalent practice where gendered bodies are enacted in relation to gametes, embryos, hormone preparations, incubators, freezers, tranquilizers, and patients' emotions. Through analyzing peer support discussions in Finland, I have argued (Meskus, 2015) that infertility treatment patients offer meticulous accounts for IVF-related drugs and technologies and their effects on embodied biological processes and affective intensities, following accounts of how everyday action is encompassed and conditioned by these nonhuman but thoroughly social actors. Drugs awaiting in the home fridge and embryos awaiting in the incubator or the freezer of the fertility clinic affect the bodies and actions of people trying to conceive a child and form a family (Meskus 2015; Helosvuori, 2020). Entangled with these experiences, biomedical knowledge is generated at the IVF clinics. From identifying and selecting the most 'suitable' gametes in terms of kin and race in gamete donation (Homanen, 2018) to identifying and selecting the most 'viable' embryo in embryo transfer (Helosvuori, 2018), biological processes become co-constitutive of social action.

Together with existing and emerging technologies, biomedicine attempts to shape the conditions of humanity at the level of the body and biological materials. Biomedical research, technologies, and clinical practices collect, use, exchange, and commercialize human-derived materials such as blood, gametes, tissue, organs, and stem cells. One gains analytical leverage with these phenomena by applying new materialist approaches, which entails paying specific attention to 'the constitutive relations' (Haraway in Gane, 2006) between, for instance, bioscientists and their research materials. This entails, I propose, a sustained focus on what researchers do to lively research tools like reproductive tissue and stem cells, but also on what the tools do to the researchers (Meskus, 2018; Meskus and Oikkonen, 2020). Operationalizing new materialist approaches enables social scientists to theorize how social practice is entangled with and dependent on a multitude of lively entities. To paraphrase Haraway (2016), the point is not to lose human perspective, but rather to ease or lessen human exceptionalism. It is worth underscoring that attending to materiality does not imply that one does not study biopolitical practices or programs of governing. It means that one becomes more open to the complexity of agencies in explaining the scientific governing of life.

1.4 Futures

A third common theme running through research projects on the scientific governing of life is the question of how scientific knowledge invokes and enacts visions and imaginaries of futures. Biotechnologies that deploy human cells and tissue are deeply invested in formulating and promising better health, well-being, and happiness for future societies. At the level of populations, scientific practices such as reproductive biomedicine, biogerontology, epidemiology, and environmental and public health propose scenarios about how life is expected to unfold in the decades to come. The scientific governing of life is also dependent on generating and harnessing imaginaries of the future at people's personal, experiential, and embodied levels. As with the two other themes discussed above, studies that investigate biomedicine and biotechnologies from the temporal perspective engage with Foucauldian ideas on biopower yet also develop these further and/or turn towards other philosophical approaches to theorize the relationship between bioscience and the future. I will first discuss Foucault-inspired research on cryotechnologies in biomedicine to illustrate my point, and then introduce speculative research conducted on, for instance, biomedical practices and technologies.

Freezing and thawing biological substances for the study, management, and commercialization of life processes has become a central practice linking biomedicine to societal power relations with a distinctive orientation to the future. Research has shown how so-called cryotechnologies contribute to making particular pasts, presents, and futures (Radin and Kowal, 2017; Kroløkke et al., 2019; Katz et al., 2020; Braun et al., 2023). Refrigerators, freezers, dry ice, and liquid nitrogen constitute cryopreservation techniques that emerge and are marketed in reference to securing future biomedical research and treatment options. Biobanking, introduced in the previous section, is a central means to facilitate present and future biomedicine by storing biological materials collected sometimes even in the quite distant past. Biobanking has emerged from technologies of cold preservation to 'hold still' biological matter and to manipulate, relocate, and recombine this matter to answer a multitude of biomedical questions, as well as those that were not anticipated when the original samples were collected from human bodies (Radin, 2017).

For Foucault (1990, p. 138), power over the living is essentially about 'power to *foster* life or *disallow* it to the point of death'. Referring to Foucault's work on biopolitics – governmental activities aimed at shaping human vitality, morbidity, and mortality – scholarship on cryopreservation argues that with this technoscientific practice, humans and nonhumans are made to live and are *not allowed to die* (Radin and Kowal, 2017). Thus, 'cryopolitics' describes a form of biopolitics that suspends, or freezes, life through technoscientific means and thereby defers death. Among the freezing practices of biological materials are cold storage of laboratory mice gametes (Myelnikov and Peres, 2023), embryos created in IVF clinics (Lafuente-Funes, 2023), gametes of cancer treatment patients (Barlevy et al., 2020), human organs used in transplantation medicine (Hoeyer, 2017), and pathogens such as bacteria and viruses (Oikkonen, 2024). Notably, studies on cryopreservation and biobanking have been vigilant to highlight how the freezing techniques and the collection of blood samples have been ways to extract biomedical knowledge and future population health imaginaries from indigenous peoples. In the name of future research, indigenous peoples have been regarded as raw materials and 'baseline' bodily evidence on, for instance, the scope of environmental contamination (Radin, 2017; TallBear, 2017).

Future imaginaries on biomedicine and biotechnologies have recently also been studied with a different theoretical orientation, namely speculative approaches that draw on the philosophical thinking of Isabelle Stengers. Stengers draws from A. N. Whitehead's speculative philosophy so as 'to be able to think about the creative power of the sciences', but also 'about their catastrophic indifference to what they judge "non-scientific"' (Stengers, 2011a, p. 11). My own research on the co-constitution of biomedicine, biotechnologies, and society has navigated between Foucauldian, new materialist, and speculative theorization, and I wish to use the rest of this section to introduce what speculative research has to offer in studying the interconnections between biomedicine and society.

Speculative social research can give new insight into the investigation of different forms of knowledge production – on, for instance, biologies of the body and technologies that shape the human condition. Here, the notion of speculation is detached from actuarial and economics-based analytical frameworks and taken into use in studying the relation between scientific and social practices and the imaginary in those practices (Savransky et al., 2017). Drawing from Stengers' work (2005, 2010, 2011a, 2011b), scholars engaging with speculative methodology study sociotechnical developments and related futures often in collaboration with research participants. That is, this theoretical-methodological orientation caters to social research that aims to engage in the co-production of knowledge, as is often done in design research. Design research that builds on speculation aims to open up different kinds of possibilities of sociotechnical development for discussion and debate (Dunne and Raby, 2013, 2019; Escobar, 2017). In social sciences, speculative methodology has been applied in the empirical research contexts of, for example, emergency provision (Guggenheim et al., 2017) and energy transition (Wilkie and Michael, 2018).

In studying the biomedical governing of life, the speculative approach has allowed me to address sociotechnical uncertainties apparent in emerging biotechnologies. To be more specific, it has enabled the collaborative imagining with study participants of deriving egg and sperm cells from stem cells through in vitro gametogenesis, which is an emerging field of study in bioscience. My ethnographic research engagements with bioscientists in Finland, Sweden, the United Kingdom, and Italy show that the revolutionary technique of cellular reprogramming in stem cells has opened up the possibility of crafting synthetic gametes in the laboratory, which in the future could create new options for treating infertility and involuntary childlessness (Meskus, 2023). Meanwhile, speculative engagements with elderly people in Southern Finland allowed for investigating the prospect of using genetic and epigenetic knowledge to shape biological aging. This engagement produced various alternative perspectives into what is considered 'normal' aging, thus pointing to how the scientific governing of life may be resisted and reshaped. Together with research group members, we argued that as speculative thinking foregrounds experiential knowledge, it provides for unruliness and freedom that allows other types of aging futures to emerge alongside biomedical ones (Hautamäki and Meskus, 2024; Meskus and Tikka, 2024).

The motivation to explore speculative research arises often from the fact that while, for instance, cryotechnologies already operate in the present and shape futures, one might end up studying not-yet-realized technologies and treatments-to-be, as with the case of in vitro gametogenesis. It is challenging to grasp empirically that which is only emerging and circulates through visionary discussions and tentative practices. Having worked with Foucauldian analysis of textual documents and new materialist ethnographic research, speculative knowledge production is an intriguing methodological addition because it entails shifting positions in research engagements between researchers and informants. It appreciates the suppression of hierarchies of knowledge and the uncertainties or not-knowing involved in envisioning shared futures.

In terms of researching the scientific governing of life, developing speculative methodology involves, in my use, attempts to bring together the perspectives of power relations, scientific knowledge, and the embodied and personal in people's lived experiences. Speculative methodology foregrounds the interconnectedness of knowledge and experience and the perceiving body as the focal site of experience. Here we return to the point made in the introduction of this chapter, namely that social research on biomedicine and society also needs to pay attention to how and when life in its multiple processes and forms 'kicks back', to use Barad's (2007) expression, so that the premises of scientific and policy practices become problematized and reshaped. Thus, a speculative approach to the biomedical governing of life may allow the critical investigation and bottom-up problematization of existing biopolitical and bioscientific rationalities. These problematizations can concern valuations of worthy life in the face of novel technologies and differential orderings of groups (or populations) of humans and nonhumans in developing new biomedical therapies.

1.5 Conclusion

In this chapter I have proposed that a central area of study on biomedicine and society is one that could be called the scientific governing of life. It arises from Foucault's thinking but goes also beyond the Foucauldian analysis of power and knowledge. I have given examples of studies that show how biomedical research and treatment practices orientate towards human life as an object of governing. However, I have also introduced studies that expand and explore further the relationship between knowledge and governing through foregrounding the agency of biological entities as material, more-than-human participants in social practices. These agencies may and often do resist acts of governing, generating effects in human action, values, and aspirations. Furthermore, I argued that as some studies on the scientific governing of life focus on technologies that are highly experimental and only at the stage of early envisioning and emergence, this calls for different kinds of engagements with technoscientific futures and novel theoretical and methodological explorations that highlight the experiential, non-hierarchical understanding of biomedical knowledge and related technological applications.

I divided the study of the scientific governing of life into three themes: populations, biologies, and futures. Many of the studies that were introduced under one theme could have belonged also to one of the others. When research involves the study of societal conditions and the implications of biomedicine, issues to be discussed often cut across several scales from populations to the cellular and microscopic, as they also extend across the temporal axis of the past, present, and future. This means that the three thematic approaches to biomedicine and society are linked in several ways. Whether the emphasis is on populations, biologies, or futures, biomedical practice is seen not only to know but also to shape the conditions of life, that is, biological mechanisms and processes in the body over time and in relation to the environment. This activity is based on scientifically produced knowledge by various bioscience and other experts. Yet, the approaches are connected also through acknowledging the importance of persons' and groups' embodied, affective experiences. Experiential knowledge is studied to understand how the scientific governing of life becomes effective in people's lives but also how it is resisted and ignored.

The studies discussed have engaged with Foucauldian analytics of power to study the scientific governing of life. Some have incorporated new materialist theorizing into their analyses of biomedical care and control. Finally, speculative approaches have been tested and deployed to explore uncertain futures connected to bioscience and biotechnology. Depending on the theoretical emphasis, research on biomedicine and society attends to various research 'subjects'. Some studies focus on scientific and policy experts such as bioscience researchers and public health and population policy authorities, while others engage with citizen-informants such as patients of a given condition or members of a certain population group. In some studies, attention is given to nonhumans or more-than-humans such as cell lines, laboratory animals, and biomedical devices and techniques.

In terms of developing the study of the scientific governing of life further, conceptual development is needed. How can we understand 'science' through its multifaceted, affective effects critically yet with acceptance of changing forms of knowledge production? What are the shifting forms of 'governing' and how could these be theorized further? Finally, what does the idea of 'life' refer to and what does it mediate in present and future technological development that is accompanied by increasing concern over other forms of life than humans? These questions invite researchers of biomedicine and society to push their work beyond existing theoretical boundaries.

The conceptual development is interconnected with methodological work. The task at hand is finding ways to construct empirical research settings, document analysis, interview questions, questionnaires, ethnographic observation, and other forms of data gathering that boldly address the scope of biomedical knowledge in society. That humans speak for nonhumans is a starting point one must accept. This means that language is always at play in researching the material-discursive dimensions of biomedicine. Constitutive relations include meanings, interests, and affects that co-evolve together with material practices. Moreover, constitutive relations open up and enfold also on ourselves as researchers. Social scientists become engaged in the co-production of knowledge with study participants, which adds challenges to and is a point of intrigue for the study of the scientific government of life.

References

Alaimo, S. and Hekman, S. (2008). Introduction: Emerging models of materiality in feminist theory. In: Alaimo, S. and Hekman, S. (Eds.), *Material Feminisms*. Bloomington and Indianapolis: Indiana University Press, pp. 1–19.

Alastalo, M. and Homanen, R. (2018). Yksilöfaktaa ja väestötietoa. Väestökirjanpito ulkomaalaisten hallinnan ja tietämisen teknologiana [Facts about individuals and knowledge about populations. Population bookkeeping as a technology of governance and knowledge production]. *Sosiologia*, 55(2), pp. 147–166.

Anderson, B. (2012). Affect and biopower: Towards a politics of life. *Transactions – Institute of British Geographers*, 37(1), pp. 28–43.

Andersson, H., Brandstedt, E., and Torpman, O. (2021). Review article: The ethics of population policies. *Critical Review of International Social and Political Philosophy*, 27(4), pp. 635–658.

Åsberg, C., Koobak, R., and Johnson, E. (2011). Beyond the humanist imagination. *Nordic Journal of Feminist and Gender Research*, 19(4), pp. 218–230.
Barad, K. (2007). *Meeting the Universe Halfway: Quantum Physics and the Entanglement of Matter and Meaning*. Durham: Duke University Press.
Barlevy, D., Werren, S., and Ravitsky, V. (2020). Posthumous planning following fertility preservation: A study of adolescent cancer patients in Israel. *New Genetics and Society*, 39(3), pp. 271–287.
Bennett, J. (2010). *Vibrant Matter: A Political Ecology of Things*. Durham: Duke University Press.
Birch, K. (2017). Rethinking value in the bio-economy: Finance, assetization, and the management of value. *Science, Technology, & Human Values*, 42(3), pp. 460–490.
Birke, L. (1986). *Women, Feminism and Biology*. Brighton: Wheatsheaf Books.
Braidotti, R. (2013). *The Posthuman*. Cambridge: Polity.
Braun, V., Lafuente-Funes, S., Lemke, T., and Liburkina, R. (2023). Making futures by freezing life: Ambivalent temporalities of cryopreservation practices. *Science, Technology & Human Values*, 48(4), pp. 693–699.
Bunton, R. and Petersen, A. (Eds.) (1997). *Foucault, Health and Medicine*. London and New York: Routledge.
Clarke, A. E. (2018). Introducing making kin not population. In: Clarke, A. E. and Haraway, D. (Eds.), *Making Kin Not Population: Reconceiving Generations*. Chicago: Prickly Paradigm Press, pp. 1–39.
Clarke, A. E. and Haraway, D. (Eds.) (2018). *Making Kin Not Population: Reconceiving Generations*. Chicago: Prickly Paradigm Press.
Cooper, M. and Waldby, C. (2014). *Clinical Labor: Tissue Donors and Research Subjects in the Global Bioeconomy*. Durham: Duke University Press.
Dean, M. (1999). *Governmentality: Power and Rule in Modern Society*. London: Sage.
Dolphijn, R. and van der Tuin, I. (2012). *New Materialism: Interviews & Cartographies*. University of Michigan Library, Ann Arbor: Open Humanities Press.
Dow, K. and Lamoreaux, J. (2020). Situated kinmaking and the population 'problem'. *Environmental Humanities*, 12(2), pp. 475–491.
Dunne, A. and Raby, F. (2013). *Speculative Everything: Design, Fiction, and Social Dreaming*. Cambridge: The MIT Press.
Dunne, A. and Raby, F. (2019). Designers need to recognise their limitations and work with them: James Auger in conversation with Anthony Dunne and Fiona Raby, pioneers of Critical Design. *SpeculativeEdu*. https://speculativeedu.eu/interview-dunne-raby/
Escobar, A. (2017). *Designs for the Pluriverse: Radical Interdependence, Autonomy, and the Making of Worlds*. Durham: Duke University Press.
Foucault, M. (1990). *The History of Sexuality. Vol. 1. An Introduction*. London: Penguin Books.
Foucault, M. (1997). The birth of biopolitics. In: Rabinow, P. (Ed.), *Ethics, Subjectivity and Truth. The Essential Works of Michel Foucault 1954–1984, Vol. 1*. London: Allen Lane.
Foucault, M. (2003). *Society Must Be Defended. Lectures at the Collège de France 1975–1976*. New York: Picador.
Foucault, M. (2007). *Security, Territory, Population. Lectures at the Collège de France, 1977–1978*. New York: Palgrave Macmillan.
Foucault, M. (2008). *The Birth of Biopolitics. Lectures at the Collége de France 1977–1978*. Basingstoke: Palgrave Macmillan.
Franklin, S. (2013). *Biological Relatives: IVF, Stem Cells, and the Future of Kinship*. Durham: Duke University Press.
Friese, C. (2013). Realizing potential in translational medicine: The uncanny emergence of care as science. *Current Anthropology*, 54(S7), pp. 129–138.

Gane, N. (2006). When we have never been human, what is to be done? Interview with Donna Haraway. *Theory, Culture & Society*, 23(7/8), pp. 135–158.

Guggenheim M., Kraftner, B., and Kroll, J. (2017). Creating idiotic speculators: Disaster cosmopolitics in the sandbox. In: Wilkie, A., Savransky, M., and Rosengarten, M. (Eds.), *Speculative Research: The Lure of Possible Futures*. London: Routledge, pp. 145–162.

Haraway, D. (2016). *Staying with the Trouble: Making Kin in the Chthulucene*. Durham and London: Duke University Press.

Haraway, D. (2018). Making kin in the Chthulucene: Reproducing multispecies justice. In Clarke, A. E. and Haraway, D. (Eds.), *Making Kin Not Population: Reconceiving Generations*. Chicago: Prickly Paradigm Press, pp. 67–99.

Hautamäki, L. and Meskus, M. (2024). Living temporality: Speculative engagements with elderly people on bioscience and the body. *Time & Society*, 33(2), pp. 191–211.

Helén, I. (2014). Biological citizenship across the borders: Politics of DNA profiling for family reunification. *Distinktion*, 15(3), pp. 343–360.

Helosvuori, E. (2018). Assembling viability: The art of mundane embryo selection in IVF. *BioSocieties*, 14(1), pp. 1–22.

Helosvuori, E. (2020). Lingering technological entanglements: Experiences of childlessness after IVF. *European Journal of Women's Studies*, 27(3), pp. 267–281.

Helosvuori, E. and Homanen, R. (2022). When craft kicks back: Embryo culture as knowledge production in the context of the transnational fertility industry. *Social Studies of Science*, 52(3), pp. 425–446.

Hinterberger, A. (2012). Investing in life, investing in difference: Nations, populations and genomes. *Theory, Culture & Society*, 29(3), pp. 72–93.

Hird, M. J. (2009a). *The Origins of Sociable Life: Evolution after Science Studies*. Houndmills, Basingstoke: Palgrave Press.

Hird, M. J. (2009b). Feminist engagements with matter. *Feminist Studies*, 35(2), pp. 329–346.

Hoeyer, K. (2017). Suspense: Reflections on the cryopolitics of the body. In: Radin, J. and Kowal, E. (Eds.), *Cryopolitics: Frozen Life in a Melting World*. Cambridge and London: The MIT Press, pp. 205–214.

Holmberg, T. (2011). Mortal love: Care practices in animal experimentation. *Feminist Theory*, 12(2), pp. 147–163.

Homanen, R. (2018). Reproducing whiteness and enacting kin in the Nordic context of transnational egg donation: Matching donors with crossborder traveller recipients in Finland. *Social Science & Medicine*, 203, pp. 28–34.

Homanen, R. and Meskus, M. (2024). Population anxieties in constituting Nordic welfare state futures: Affective biopolitics in the age of environmental crises. *BioSocieties*, 19(2), pp. 232–258.

Jent, K. (2017). *Making Stem Cell Niches: An Ethnography of Regenerative Medicine in Scotland and the United States*. Doctoral dissertation, St Catharine's College, University of Cambridge.

Katz, O., Hashiloni-Dolev, Y., Kroløkke, C., and Raz, A. (2020). Frozen: Social and bioethical aspects of cryopreservation. *New Genetics and Society*, 39(3), pp. 243–249.

Kirby, V. (2008). Natural convers(at)ions: Or, what if culture was really nature all along? In: Alaimo, S. and Hekman, S. (Eds.), *Material Feminisms*. Bloomington and Indianapolis: Indiana University Press, pp. 214–236.

Koichi, M. and Stephens, N. (2016). Local biologicals and the politics of standardization: Making ethical pluripotent stem cells in the United Kingdom and Japan. *BioSocieties*, 11(2), pp. 220–239.

Krarup, T. M. and Blok, A. (2011). Unfolding the social: Quasi-actants, virtual theory, and the new empiricism of Bruno Latour. *The Sociological Review*, 59(1), pp. 42–63.

Kroløkke, C., Petersen, T. S., Herrmann, J. R., Bach, A. S., Adrian, S. W., Klingenberg, R., and Petersen, M. N. (2019). *The Cryopolitics of Reproduction on Ice: A New Scandinavian Ice Age.* Leeds: Emerald Publishing Limited.

Lafuente-Funes, S. (2023). The role of vitrification in Spanish reproductive labs: A cryo-revolution led by strategic freezing. *Science, Technology, & Human Values*, 48(4), pp. 752–776.

Lappé, M., Hein, R. J., and Landecker, H. (2019). Environmental politics of reproduction. *Annual Review of Anthropology*, 48, pp. 133–150.

Latour, B. (1987). *Science in Action: How to Follow Scientists and Engineers through Society.* Cambridge: Harvard University Press.

Latour, B. (2003). The promises of constructivism. In: Ihde, D. and Selinger, E. (Eds.), *Chasing Technoscience: Matrix for Materiality.* Bloomington: Indiana University Press, pp. 27–46.

Latour, B. (2004). *Politics of Nature: How to Bring the Sciences into Democracy.* Cambridge and London: Harvard University Press.

Latour, B. (2005). *Reassembling the Social: An Introduction to Actor-Network-Theory.* Oxford: Oxford University Press.

Lehtonen, T.-K. (2009). How does materiality matter for the social sciences? In: Colas, D. and Kharkhordin, O. (Eds.), *The Materiality of Res Publica: How to Do Things with Publics.* Newcastle upon Tyne: Cambridge Scholars Publishing, pp. 271–288.

Lemke, T. (2010). From state biology to the government of life: Historical dimensions and contemporary perspectives of 'biopolitics'. *Journal of Classical Sociology*, 10(4), pp. 421–438.

Lemke, T. (2015). New materialisms: Foucault and the 'government of things'. *Theory, Culture & Society*, 32(4), pp. 3–25.

Lewis, S. (2017). Cthulhu plays no role for me. *Viewpoint Magazine*, 8 May 2017. https://www.viewpointmag.com/2017/05/08/cthulhu-plays-no-role-for-me/

MacLure, M. (2013). Researching without representation? Language and materiality in post-qualitative methodology. *International Journal of Qualitative Studies in Education*, 26(6), pp. 658–667.

M'charek, A., Schramm, K., and Skinner, D. (2014). Topologies of race: Doing territory, population and identity in Europe. *Science, Technology, & Human Values*, 39(4), pp. 468–487.

M'charek, A. and Wade, P. (2020). Doing the individual and the collective in forensic genetics: Governance, race and restitution. *BioSocieties*, 15(3), pp. 317–328.

Merleau-Ponty N., Vertommen, S., and Pucéat, M. (2018). I6 passages: On the reproduction of a human embryonic stem cell line from Israel to France. *New Genetics and Society*, 37(4), pp. 338–361.

Meskus, M. (2015). Agential multiplicity in the assisted beginnings of life. *European Journal of Women's Studies*, 22(1), pp. 70–83.

Meskus, M. (2018). *Craft in Biomedical Research: The iPS Cell Technology and the Future of Stem Cell Science.* Basingstoke & New York: Palgrave Macmillan.

Meskus, M. (2023). Speculative feminism and the shifting frontiers of bioscience: Envisioning reproductive futures with synthetic gametes through the ethnographic method. *Feminist Theory*, 24(2), pp. 151–169.

Meskus, M. and Oikkonen, V. (2020). Embodied material encounters and the ambiguous promise of biomedical futures: The case of biologically derived medicines. *New Genetics and Society*, 39(4), pp. 441–458.

Meskus, M. and Tikka, E. (2024). Speculative approaches in social science and design research: Methodological implications of working in 'the gap' of uncertainty. *Qualitative Research*, 24(2), pp. 209–228.

Mittra, J. (2016). *The New Health Bioeconomy: R&D Policy and Innovation for the Twenty-First Century.* London: Palgrave Macmillan.

Murphy, M. (2017). *The Economization of Life.* Durham and London: Duke University Press.

Murphy, M. (2018). Against population, towards afterlife. In: Clarke, A. E. and Haraway, D. (Eds.), *Making Kin Not Population*. Chicago: Prickly Paradigm Press, pp. 101–124.
Myelnikov, D. and Peres, S. (2023). The cold futures of mouse genetics: Modes of strain cryopreservation since the 1970s. *Science, Technology, & Human Values*, 48(4), pp. 727–751.
Oikkonen, V. (2020). Belonging: Population genetics, national imaginaries, and the making of European genes. In: Luccarelli, M., Forlenza, R., and Colatrella, S. (Eds.), *Bringing the Nation Back In: Cosmopolitanism, Nationalism, and the Struggle to Define a New Politics*. New York: SUNY Press, pp. 89–106.
Oikkonen, V. (2024). Past pathogens and precarious futures. In: Strand, D., Källén, A., and Mulcare, C. (Eds.), *Critical Perspectives on Ancient DNA*. Cambridge: MIT Press. https://doi.org/10.7551/mitpress/15190.001.0001
Ojeda, D., Sasser, J. S., and Lunstrum, E. (2019). Malthus's specter and the anthropocene. *Gender, Place & Culture*, 27(3), pp. 316–332.
Osborne, T. and Rose, N. (2008). Populating sociology: Carr-Saunders and the problem of population. *The Sociological Review*, 56(4), pp. 552–578.
Pyyhtinen, O. and Meskus, M. (2025). Relationality in posthuman feminism. In: Vandenberghe, F. and Papilloud, C. (Eds.), *New Directions in Relational Sociology, Vol 2*. London: Palgrave Macmillan.
Rabinow, P. and Rose, N. (2006). Biopower today. *BioSocieties*, 1(2), pp. 195–217.
Radin, J. (2017). *Life on Ice: A History of New Uses for Cold Blood*. Chicago and London: The University of Chicago Press.
Radin, J. and Kowal, E. (Eds.) (2017). *Cryopolitics: Frozen Life in a Melting World*. Cambridge and London: The MIT Press.
Rose, N. (1999). *Powers of Freedom: Reframing Political Thought*. Cambridge: Cambridge University Press.
Rose, N. (2007). *The Politics of Life Itself: Biomedicine, Power and Subjectivity in the Twenty-First Century*. Princeton: Princeton University Press.
Roy, D. (2018). *Molecular Feminisms: Biology, Becomings, and Life in the Lab*. Seattle: University of Washington Press.
Sasser, J. (2018). *On Infertile Ground: Population Control and Women's Rights in the Era of Climate Change*. New York: NYU Press.
Savransky, M., Wilkie, A., and Rosengarten, M. (2017). The lure of possible futures: On speculative research. In: Wilkie, A., Savransky, M., and Rosengarten, M. (Eds.), *Speculative Research: The Lure of Possible Futures*. London: Routledge, pp. 1–17.
Schuller, K. (2018). *The Biopolitics of Feeling. Race, Sex, and Science in the Nineteenth Century*. Durham: Duke University Press.
Schultz, S. (2015). Reproducing the nation: The new German population policy and the concept of demographization. *Distinktion: Scandinavian Journal of Social Theory*, 16(3), pp. 337–361.
Stengers, I. (2005). The cosmopolitical proposal. In: Latour, B. and Weibel, P. (Eds.), *Making Things Public: Atmospheres of Democracy*. Cambridge: MIT Press, pp. 994–1003.
Stengers, I. (2010). *Cosmopolitics I. Posthumanities 9*. Trans. Robert Bononno. Minneapolis: University of Minnesota Press.
Stengers, I. (2011a). *Thinking With Whitehead: A Free and Wild Creation of Concepts*. Trans. Michael Chase. Cambridge and London: Harvard University Press.
Stengers, I. (2011b). *Cosmopolitics II. Posthumanities 10*. Trans. Robert Bononno. Minneapolis: University of Minnesota Press.
Stephens, N., Atkinson, P., and Glasner, P. (2008). The UK Stem Cell Bank as performative architecture. *New Genetics & Society*, 27(2), pp. 87–98.
Stephens, N., Morrison, M., Martin, P., and Hogle, L. (2021). Spatiotemporal readiness is key to preparing regenerative medicine for the clinic. *Regenerative Medicine*, 16(3), pp. 229–235.

Sunder Rajan, K. (2007). *Biocapital: The Constitution of Postgenomic Life.* Durham and London: Duke University Press.
Suzuki, W. (2015). The care of the cell: Onomatopoeia and embodiment in a stem cell laboratory. *NatureCulture*, 3, pp. 87–105.
TallBear, K. (2017). Beyond the life/not-life binary: A feminist-Indigenous reading of cryopreservation, interspecies thinking, and the new materialisms. In: Radin, J. and Kowal, E. (Eds.), *Cryopolitics: Frozen Life in a Melting World.* Cambridge and London: The MIT Press, pp. 179–202.
TallBear, K. (2018). Making love and relations beyond settler sex and family. In: Clarke, A. E. and Haraway, D. (Eds.), *Making Kin Not Population: Reconceiving Generations.* Chicago: Prickly Paradigm Press, pp. 145–164.
van Dooren, T., Kirksey, E., and Münster, U. (2016). Multispecies studies: Cultivating arts of attentiveness. *Environmental Humanities*, 8(1), pp. 1–23.
Wahlberg, A. (2018). *Good Quality: The Routinization of Sperm Banking in China.* Oakland: University of California Press.
Waldby, C. (2002). Stem cells, tissue cultures and the production of biovalue. *Health*, 6(3), pp. 305–323.
Webster, A., Haddad, C., and Waldby, C. (2011). Experimental heterogeneity and standardisation: Stem cell products and the clinical trial process. *BioSocieties*, 6(4), pp. 401–419.
Whatmore, S. (2006). Materialist returns: Practising cultural geography in and for a more-than-human world. *Cultural Geographies*, 13(4), pp. 600–609.
Wilkie, A. and Michael, M. (2018). Designing and doing: Enacting energy-and-community. In: Marres, N., Guggenheim, M., and Wilkie, A. (Eds.), *Inventing the Social.* Manchester: Mattering Press, pp. 125–147.

2 Health under climate pressure: An emerging research agenda

Isabella M. Radhuber, Amelia Fiske, and Barbara Prainsack

2.1 Introduction

As the health effects of climate change increase, the shortfalls of narrow biomedical understandings of health are becoming even more evident (e.g. IPCC 2023; WHO 2021b; Costello et al. 2009; Millennium Ecosystem Assessment 2005; Lock & Nguyen 2018). An emerging research agenda is crystallising around the connections between climate and health (Romanello et al. 2023; Whitmee et al. 2015; Horton & Lo 2015). This agenda gained momentum with the launch of the Lancet Countdown on Health and Climate Change in 2015, initiated in the wake of the quantitative risk assessment of climate change effects on selected causes of death by the World Health Organization (WHO 2014). By 2023, this initiative represented the most comprehensive research effort to date that 'independently monitors the evolving impacts of climate change on health, and the emerging health opportunities of climate action' (Romanello et al. 2023, p. 1).

One major challenge in understanding these impacts stems from the complex, often indirect and dynamic interactions between climate and health. In this context, Butler (2014, 2018) distinguishes between primary, secondary, and tertiary health effects of climate change: primary effects occur when extreme weather events, such as heatwaves and floods, directly cause deaths, injuries, and diseases;[1] secondary effects arise from changing ecosystem conditions including infectious diseases, vector-borne diseases, food- and water-borne infections, and air quality issues such as allergic reactions (Butler 2018, 2014); and tertiary effects result from contextual dynamics where 'health consequences are modified by numerous cultural, political, economic, social and other effects such as poverty, inequality, population growth, resource scarcity and governance' (Butler 2014, p. 2). Butler and colleagues (Butler et al. 2005; Butler 2014; Smith et al. 2014; Whitmee et al. 2015) argue that tertiary health impacts of climate change require the most urgent attention. They caution that by mid-century, these impacts could surpass the combined effects of primary and secondary health impacts. Despite growing concern across various disciplines, tertiary impacts remain underexplored in the fields of biomedicine, healthcare, and climate sciences.

In this chapter, we ask: How can the health effects of climate change be understood in a way that does justice to the diverse natural, ecosystemic, and societal dynamics[2] shaping these effects? Here—drawing on previous work (Radhuber et al. 2023; Radhuber et al. 2024; Radhuber et al. 2025)—we explore the health impacts of climate change using the example of extreme weather events. Given the lack of research on tertiary health impacts, we pay particular attention to how social, political, and economic dynamics shape the impact that climate change has on health. We propose a multidimensional understanding of health amidst climate change and discuss how complex problems can be analysed through a mixed methods approach that incorporates both qualitative research and transdisciplinary perspectives.

As climate change increases the risk of extreme weather events,[3] ever more people experience the health impacts of heatwaves,[4] heavy rainfall, floods, droughts, storms, and compound events (IPCC 2023; WMO 2022; Seneviratne et al. 2021). Heatwaves and floods are the two most common climate change-induced extreme weather events, both of which can increase health impacts of climate change, such as the transmission of communicable diseases (by microbes, vectors, and reservoir animals), as well as non-communicable diseases, and vulnerability due to displacement, loss of work, or ruptures to the social fabric. According to Talukder et al. (2021), diseases associated with flooding include food- and water-borne infections, conjunctivitis, schistosomiasis, skin and soft tissue infections, and dermatitis. These health issues are further aggravated by contamination of freshwater sources, inadequate sanitation, disrupted healthcare access, infrastructure breakdown, and related challenges (i.e., the tertiary health impacts of climate change). In contrast, droughts can trigger infectious diseases through groundwater contamination by viruses, protozoa, and bacteria, along with pests and diseases introduced by mulching processes. Droughts also raise critical concerns about food insecurity, contamination of agricultural products, and much more. Moreover, these events contribute to non-communicable diseases such as cardiovascular diseases, cancers, respiratory problems, and neurological disorders, due to exposure to algal and fungal biotoxins in contaminated water and food, as well as increased mental health and occupational safety concerns.

Floods (see Table 2.1 for recent examples) have received relatively little scholarly attention, which is why they have been selected as the main focus of this chapter. Most examples—cited throughout the chapter in discussions of tertiary health impacts—concentrate on flash floods, which are sudden, intense events that can occur within minutes or hours of heavy rainfall or rapid snowmelt.

2.2 A multidimensional understanding of health amid climate change

Understanding health in relation to climate change draws attention to the ecological processes that influence the well-being of all living species. Here we take inspiration from advocates of the Rights of Nature, who argued for an ‘Earth jurisprudence that allows us once more to assume our rightful place as an integral part of the larger

Table 2.1 Recent examples of flooding

Case	Description
Floods in Bangladesh, June 2022	Bangladesh is one of the countries most affected by climate change, facing increasing risks of flash floods (Germanwatch 2021; LSE 2023). In June 2022, the country experienced its worst floods in living memory, with 80% of the northeastern districts submerged, resulting in at least 141 fatalities and millions of others in the region injured, impoverished, or displaced (Human Rights Watch 2023).
Floods in Pakistan, June 2022	From June to August/September 2022, Pakistan experienced the worst floods in its history. More than 1,700 people died, 22 million people lost their homes, land, and jobs, 800,000 cattle and other livestock perished, and 28,999 schools and clinics were damaged (*The Guardian* 2023).
Floods in Western Germany, July 2021	In July 2021, the low-pressure system Bernd caused flooding in Western Germany. Despite warnings from weather experts and the European Flood Warning System, only residents within 50 metres of the river were asked to leave their homes. However, the floods affected people up to 250 metres away, claiming over 180 lives in addition to a €4.5 to 5.5 billion damage (BPB 2022; GDV 2022).
Floods in Southern Austria, August 2023	In early August 2023, heavy flooding affected parts of Southern Styria and Lower Carinthia due to the Zacharias Low. Rainfall reached 200 litres per square metre in five days, with almost 300 litres recorded in Slovenia. Evacuations took place, and at least six people died in Slovenia and Austria (*Die Zeit* 2023; BML 2024).
Update: Floods in Central Europe, September 2024	In September 2024, Storm Boris caused severe flooding in Austria, the Czech Republic, Hungary, Poland, Romania, and Slovakia. With up to five times the average September rainfall in just four days, the storm led to widespread evacuations and claimed the lives of at least 21 people, with several still missing.
Floods in East Africa, April 2024	In April 2024, East Africa experienced heavy rainfall and flooding, particularly Kenya, Tanzania, and Burundi. More than 200 people died, 100,000 were displaced, and damage to farmland and infrastructure was reported (*The Guardian* 2024). As of 30 May 2024, reports even indicated that 528 people had lost their lives, over 480,000 people had been displaced, and 1.6 million were affected by the flooding event, primarily in Kenya, Ethiopia, and Somalia (UNOCHA 2024).
Floods in Brazil, February 2022	On 15 February 2022, the city of Petrópolis in the highlands of the state of Rio de Janeiro experienced unusually heavy rainfall of 258 millimetres in three hours. Severe flash floods and subsequent landslides led to the deadliest landslide disaster ever recorded in the city, with 231 fatalities (Alcântara et al. 2022).
Floods in Ecuador, March 2020	In March 2020, Indigenous communities in Sarayaku were flooded following a historic storm in the Ecuadorian Amazon. Amid the COVID-19 pandemic, the floods destroyed infrastructure such as bridges, homes, schools, and gardens for growing food and medicine (Sarayaku 2020).

Source: Authors.

community of beings' (Cullinan 2003, p. 203). In line with this reasoning, Tănăsescu (2022) used the term 'Ecocene' to denote an era that is no longer solely about humans, but about accommodating, making peace with, and negotiating with everything that is non-human. This shift in focus away from human-centred to ecological processes indicates, in Tănăsescu's view, the broader context in which public health is pursued. This is also emphasised by One Health and Planetary Health scientists (Myers 2017, p. 2866; Whitmee et al. 2015, p. 1978; Redvers 2021, p. 2), with Redvers (2021) distinguishing between environmental determinants of human health, ecological determinants that influence both human and planetary health, and a more ecocentric approach that considers the conditions that affect the health of the planet as a whole (i.e., planetary determinants of health). Such work offers an invitation to expand the WHO's 1946 definition of health as 'a state of complete physical, mental and social well-being and not merely the absence of disease and infirmity' in relation to climate change.

In this context, 'natural' factors,[5] that is physical, biological, environmental, ecological, and planetary factors, should be analysed in conjunction with socio-political-economic dimensions that determine the health impacts of climate change. In Figure 2.1 we present a visualisation to assist researchers and policymakers in examining how factors within natural, biological, ecological, social, economic, political, and other previously unknown dimensions do not merely add up to affect health, but also interact in complex ways. This illustration also shows how these interactions span temporal and spatial dimensions, indicating that health impacts are produced and materialise in the past, present, and future, influenced by factors that overlap with acute, persistent, and chronic issues and evolving across geographical scales from local to global.

As Figure 2.1 illustrates, climate-related health impacts are not solely caused by natural disasters. Changing ecosystem conditions also make vector-borne diseases, such as malaria, and water-borne diseases, such as diarrhoeal diseases, more frequent. In the case of the floods in Bangladesh in 2022, for example, the WHO (2022) had recorded 2,492 cases of illness and injuries by 20 June, including instances of near-drowning, injuries, lightning, acute watery diarrhoea (AWD), skin, respiratory and eye infections with further outbreaks of disease expected after the water receded. In the case of the 2022 floods in Pakistan, the country was set back in its efforts to combat malaria (WHO 2023). In addition to these natural, physical, biological, and ecological dimensions that shape the health impacts of extreme weather events, people also vary in their ability to protect themselves from and deal with the health consequences.

Impacts from extreme weather events can exacerbate existing socio-economic vulnerabilities, with heatwaves, for instance, affecting people differently depending on their housing conditions, access to air conditioning, and the efficiency of emergency services. Floods, meanwhile, have a particularly severe impact on those with limited resources to cope with the loss of homes, jobs, or farmland, forced relocation, or the interruption of children's education. It becomes difficult to afford nutritious food or medical care, and on top of this, social services can be disrupted and public infrastructure destroyed, which can trigger famine, migration, and conflict (cf. Jungmann

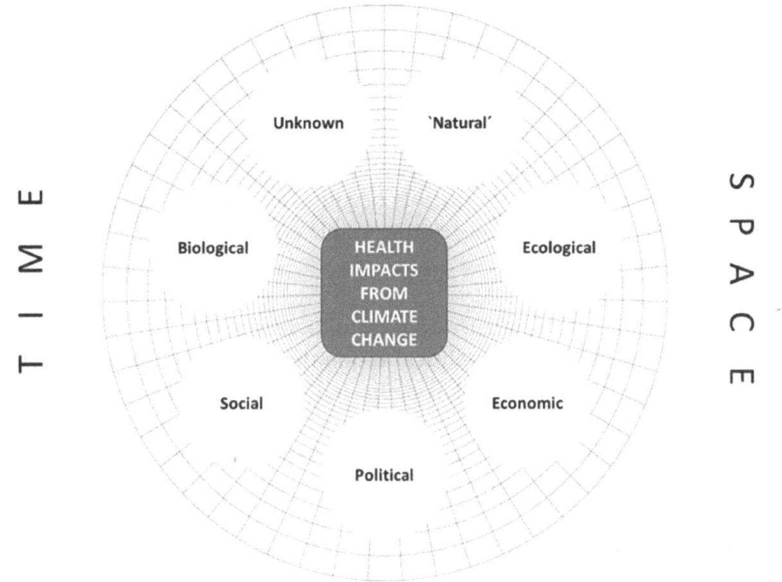

Source: Authors.

Figure 2.1 Multidimensional understanding of health amid climate change

2021, p. 15). The 2020 floods in Ecuador affected the Indigenous Sarayaku people, who—already struggling with the COVID-19 pandemic—had long been neglected by the state. The 2022 floods in Bangladesh hit those affected by long-standing inequalities related to race, ethnicity, religion, gender, and age the hardest (Chakraborty et al. 2024; *The Guardian* 2023). The results were drownings, injuries, lightning strike-related consequences, snake bites, shortages of drinking and bathing water, waterborne diseases, an increased disease burden among vulnerable people, a rising prevalence of mental health issues, food insecurity, and disruptions to health services. Health status, mental health, ecosystemic changes, poverty, inequalities, economic hardship, and the breakdown of infrastructure interacted very closely.

Moreover, health impacts from extreme weather events are not only caused directly by climate factors, but they are enabled also from harmful practices in the construction and extractive industries. For instance, the 2022 floods in Bangladesh were enabled not only by the country's topographical characteristics including its extensive floodplains formed by the Ganges, Brahmaputra, and Meghna rivers (80% of the country is floodplain), but also by deforestation, soil erosion from agriculture, and the damming of rivers (Human Rights Watch 2023; *The Guardian* 2023). Similarly, the 2024 East African floods were driven not only by human-induced climate change but also by rapid urbanisation, resource scarcity, and activities such as deforestation and agriculture (World Weather Attribution 2024). In Petrópolis, Brazil, unplanned urban growth on steep slopes, vegetation removal, and inadequate controls also contributed to flash flooding (Alcântara et al. 2022). In this context, construction, deforestation, agriculture, and other extractive industries are significant political-economic factors driving the health impacts of climate change. Considering multiple levels of health analysis into Environmental Impact Assessments (EIAs) and Strategic Environmental Assessments (SEAs) could be a strategy to mitigate the harmful impacts of extractive activities (Olalekan et al. 2020). In practice, however, this strategy has often proven problematic: these assessments frequently become formal tools to legitimise state-led extractive agendas (Fiske 2017), neglecting viable environmental, political, and economic alternatives.

Such debates regarding the influence of harmful industries on climate-health dynamics underscore the critical role of political action that tackles structural factors. There is a growing recognition that it takes dedicated political initiatives, measures, and policies to address the health impacts of climate change. International organisations have established knowledge hubs such as the WHO's focal point for climate and health (WHO 2021a), and the European Commission (EC) and the European Environment Agency (EEA) have launched the European Climate and Health Observatory (ECHO) (EC 2020; EEA 2021; ECHO 2023). Moreover, an emerging legislative body linking environmental and health aspects is evolving (see LSE 2022; Wu 2021): Some countries are integrating health-related goals and measures into climate legislation and, vice versa, incorporating environmental and climate considerations into health legislation. In 2021, 86% of countries included health concerns in their climate protection targets (Romanello 2022, p. 1622), and there are also calls to include climate protection as a fundamental right in constitutional law (for Austria, see Bioethikommission 2022).[6]

Furthermore, policy problems are increasingly framed in terms of health and climate. Echoing the plea for health-in-all-policies (Hall & Jacobson 2018, p. 364), One Health and Planetary Health scholars have called for governments to develop, implement, and assess 'ambitious, integrated policies to address the social, economic, and environmental determinants of health' (Whitmee et al. 2015, p. 1978; cf. de Castañeda et al. 2023; Haas et al. 2023; Batawalage et al. 2023). Here, we believe that it is useful to distinguish between precautionary, preventive, and adaptive measures. Precautionary measures are enacted even in the absence of full scientific certainty to prevent anticipated harm, and also because risks can become unmanageable once triggered. In contrast, preventive measures focus on addressing recognised risks, while adaptive measures respond to impacts that have already occurred. Environmental health scholars have long argued that a precautionary principle should shape a new public paradigm in terms of 'a set of guidelines that contend that society should take preventive action in the face of uncertainty in order to safeguard human health' (Mayer et al. 2002, p. 575; Brown 2007). Yet conversations about precautionary[7] and preventive measures related to climate and health remain sparse, while adaptation policies have garnered some attention. Jungmann's (2021) Climate Change Health Adaptation Index (CHAIn), for example, gauges countries' readiness to adapt to health impacts posed by climate change, factoring in risk recognition, adaptive capacity, and adaptation efforts. At the same time, the author cautions that these adaptation measures may carry the risk of unintended side effects.

Political initiatives aimed at mitigating the health impacts of climate change can have unintended side effects if the complexity of the situation is not sufficiently considered (cf. Wagenaar & Prainsack 2021; Wagenaar 2007; Prainsack 2023). Adaptation initiatives targeting heatwaves, drought, and desertification can exhibit such unintended consequences. For example, the provision of air conditioning in response to heatwaves can increase the demand for energy from fossil fuels and thus exacerbate 'the root problem of climate change' (Jungmann 2021, p. 29), which in turn has knock-on impacts on health. Conversely, improved water harvesting technologies can not only provide immediate relief during periods of drought and desertification but also reduce water-related health risks and support more sustainable management of natural resources in the long term.

People affected by the adverse health impacts of flooding have gained insight into the different dimensions that need to be considered when responding to the complex interactions between climate and health. The people affected by the 2023 floods in Carinthia (Austria) were keenly aware of how various factors interacted to create the situation.[8] Government-initiated projects to assist municipalities, communities, and residents in preparing for heavy rainfall events focused on housing planning, community flood defences, and citizen preparedness (Umweltbundesamt 2020). Despite these efforts, the residents of Guntschach expressed dissatisfaction with the political support at the municipal, state, and federal levels—arguably because they recognised that these measures did not get to the root causes of the problem. Residents pointed to factors such as soil sealing[9] in neighbouring villages, which they believed contributed to the increased flooding but were not adequately addressed (*Der Standard* 2024).[10] They criticised the political responses for failing to sufficiently consider the interacting factors that led to the flooding (cf. *Die Zeit* 2023; BML 2024) and knock-on health impacts—factors/dimensions that can have an impact across temporal and spatial boundaries.

When the impact of a single weather event does not stop at political borders, spatial interdependencies are becoming tangible. The inhabitants of villages such as Guntschach feel the health repercussions of floods that have been exacerbated by soil sealing in neighbouring areas. Moreover, as floods often affect more than one country, flood and water management in one country can affect the severity of flooding in another. These spatial interdependencies become more intricate when intertwined with global inequalities, as seen in situations where anthropogenic climate change originates in one area but influences populations in far-off locales. In 2022, floods in Bangladesh and Pakistan claimed thousands of lives and displaced millions of people. Despite being low-emission countries—Bangladesh produced only 0.25% of the world's total greenhouse gas emissions in 2021 and Pakistan accounted for less than an eighth of the per capita emissions of the US and a third of the emissions of the UK in 2020 (*The Guardian* 2023)—they faced widespread devastation from increasing extreme weather events such as flash floods. These countries are in a position of utter dependence on global efforts to mitigate climate change, particularly those of high-emission industrialised nations. This situation highlights the unequal distribution of disease burdens globally, which has historically been shaped by the interplay of violence, power, and colonialism (King & Koski 2020; Affun-Adegbulu & Adegbulu 2020; Hommes et al. 2021). As shown in the illustration (see Figure 2.1), the health impacts of climate change stem from chronic, persistent, and acute problems and are unevenly distributed across global, national, and local scales.

The illustration—depicting how various factors influencing health amid climate change interact across time and space—could be a helpful orientation for both policymakers and researchers. For the former, this figure could help to avoid the trap of reductionist problem framings, and the associated problems of solutions remaining within single policy fields, thereby encouraging integrated or at least coordinated action across multiple policy areas. For researchers, it could help locate existing evidence and identify research gaps, while prompting an exploration of methodological approaches that can yield insights for effective policy interventions. In this context, natural, biological, ecological, and socio-political-economic dimensions should be treated as analytical categories in climate-health research, serving as integral components of the situation or problem being studied. The following section examines how employing a mixed-methods approach that integrates inductive, qualitative, and transdisciplinary research can enhance our multidimensional understanding of health in relation to climate change.

2.3 How to research complex interactions? Mixed approaches, qualitative research, and transdisciplinarity

2.3.1 Unpacking the Politics Behind Evidence

Health effects from climate change are the result of a complex network of different interconnected and interacting factors that have not yet been fully explored. To date, much of the empirical work investigating the effects of climate change on health has consisted of quantitative model predictions (Whitmee 2015, p. 2018; *The Lancet Planetary Health* 2021; Betts & Sawyer 2015). As outlined in Table 2.2, these initiatives show that modelling work has addressed both the direct health impacts of climate change and those stemming from shifting ecosystem conditions. However, relatively little attention has been paid to the socio-political-economic factors that influence the health impacts of climate change.

Quantitative assessments of the health impacts of climate change are not ideal for capturing the interplay of the various social, economic, and political factors that influence these impacts. Whitmee et al. (2015, p. 1976) argued that '[m]any effects of global environmental change are difficult to quantify because they are mediated through complex systems that might have feedback loops and non-linear relationships between environmental change and health outcomes'. This raises the question of how mixed methods approaches that include qualitative methods could help to understand the complexity of tertiary health impacts specifically. Could such approaches improve

Table 2.2 Climate-health modelling

Initiative	Description
Coupled Model Intercomparison Project (CMIP), launched in 1995 by the Working Group on Coupled Modelling (WGCM) of the World Climate Research Programme (WCRP)	• Collaborative initiative to improve our understanding of climate change. • Brings together computer-based coupled climate models, which simulate complex interactions between different components of the Earth, such as the atmosphere, oceans, land, and ice. • Serves as a crucial data infrastructure for the Intergovernmental Panel on Climate Change (IPCC) and various national and supranational climate assessment initiatives (CMIP 2023; *The Lancet Planetary Health* 2021; *The Lancet* 2014).
Inter-Sectoral Impact Model Intercomparison Project (ISIMIP), launched in 2012 by the Potsdam Institute for Climate Impact Research (PIK) and the International Institute for Applied Systems Analysis (IIASA)	• Engaging 100 modelling groups worldwide by 2023. • Integrates socio-economic factors into the analysis of factors influencing the impacts of climate change and specifies these impacts in different sectors such as water, lakes, forests, and biodiversity at both global and regional levels. • Includes health-related issues such as temperature-related mortality, vector-borne and waterborne diseases, and food security and nutrition (ISIMIP 2023).
Environment and Health Modelling Lab (2023), at the Department of Public Health, Environment, and Society at the London School of Hygiene & Tropical Medicine	• Led by a multidisciplinary team of researchers specialised in biostatistics, environmental epidemiology, data science, statistical data processing, climatology, and other fields. • Develops pioneering innovative study designs, statistical methods, and modelling techniques for research on environmental health risks. • Has a specific focus on projecting the health effects of climate change. • Provides analysis of the time- and location-specific implications of temperature variations on health.
Special issue of *The Lancet Planetary Health* from 2021, titled: 'Taking globally consistent health impact projections to the next level' (Rocklöv et al. 2021; for a participatory modelling initiative, also see Olabisi et al. 2018)	• Analyses harmonised data and simulation protocols from ISIMIP. • Explores the specific health consequences of rising temperatures and disease spread across diverse locations. • Discusses the risks posed by specific vector-, food-, and water-borne diseases. • Also addresses occupational health risks such as anticipated declines in labour supply and productivity.

Source: Authors.

understandings of how the health impacts of climate change unfold unevenly across socio-spatial divides? McMichael and Lindgren (2011, p. 410) underscore that people's vulnerability to the health effects of climate change is contingent upon their geographical and social positioning. For instance, the Notre Dame Global Adaptation Initiative ND-GAINs ranking highlights general health risks across various sectors at the national level. Within this framework, when assessing water risks—specifically the vulnerability of freshwater supplies to climate change—India ranks 9th most vulnerable among 169 countries, Mexico 59th, and Austria 136th (GAIN 2023). However, preconceived categories such as people's national location are not enough, as we do not know how socio-spatial divides play out in people's everyday lives and what categories of difference lie behind the emerging areas of inequality that need to be addressed.

Insights garnered from everyday experiences may offer pathways to a better understanding in two ways. First, by enriching our understanding of how people perceive, experience, and understand the health impacts of climate change across socio-geographical boundaries. Second, these insights may shed light on how people experience the complex interactions between natural, biological, ecological, and socio-political-economic dimensions in their lives. Additionally, they may reveal other, previously unknown, unaccounted-for dimensions that influence, amplify, or limit the health impacts of climate change. While analysing the causal relationships between predefined categories may prove insufficient, an inductive qualitative research approach could yield unexpected results that recognise the complexity of the situation. Situational Analysis, which complements Constructivist Grounded Theory, stands out as a suitable approach because it breaks downs the division between a phenomenon and its context (Clarke et al. 2022). This method enables a holistic examination of all entities involved, encompassing individuals and groups as well as additional factors like meaning, power dynamics, material resources, and the involvement of non-human actors in a specific situation (Kalenda 2016; Timmermans & Tavory 2012; Charmaz 2006).[11] Thus, inductive as well as abductive approaches such as Situational Analysis offer the potential to integrate existing knowledge about how people perceive environmental changes, experience related health impacts, and navigate complex socio-political-economic dynamics within a transdisciplinary approach.

2.3.2 The Need for Transdisciplinary Research

Qualitative social science can play a crucial role in bringing to the fore a broad range of evidence on how people experience the health impacts of climate change. Such evidence can be gathered, for example, from civil society, Indigenous peoples, and personal accounts of affected communities. This is particularly important given the historical context where vested interests opposed to climate action, such as oil companies, have actively undermined scientific knowledge. They have disingenuously argued that alternatives to oil would be economically disastrous (Dembicki 2022). A group of scientists with close connections to the oil industry misled the public about global warming, tobacco smoke, acid rain, and insecticides (Oreskes & Conway 2010). There is an urgent need to scrutinise, challenge, and change the underlying politics of evidence: this could be achieved by shifting the burden of proof to proponents of extractive activities such as oil drilling and mineral extraction, and by engaging a broad range of stakeholders in efforts to protect human health and the environment (Mayer et al. 2002, p. 117; Fiske 2023). Such calls for integrating perspectives, experiences, and knowledge from various stakeholders at local, national, and international levels have also been articulated in the field of climate and health in recent years by The Lancet Countdown to Health and Climate Change and the Rockefeller Foundation-Lancet Commission on Planetary Health (Romanello et al. 2023, p. 2353; 2022, p. 1622; Whitmee et al. 2015, p. 2018; cf. Myers 2017).

But what could transdisciplinary climate and health research look like? Sustainability scientists have described transdisciplinarity as a third epistemic pathway beyond the binary emphasis on either scientific research or practical application; one that involves 'research collaborations among scientists from different disciplines and non-academic stakeholders from business, government, and the civil society to address sustainability challenges and develop solution options' (Lang et al. 2021, p. 26; cf. Lang et al. 2012). It shares characteristics with other collaborative research approaches such as community-based, interactive, and participatory approaches and encounters similar challenges—including the fact that collaborating partners may interpret the problem at hand differently, that they may lack a shared vocabulary for discussing the topic, and that they adhere to distinct forms of organising their work.

One of the key questions thus is how collaborators perceive, experience, and address the challenges arising from the interactions between climate and health. Engaging flood-affected residents in Guntschach, Austria, in research collaborations with scientists could generate valuable knowledge. Likewise, partnering with business, government, and civil society stakeholders from flood-prone regions such as Bangladesh and Pakistan could help rethink policy interventions, strengthen institutional commitments, and foster global responsibility. In their analysis of the 2023 floods in Bangladesh, scholars underscored the importance of coordinating among various stakeholders, such as global players, national governments, local governments, civil society organisations, the private sector, and research institutions. The 2021 floods in Germany were attributed to a lack of responsibility on the part of the federal states in addition to inadequate risk maps, inefficient crisis communication, and insufficient siren infrastructure (see e.g., Decker et al., 2021). Regarding the 2023 floods in Bangladesh, scholars have also highlighted the need to collect knowledge about vulnerabilities and local needs, and to integrate local knowledge into policies, plans, and decision-making processes (LSE 2023; Chakraborty et al. 2024). This means that in addition to improving early warning systems, flood hazard maps, flood monitoring tools, and nature-based solutions such as mangrove planting, reforestation, and afforestation, it is necessary to pay close attention to people's experiences during floods: what happens when people lose their homes? How do they depict these processes (e.g., drawing community maps)? How do they observe environmental change over time (e.g., marking high water levels during floods)? What kind of health impacts do they experience, including mental health challenges such as dislocation, Post-Traumatic Stress Disorder (PTSD), or difficulty getting health needs met during times of crisis? What kinds of local knowledge do they apply (e.g., Indigenous knowledge on tidal river management, changes in building or community design)? Such collaboratively created knowledge can be of utmost importance for identifying possible interventions against the health effects from climate change.[12]

There is considerable potential for researchers, scientific communities, and academia to address the most pressing health challenges of the twenty-first century through transdisciplinary collaboration. At the same time, however, transdisciplinary research faces significant institutional barriers. Academic institutions, despite rhetoric around the importance of transdisciplinary and interdisciplinary research, still give incentives to disciplines operating in silos. Discipline-specific evaluation criteria and educational curricula that marginalise collaborative, inter-, and transdisciplinary output (cf. Frickel & Gross 2005; Frickel & Moore 2006) are still the norm in universities in most world regions. Additionally, institutional support structures, encompassing administrative services, infrastructure, and professional development opportunities, are typically tailored to traditional disciplinary research paths, lacking the flexibility required for transdisciplinary work. With only a few exceptions, funding mechanisms often exacerbate this challenge, as grant agencies and institutional funding bodies typically favour well-established disciplinary research, which discourages transdisciplinary initiatives that may seem riskier or less conventional. We argue that this fragmentation still holds in place a research culture that prioritises disciplinary depth over inter- and transdisciplinary breadth, making it difficult for researchers to engage in collaborative efforts across disciplines, fields, and sectors. A systemic overhaul is necessary to shift this culture towards integrative and co-produced knowledge, which is necessary for the advancement of transdisciplinary climate and health research.

Transdisciplinary insights, knowledge, and research can illuminate the complex dynamics among various factors influencing the health impacts of climate change. Such an understanding can also pinpoint leverage points, meaning 'places within complex systems ... where a small shift in one thing can produce big changes in everything' (Meadows 1999, p. 1; cf. Abson et al. 2017, p. 30; Lang et al. 2021, p. 32). Identifying these leverage points is crucial for devising effective strategies to address, mitigate, and adapt to the health effects of climate change. However, Abson et al. (2017) have highlighted that leverage points which are easily influenced, intuitively conceived, and seemingly 'quick fixes' are often too weak for urgent issues like the climate crisis. More impactful leverage points are typically less obvious, sometimes harder to influence, but ultimately more effective. In the realm of climate-health interventions, these may involve sustainable land use, rewilding initiatives, cultural heritage preservation, respect for socio-communitarian relations, addressing existing inequalities, legal and policy measures, and much more. Within the complex interplay of climate and health, such dynamics could serve as crucial leverage points with the potential to prevent, mitigate, or adapt to the health impacts of climate change.

Transdisciplinary approaches to understanding the multidimensional constitution of health in a changing climate hold the potential to identify profound leverage points for political interventions that may be less obvious but often prove more effective. They moreover prompt a reassessment of the strategies employed in public health delivery in safeguarding public health amidst a changing climate.

Notes

1. The Millennium Ecosystem Assessment (commissioned by the United Nations in 2000 and published in 2005) encapsulates the direct health impacts succinctly as 'flooding, heat waves, water shortage, landslides, exposure to ultraviolet radiation, exposure to pollutants' (Millennium Ecosystem Assessment 2005).
2. Here, the term 'natural' tends to refer to the primary, the term 'eco-systemic' to the secondary, and the term 'societal dynamics' to the tertiary health effects of climate change.
3. While research has established a broad correlation between convective precipitation and air temperature (Fowler et al. 2021), the recently developed attribution theory for extreme weather can show the extent to which extreme weather events can be attributed to anthropogenic climate change and/or other factors (Otto & von Brackel 2019).
4. Heatwaves are often associated with drought, poor air quality, and forest fires, which may make flash flooding more likely when rains come (WMO 2022).
5. 'Natural', written here in inverted commas, is an indicator of dynamics that may appear natural in the sense of externally given influences, but which could later be understood more deeply in their biological, ecological, socio-political-economic, and other constitution.
6. As is widely recognised, supranational entities have enacted climate change legislation, such as the European Climate Change Law (EC 2021) and the climate strategy of the African Union (2022).
7. We believe that this is a crucial starting point for scientific, political, and social action, but it requires a broader discussion that we cannot provide in this chapter.
8. In the municipality of Bad Eisenkappel, emergency aid was provided to 200 residents who were supplied with food and medicine after the access road was destroyed by the flood. In Guntschach, 70 inhabitants were isolated from December 2022 to May 2024 due to a rockfall in 2022 and landslides during the 2023 floods that washed away an emergency road. Despite predictions of increased extreme weather, Guntschach residents chose to stay, using a ferry and forest trails to leave the village.
9. Soil sealing means that natural soil is covered with materials such as concrete, asphalt, or buildings, which prevents water from infiltrating into the ground.
10. In Europe, the European Commission launched a Floods Directive in 2007 to reduce the risk of flood damage through '[i]ntegrated flood risk management [that] must focus on sustainable water management and measures that strengthen the resilience of nature and society to extreme weather events' (EC 2024).
11. Actor Network Theory is another approach for this purpose.
12. Here, it is important to note that such interventions can address both health impacts and climate change to varying degrees.

References

Abson, D. J., Fischer, J., Leventon, J., Newig, J., Schomerus, T., Vilsmaier, U., et al. (2017) 'Leverage points for sustainability transformation'. *Ambio*, 46, pp. 30–39.

Affun-Adegbulu, C., & Adegbulu, O. (2020) 'Decolonising global (public) health: From western universalism to global pluriversalities'. *BMJ Global Health*, 5(8). https://doi.org/10.1136/bmjgh-2020-002947

African Union (2022) *African Union Climate Change and Resilient Development Strategy and Action Plan (2022–2032).* (Online) https://au.int/en/documents/20220628/african-union-climate-change-and-resilient-development-strategy-and-action-plan

Alcântara, E., Marengo, J. A., Mantovani, J., Londe, L., San, R. L. Y., Park, E., et al. (2022) 'Deadly disasters in southeastern South America: Flash floods and landslides of February 2022 in Petrópolis, Rio de Janeiro'. *Natural Hazards and Earth System Sciences Discussions*, 23(3), pp. 1157–1175.

Batawalage, L. H. F., Williams, B., & Wijegoonewardene, M. N. Y. F. (2023) 'A climate health policy: Will it be a better approach to overcome the greatest global challenge of the 21st century? A review to explore public and public health officials' perceptions towards policy development'. *The Journal of Climate Change and Health*, 13. https://doi.org/10.1016/j.joclim.2023.100257

Betts, K., & Sawyer, K. (2015) *Modeling the Health Risks of Climate Change: Workshop Summary. Standing Committee on Emerging Science for Environmental Health Decisions; Board on Life Sciences; Division on Earth and Life Studies; National Research Council, Academic Press (US).* (Online) https://www.ncbi.nlm.nih.gov/books/NBK305533/

Bioethikkommission (2022) *Die Klimakrise als ethische Herausforderung. Stellungnahme der Bioethikkommission, Wien.* (Online) https://www.bundeskanzleramt.gv.at/dam/jcr:d0e336aa-db97-4833-b0a5-e2d51e9eca7d/klimakrise_ethische_herausforderung.pdf

BML (2024) 'Die Hochwasserereignisse vom 03. bis 07. August 2023 im Süden und Südosten Österreichs'. (Online)https://info.bml.gv.at/themen/wasser/wasser-oesterreich/hydrographie/chronik-besonderer-ereignisse/hochwasser-august-2023.html

BPB (2022) 'Jahrhunderthochwasser 2021 in Deutschland. Bundeszentrale für politische Bildung'. (Online) https://www.bpb.de/kurz-knapp/hintergrund-aktuell/337277/jahrhunderthochwasser-2021-in-deutschland

Brown, P. (2007) *Toxic Exposures: Contested Illnesses and the Environmental Health Movement.* Columbia University Press.

Butler, C. D. (2014) 'Climate change and global health: A new conceptual framework-Mini Review'. *CABI Reviews*, 9(27), pp. 1–3.

Butler, C. D. (2018) 'Climate change, health and existential risks to civilization: A comprehensive review (1989–2013)'. *International Journal of Environmental Research and Public Health*, 15(10), p. 2266.

Butler, C. D., Corvalan, C. F., & Koren, H. S. (2005) 'Human health, well-being, and global ecological scenarios'. *Ecosystems*, 8, pp. 153–162.

Chakraborty, D., Mondal, K. P., Jubaer, A., Islam, S. T., & Talukder, B. (2024) 'Health impacts of rapid-onset event: 2022 flash flood in Bangladesh.' In Letcher, T. M. (Ed.), *Living with Climate Change*, Elsevier, pp. 199–212.

Charmaz, K. (2006) *Constructing Grounded Theory: A Practical Guide Through Qualitative Analysis.* Sage.

Clarke, A. E., Washburn, R., & Friese, C. (Eds.) (2022) *Situational Analysis in Practice: Mapping Relationalities Across Disciplines.* Routledge.

CMIP (2023) *Coupled Model Intercomparison Projects (CMIP).* (Online) https://wcrp-cmip.org/

Costello, A., Abbas, M., Allen, A., Ball, S., Bell, S., Bellamy, R., et al. (2009) 'Managing the health effects of climate change'. *The Lancet*, 373(9676), pp. 1693–1733.

Cullinan, C. (2003) *Wild Law: A Manifesto for Earth Justice.* Green Books in association with the Gaia Foundation.

de Castañeda, R. R., Villers, J., Guzmán, C. A. F., Eslanloo, T., de Paula, N., Machalaba, C., et al. (2023) 'One Health and planetary health research: Leveraging differences to grow together'. *The Lancet Planetary Health*, 7(2), pp. e109–e111.

Decker, M., Heinze, S., & Cleven, T. (2021) 'Unwetter-Katastrophe in NRW und RLP: Was lief beim Hochwasser schief?' (Online) https://www.rnd.de/politik/unwetter-katastrophe-in-nrw-und-rlp-was-lief-beim-hochwasser-schief-Q56JBKWS6VDPZDCLKBI44BLJMQ.html

Dembicki, G. (2022). *The Petroleum Papers: Inside the Far-Right Conspiracy to Cover Up Climate Change*. Greystone Books Ltd.

Der Standard (2024) 'Mitten in Österreich, abgeschnitten von der Welt: Guntschach kämpft um seine Zukunft'. (Online) https://www.derstandard.at/story/3000000201432/mitten-in-oesterreich-abgeschnitten-von-der-welt-guntschach-kaempft-um-seine-zukunft

Die Zeit (2023) 'Die Geräusche waren das Schlimmste'. (Online) https://www.zeit.de/gesellschaft/2023-08/oesterreich-slowenien-unwetter-ueberschwemmungen-hochwasser

EC (2020) 'Adaptation to health effects of climate change in Europe'. (Online) https://op.europa.eu/en/web/eu-law-and-publications/publication-detail/-/publication/e885e150-c258-11ea-b3a4-01aa75ed71a1

EC [European Commission] (2021) *European Climate Change Law*. (Online) https://climate.ec.europa.eu/eu-action/european-green-deal/european-climate-law_de

EC (2024) 'Floods. EU measures to manage the risks floods pose to human health, the environment, the economy and cultural heritage'. (Online) https://environment.ec.europa.eu/topics/water/floods_en

ECHO [European Climate and Health Observatory] (2023). *European Climate and Health Observatory*. (Online) https://climate-adapt.eea.europa.eu/en/observatory

EEA [European Environment Agency] (2021) 'Europe's changing climate hazards — an index-based interactive EEA report'. (Online) https://www.eea.europa.eu/publications/europes-changing-climate-hazards-1/wet-and-dry-1/wet-and-dry-heavy

Fiske, A. (2017) 'Bounded impacts, boundless promise: Environmental impact assessments of oil production in the Ecuadorian Amazon'. In Jalbert, K., Willow, A., Casagrande, D., & Paladino, St. (Eds.), *ExtrACTION*, Routledge, pp. 63–76.

Fiske, A. M. (2023) *Reckoning with Harm: The Toxic Relations of Oil in Amazonia*. University of Texas Press.

Fowler, H. J., Lenderink, G., Prein, A. F., Westra, S., Allan, R. P., Ban, N., Barbero, R., Berg, P., Blenkinsop, S., Do, H. X., Guerreiro, S., Haerter, J. O., Kendon, E. J., Lewis, E., Schaer, C., Sharma, A., Villarini, G., Wasko, C., & Zhang, X. (2021) 'Anthropogenic intensification of short-duration rainfall extremes'. *Nature Reviews Earth & Environment*, 2, pp. 107–122. (Online) https://www.nature.com/articles/s43017-020-00128-6

Frickel, S., & Gross, N. (2005) 'A general theory of scientific/intellectual movements'. *American Sociological Review*, 70(2), pp. 204–232.

Frickel, S., & Moore, K. (Eds.) (2006) *The New Political Sociology of Science: Institutions, Networks, and Power*. University of Wisconsin Press.

GAIN (2023) *Notre Dame Global Adaptation Index, or ND-GAIN. Water/Country Rankings*. (Online) https://gain-new.crc.nd.edu/ranking/vulnerability/water

GDV (2022) 'Tiefdruckgebiet "Bernd": GDV erhöht Schadenschätzung auf 4,5 bis 5,5 Milliarden Euro'. (Online)https://www.gdv.de/de/themen/news/tiefdruckgebiet-bernd-gdv-er-hoeht-schadenschaetzung-auf-4-5-bis-5-5-milliarden-euro-69038

Germanwatch (2021) *Global Climate Risk Index 2021*. (Online) https://www.germanwatch.org/en/19777

Haas, W., Lampl, C., Aigner, E., & Schmidt, A. (2023) 'Climate mainstreaming: Climate and health policy, POLICY BRIEF February 2023, FEPS Foundation for European Progressive Studies, Brussels'. (Online) https://feps-europe.eu/publication/climate-and-health-policy/

Hall, R. L., & Jacobson, P. D. (2018) 'Examining whether the health-in-all-policies approach promotes health equity'. *Health Affairs*, 37(3), pp. 364–370.

Hommes, F., Monzó, H. B., Ferrand, R. A., Harris, M., Hirsch, L. A., Besson, E. K., et al. (2021) 'The words we choose matter: Recognising the importance of language in decolonising global health'. *The Lancet Global Health*, 9(7). https://doi.org/10.1016/S2214-109X(21)00197-2

Horton, R., & Lo, S. (2015) 'Planetary health: A new science for exceptional action'. *The Lancet*, 386(10007), pp. 1921–1922.

Human Rights Watch (2023) *Bangladesh: Protect People Most At Risk During Monsoon Season.* (Online) https://www.hrw.org/news/2023/06/19/bangladesh-protect-people-most-risk-during-monsoon-season#:~:text=Severe%20flash%20floods%20in%20northeastern,disproportionate%20difficulties%20in%20surviving%20extreme

IPCC (2023) *AR6 Synthesis Report. Climate Change 2023.* (Online) https://www.ipcc.ch/report/ar6/syr/

ISIMIP (2023) *The Inter-Sectoral Impact Model Intercomparison Project (ISIMIP).* (Online) https://www.isimip.org/

Jungmann, M. (2021) *The Politics of the Climate Change-Health Nexus.* Routledge.

Kalenda, J. (2016) 'Situational analysis as a framework for interdisciplinary research in the social sciences'. *Human Affairs*, 26(3), pp. 340–355.

King, N. B., & Koski, A. (2020) 'Defining global health as public health somewhere else'. *BMJ Global Health*, 5(1). https://doi.org/10.1136/bmjgh-2019-002172

Lang, D. J., Renn, O., Rehm, A., & Ernst, A. (2021) 'Transdisziplinäre Forschung mit transformativem Anspruch: Zehn Jahre NaWis: Rückblick und Vorausschau'. *GAIA-Ecological Perspectives for Science and Society*, 30(1), pp. 51–53.

Lang, D. J., Wiek, A., Bergmann, M., Stauffacher, M., Martens, P., Moll, P., et al. (2012) 'Transdisciplinary research in sustainability science: Practice, principles, and challenges'. *Sustainability Science*, 7, pp. 25–43.

Lock, M. M., & Nguyen, V. K. (2018) *An Anthropology of Biomedicine.* John Wiley & Sons.

LSE (2022) 'What is climate change legislation?' (Online) https://www.lse.ac.uk/granthaminstitute/explainers/what-is-climate-change-legislation/

LSE (2023) 'Policy brief. Tackling flooding in Bangladesh in a changing climate'. (Online) https://www.lse.ac.uk/granthaminstitute/wp-content/uploads/2023/08/Tackling-flooding-in-Bangladesh-in-a-changing-climate.pdf

Mayer, B., Brown, P., & Linder, M. (2002) 'Moving further upstream: From toxics reduction to the precautionary principle'. *Public Health Reports*, 117(6), pp. 574–586.

McMichael, A. J., & Lindgren, E. (2011) 'Climate change: Present and future risks to health, and necessary responses'. *Journal of Internal Medicine*, 270(5), pp. 401–413.

Meadows, D. (1999) *Leverage Points: Places to Intervene in a System.* The Sustainability Institute.

Millennium Ecosystem Assessment (2005) *Ecosystems and Human Well-being: Wetlands and Water.* World Resources Institute.

Myers, S. S. (2017) 'Planetary health: Protecting human health on a rapidly changing planet'. *The Lancet*, 390(10114), pp. 2860–2868.

Olabisi, L. S., Azhar, G. S., Abbott, M., & Lempert, R. J. (2018) 'Participatory modeling of climate change impacts on public health in Long Beach, California: Discussion from a workshop hosted by the RAND Frederick S. Pardee Center for Longer Range Global Policy and the Future Human Condition'. *Rand Health Quarterly*, 8(1), p. 4.

Olalekan, R. M., Oluwatoyin, O. A., Olawale, S. H., Emmanuel, O. O., & Olalekan, A. Z. (2020) 'A critical review of health impact assessment: Towards strengthening the knowledge of decision makers understand sustainable development goals in the twenty-first century: Necessity today; Essentiality tomorrow'. *Research and Advances: Environmental Sciences*, 1, pp. 72–84.

Oreskes, N., & Conway, E. M. (2010) *Merchants of Doubt: How a Handful of Scientists Obscured the Truth on Issues from Tobacco Smoke to Global Warming.* Bloomsbury.

Otto, F., & von Brackel, B. (2019) *Wütendes Wetter: Auf der Suche nach den Schuldigen für Hitzewellen, Hochwasser und Stürme*. Ullstein Buchverlage.

Prainsack, B. (2023) 'The roots of neglect: Towards a sociology of non-imagination'. *TECNOSCIENZA: Italian Journal of Science & Technology Studies*, 13(2), pp. 13–34.

Radhuber, I. M., Fiske, A., Galasso, I., Gessl, N., Hill, M. D., Morales, E. R., et al. (2023) 'Toward global citizenship? People (de)bordering their lives during COVID-19 in Latin America and Europe'. *Global Public Health*, 18(1). https://doi.org/10.1080/17441692.2023.2285880

Radhuber, I., El-Sayed, S., Haddad, Ch., Kieslich, K., Paul, K. T., Prainsack, B., et al. (2024) 'Citizenship in times of crises: Biosocial state-citizen relations during Covid-19 in Austria'. *BioSocieties*, 19, pp. 326–351.

Radhuber, I., Ferstl, S., Kancelová, N. V., Kieslich, K., Kraus, D., Paul, K., et al. (2025) 'Why "inclusive policymaking" is needed during crises: COVID-19 and social divisions in Austria'. *SSM – Qualitative Research in Health*, 7. https://doi.org/10.1016/j.ssmqr.2025.100539

Redvers, N. (2021) 'The determinants of planetary health'. *The Lancet Planetary Health*, 5(3), pp. e111–e112.

Rocklöv, J., Huber, V., Bowen, K., & Paul, R. (2021) 'Taking globally consistent health impact projections to the next level'. *The Lancet Planetary Health*, 5(7), pp. e487–e493.

Romanello, M., Di Napoli, C., Drummond, P., Green, C., Kennard, H., Lampard, P., et al. (2022) 'The 2022 report of the Lancet Countdown on Health and Climate Change'. *The Lancet*, 400(10363), pp. 1619–1654.

Romanello, M., Di Napoli, C., Green, C., Kennard, H., Lampard, P., Scamman, D., et al. (2023) 'The 2023 report of the Lancet Countdown on Health and Climate Change: The imperative for a health-centred response in a world facing irreversible harms'. *The Lancet*, 402(10419), pp. 2346–2394.

Sarayaku (2020) 'Sarayaku después de la inundación'. (Online) https://sarayaku.org/sarayaku-despues-de-la-inundacion/

Seneviratne, S. I., Zhang, X., Adnan, M., Badi, W., Dereczynski, C., Luca, A. D., et al. (2021) 'Weather and climate extreme events in a changing climate'. In Masson-Delmotte, V. P., Zhai, A., Pirani, S. L., & Connors, C. (Eds.), *Climate Change 2021: The Physical Science Basis: Working Group I Contribution to the Sixth Assessment Report of the Intergovernmental Panel on Climate Change*, Cambridge University Press, pp. 1513–1766.

Smith, K. R., Chafe, Z., Woodward, A., Campbell-Lendrum, D., Chadee, D. D., Honda, Y., et al. (2014) 'Human health: Impacts, adaptation, and co-benefits'. In Field, C. B., Barros, V. R., Dokken, D. J., Mach, K. J., Mastrandrea, M. D., Bilir, T. E. et al. (Eds.), *Climate Change 2014–Impacts, Adaptation, and Vulnerability. Part A: Global and Sectoral Aspects. Contribution of Working Group II to the Fifth Assessment Report of the Intergovernmental Panel on Climate Change*. Cambridge University Press, pp. 709–754.

Talukder, B., van Loon, G. W., Hipel, K. W., Chiotha, S., & Orbinski, J. (2021) 'Health impacts of climate change on smallholder farmers'. *One Health*, 13. https://doi.org/10.1016/j.onehlt.2021.100258

Tănăsescu, M. (2022) *Ecocene Politics*. Open Book Publishers.

The Environment and Health Modelling Lab (2023) *London School of Hygiene & Tropical Medicine*. (Online) https://www.lshtm.ac.uk/research/centres-projects-groups/ehm-lab

The Guardian (2023) 'A year on, the devastating long-term effects of Pakistan's floods are revealed'. (Online)https://www.theguardian.com/global-development/2023/aug/05/a-year-on-the-devastating-long-term-effects-of-pakistans-floods-are-revealed

The Guardian (2024) 'Weather tracker: Heavy rainfall causes flooding and death in east Africa'. (Online) https://www.theguardian.com/environment/2024/apr/26/weather-tracker-heavy-rainfall-flooding-death-east-africa

The Lancet (2014) 'Planetary health for the ages'. *The Lancet*, 383, p. 847.

The Lancet Planetary Health (2021) 'Modelling health futures'. *The Lancet Planetary Health*, 5(7), pp. e827–839.

Timmermans, S., & Tavory, I. (2012) 'Theory construction in qualitative research: From grounded theory to abductive analysis'. *Sociological Theory*, 30(3), pp. 167–186.

UNOCHA (2024) 'Eastern Africa: Heavy rains and flooding Flash Update #4'. (Online) https://www.unocha.org/publications/report/kenya/eastern-africa-heavy-rains-and-flooding-flash-update-4-30-may-2024#:~:text=In%20Kenya%2C%20315%20people%20have,to%20the%20National%20Disaster%20Operations

Umweltbundesamt (2020) 'RAINMAN: So geht Starkregen-Vorsorge'. (Online) https://www.umweltbundesamt.at/news200629

Wagenaar, H. (2007) 'Governance, complexity, and democratic participation: How citizens and public officials harness the complexities of neighborhood decline'. *The American Review of Public Administration*, 37(1), pp. 17–50.

Wagenaar, H., & Prainsack, B. (2021) *The Pandemic Within: Policy Making for a Better World*. Policy Press.

Whitmee, S., Haines, A., Beyrer, C., Boltz, F., Capon, A. G., de Souza Dias, B. F., Ezeh, A., Gong, P., et al. (2015) 'Safeguarding human health in the Anthropocene epoch: Report of The Rockefeller Foundation–Lancet Commission on planetary health'. *The Lancet*, 386(10007), pp. 1973–2028.

WHO [World Health Organization] (2014) *Quantitative Risk Assessment of the Effects of Climate Change on Selected Causes of Death, 2030s and 2050s*. World Health Organization. (Online) https://www.who.int/publications/i/item/9789241507691

WHO (2021a) 'Climate and health'. (Online) https://www.who.int/news-room/fact-sheets/detail/climate-change-and-health

WHO (2021b) 'Climate change and health research: Current trends, gaps and perspectives for the future'. (Online) https://www.who.int/publications/m/item/climate-change-and-health-research-current-trends-gaps-and-perspectives-for-the-future

WHO (2022) 'Bangladesh flood 2022: WHO collaboration with DGHS/MOHFW'. (Online) https://www.who.int/bangladesh/news/detail/23-06-2022-bangladesh-flood-2022-who-collaboration-with-dghs-mohfw

WHO (2023) '"It was just the perfect storm for malaria" – Pakistan responds to surge in cases following the 2022 floods'. (Online)https://www.who.int/news-room/feature-stories/detail/It-was-just-the-perfect-storm-for-malaria-pakistan-responds-to-surge-in-cases-following-the-2022-floods

WMO [World Meterological Organization] (2022) 'Rising risks'. (Online) https://wmo.int/about-us/world-meteorological-day/wmd-2022/rising-risks

World Weather Attribution (2024) 'Urban planning at the heart of increasingly severe East African flood impacts in a warming world'. (Online) https://www.worldweatherattribution.org/urban-planning-at-the-heart-of-increasingly-severe-east-african-flood-impacts-in-a-warming-world/

Wu, C. F. (2021) 'Challenges to protecting the right to health under the climate change regime'. *Health and Human Rights*, 23(2), p. 121.

3 Immunization and society: A social science agenda for pharmacovigilance

Maurizia Mezza and Stuart Blume

3.1 Introduction

Despite ready access to vaccines, in the 1980s vaccination rates were falling in many industrialized Western countries. The decline was commonly attributed to the activities of anti-vaccination groups. By the 1990s, the internet offered these groups a new channel for promoting their views. Public health researchers then started asking 'What messages might a parent encounter, searching the internet for information?' If the actual influence of anti-vaccination groups on parental decisions had been investigated, rather than simply assumed, a different picture would have emerged.

Once social scientists began to question parents, a far more complex picture did indeed emerge. The decision whether or not to vaccinate a child was generally found to be difficult, shared with family, other parents, and by no means determined by prior ideology or anti-vax propaganda. What did appear was that negative prior experience, or the negative experiences of friends and family, weighed heavily. Parents were annoyed by the one-sided nature of information provided, by the unwillingness or inability of professionals to answer their questions, and by the often-coercive nature of encounters with public health professionals (Blume, 2006).

Whether they finally decided for or against vaccination, it became clear that many parents were hesitant and uncertain. This could not easily be ascribed to anti-vaccination organizations/misinformation. Nor could it be quantified or countered with the standard tools of public health or of epidemiology. In the early 2000s, the public health community reluctantly acknowledged that the focus had to be on what became known as 'vaccine hesitancy'. In 2019, seven years after first trying to define the concept, the World Health Organization (WHO) listed vaccine hesitancy among the top ten threats to global health (Akbar, no date).

The COVID-19 pandemic dramatically amplified public anxieties surrounding vaccine safety. The speed with which COVID-19 vaccines were developed and deployed raised concerns about the adequacy of testing and the long-term safety profile of the vaccines. Given the typically limited composition of clinical trial populations, such concerns could arise particularly in (ethnically) diverse populations (Jethwa, Wong & Abraham, 2021). Fear of potential side effects was a significant barrier to vaccine acceptance (e.g., Ruiz & Bell, 2022).

The European Medicines Agency (EMA) defines pharmacovigilance as the 'science and activities relating to the detection, assessment, understanding, and prevention of adverse effects or any other medicine-related problem' (EMA, 2024). Pharmacovigilance operates across two main phases: pre-authorization and post-authorization. In the **pre-authorization phase**, extensive data on a vaccine's safety, efficacy, and quality must be collected and submitted to regulatory agencies before it can be licensed for routine use. This phase primarily involves clinical trials conducted in controlled environments and with carefully selected populations, ensuring rigorous evaluation before market approval. The **post-authorization phase**, by contrast, focuses on the surveillance of the vaccine once it is in widespread use. This stage monitors its safety and efficacy in much larger and more diverse populations, often uncovering rare or long-term side effects that may not have been evident during pre-authorization trials. National pharmacovigilance centers play a critical role in this phase by collecting data on adverse effects reported by healthcare professionals, pharmaceutical companies, and, more recently, directly from patients and consumers. As a professional field, pharmacovigilance has expanded over the past few years. A European association established in 1992 became the International Society of Pharmacovigilance in 2000, with members from around the world (ISoP, no date). One report[1] predicts that expenditure on pharmacovigilance will reach $14.95 billion by 2028. At the same time, pharmacovigilance has become increasingly sophisticated methodologically, though with little impact on the prevalence of 'vaccine hesitancy'.

Vaccine pharmacovigilance, particularly post-authorization surveillance, plays a critical role in monitoring vaccine safety and effectiveness. How it does so has been little studied, and the field remains largely unfamiliar to society at large. This chapter begins with a historical overview of the development of pharmacovigilance, with a focus on the EU. We outline its theoretical framework and the critical questions in need of study by social scientists. Pharmacovigilance has the potential to bridge the gap between public health and civil society, fostering trust and collaboration. But many questions as to how it can best do this still remain.

3.1.1 The Origins of (Vaccine) Pharmacovigilance

Pharmacovigilance systems in Europe were created in response to the thalidomide disaster of the early 1960s, when more than 10,000 children were born with a range of severe deformities as a consequence of a sedative prescribed to their mothers to treat morning sickness (Strom, 2012). This is considered the first occasion on which healthcare professionals collaborated transnationally to establish a possible causal link between a compound and side effects (McBride, 1961).

Between 1960 and 1965, most European countries established national centers and programs to monitor adverse reactions to drugs. In the UK, the Yellow Card system was launched in 1964. In the Netherlands, in 1963 the National Medicines Evaluation

Board was established (van Grootheest & van Puijenbroek, 2002). Recognizing the global need for coordinated pharmacovigilance efforts, the WHO established its Programme for International Drug Monitoring in 1968, initially involving ten member states (WHO, 2022). The program was immediately effective. The following year it emerged that Clioquinol, a drug used to treat fungal infections, could lead to impaired vision (a condition known as retrobulbar optic neuritis) in Japan (Meade, 1975). In 1971, it was found that diethylstilbestrol, a synthetic estrogen given to pregnant women since the 1940s to prevent spontaneous abortions and to relieve nausea, could cause genital tumors in female offspring (Veurink et al., 2005). Not only can there be an ethnic susceptibility to drugs, but adverse drug effects can occur years later, or even in the next generation.

3.2 The pharmacovigilance landscape

Fearing that liability claims could drive manufacturers out of vaccine production, in 1986 the US Congress passed a National Childhood Vaccine Injury Act (NCVIA) (HRSA, no date). This both established a no-fault compensation program for vaccine-related injuries and mandated the creation of a national vaccine safety monitoring system. In 1990, the United States established its vaccine adverse events reporting system (VAERS) managed jointly by the Food and Drug Administration (FDA) and the Centers for Disease Control (CDC). In 1997, the FDA Modernization and Accountability Act aimed to streamline approval processes, while creating a more efficient and patient-centered approach to drug and device regulation. However, the Prescription Drug User Fee Act of 1992 also sought to facilitate the entry of new drugs into the market and keep the paid services that the agency provided to the industry. This is a controversial issue, since 'it implies that the regulator depends financially on the industry it intends to regulate, an issue that recent evaluations see as inconvenient' (Orozco, 2012, p. 110, authors' translation). While aiming to expedite drug access, the changes advanced by the Modernization and Accountability Act have sparked debates regarding potential conflicts of interest due to the agency's reliance on industry fees for services.

Orozco (2012, p. 41, authors' translation) highlighted how pharmacovigilance expanded and was transformed as the result of accelerated production and use of drugs, the so-called 'pharmaceutical explosion era', the vertiginous growth of the pharmaceutical industry and concerns of various social sectors to avoid new 'tragedies'. Today, most industrialized countries have national regulatory authorities, responsible for overseeing pharmacovigilance activities within their borders. These agencies manage the surveillance systems that collect data coming from healthcare professionals and (more recently) from healthcare consumers. The national agencies try to ensure that pharmaceutical companies operating in the country establish pharmacovigilance systems and report any adverse events associated with their products. The organization of pharmacovigilance differs between countries. In some, including the Netherlands, pre- and post-marketing pharmacovigilance are conducted in separate institutions. In others, including the UK, the US, and Italy, the same agency is responsible. How institutional structure, funding, and agencies' independence from government affect their functioning are questions worthy of study. So too are differences at the sub-national level.

In Italy, for example, the National Pharmacovigilance Network, a system for collecting reports of suspected adverse reactions organized by AIFA (Italian Medicines Agency), relies on the collaboration of regions and autonomous provinces, local health authorities, and hospitals. The Local Pharmacovigilance Contact Points, the Regional Pharmacovigilance Centres, and AIFA check the reports on a daily basis, request any additional information, and evaluate the causal link, each according to their own competences (AIFA, 2021).

At the European level, the foundation of the European Medicines Agency (EMA) in 1995 reflected a commitment to the harmonization of pharmacovigilance procedures. In 2001, the EMA established EudraVigilance, the database that collects and pools reports of adverse drug reaction data from EU member states. The much larger data set meant that rare events, which might escape attention at the national level, were more likely to be noticed. In the EU, since 2017, pharmaceutical companies and national competent authorities have been required to report adverse reactions to medicinal products to EudraVigilance (Sienkiewicz et al., 2022). Whilst national authorities assess potential adverse events of nationally authorized products, the EMA does the same for products authorized for the EU as a whole.

For example, COVID-19 vaccines were centrally authorized by the EMA for all EU member states, hence they were centrally monitored and assessed by the EMA's Pharmacovigilance Risk Assessment Committee (PRAC). The PRAC meets every month to assess the safety signals of medicines and vaccines coming from EudraVigilance, as well as from Vigibase, the global database managed by the Uppsala Monitoring Centre on behalf of the WHO. Based on these assessments, the PRAC makes recommendations to the EMA regarding any changes in product information, administration, and risk management that it considers necessary (EMA, 2021). From 2012 to 2018, the PRAC issued 453 recommendations, of which more than half involved changes to drug labelling (Potts et al., 2020)

By 2000, changes at the regulatory level in Europe, the US, and Canada had led to a shift from the traditional regulatory model, in which state interventions regulate market activities, to a 'harmonized' model in which the industry and regulators were regarded as two parties with overlapping interests in the drug development and surveillance process. Critics see in this shift a regulatory process increasingly influenced by the pharmaceutical industry (Abraham & Lewis, 1999; Orozco, 2012).

Over recent decades, multinational collaboration in pharmacovigilance has expanded, and the structures within which standards and protocols are established and data exchanged have multiplied. Two interesting examples are the International Conference for Harmonization (ICH) and the Brighton Collaboration. Since 1991, the regulatory authorities from Europe, Japan, and the United States and experts from the pharmaceutical industry have been meeting in the context of the ICH. The aim was to unify drug regulation standards and streamline development while ensuring safety and quality (Baber, 1994). The Brighton Collaboration was founded in 2003. Funded by seed capital from the University Children's Hospital Basel, Switzerland, its goal is developing standardized definitions and methods in assessing adverse events following immunization (AEFI). The Brighton Collaboration has grown into a global network with active participation from researchers and public health professionals from around the world. The organization develops and disseminates standardized case definitions for vaccine-related adverse events, promoting consistent reporting and data analysis across countries and healthcare systems. For COVID-19 vaccines, for instance, they worked with CEPI (Coalition for Epidemic Preparedness Innovations) to identify and prioritize a list of potential adverse events of special interest (AESI) specific to these vaccines. This list considered factors like the novel nature of the vaccines and the known biology of the SARS-CoV-2 virus, and it allowed a faster assessment of the huge bulk of data submitted to pharmacovigilance agencies during the pandemic (Black et al., 2021).

Specific initiatives have also been undertaken to address emerging challenges. The 2009 influenza pandemic led to the creation of the Accelerated Development of VAccine beNefit-risk Collaboration in Europe (ADVANCE) project (2013–2018). Funded by the Innovative Medicines Initiative, a public-private partnership between the European Union and the European Federation of Pharmaceutical Industries and Associations (EFPIA), it aimed to develop a framework for rapid and reliable vaccine safety and benefit data collection (Jeong et al., 2021). Through its work, ADVANCE developed best practices and methodologies for collaborative vaccine pharmacovigilance studies. VAC4EU (Vaccine monitoring Collaboration for Europe), launched in 2019, serves as the sustainable successor to the ADVANCE project. VAC4EU functions as an international, non-profit scientific community that builds upon the groundwork laid by ADVANCE. It serves as a platform for researchers to collaborate on vaccine safety studies and share data, ultimately aiming to provide robust and timely evidence on vaccine benefits and risks for informed decision-making. As in other policy fields, this multiplication of global fora raises questions of possible jurisdictional disputes, and differences in procedures and outcomes.

Today, the global harmonization of pharmacovigilance absorbs substantial effort and considerable resources: public and private. Guidelines and standards flow down from international organizations to national pharmacovigilance systems, adapted to specific regulatory environments, healthcare systems, and resources. Patients' and consumers' data flow back up, from national pharmacovigilance centers and regulatory agencies to regional and global organizations that collect, compare, and assess ever-larger quantities of data. How effectively, and with what effect these flows occur in practice are questions in need of study.

3.3 The production of vaccine pharmacovigilance data

The process through which individual symptoms or experiences are turned into pharmacovigilance data is a complex one, its various steps mediated by different technologies, systems, and stakeholders at the local, national, and international levels (WHO, 2022).

In pharmacovigilance, an AEFI is any untoward medical occurrence which follows immunization, whether or not as a result of the immunization. An adverse event may be any unfavorable or unintended sign, abnormal laboratory finding, symptom, or disease. Reported adverse events can either be true adverse events (AE), i.e. really a result of the vaccine or immunization process, or coincidental events that are not due to the vaccine or immunization process but are temporally associated with immunization (WHO, 2016).

AEFIs are monitored and assessed through both 'active' and 'passive' surveillance. The former involves actively looking for AEFIs in hospitals, through electronic health records, and/or in specific studies. The latter, which is more common, makes use of the large national, regional, or global databases discussed earlier. However, their effectiveness depends on the upward flow of data. This in turn depends on health professionals' (and perhaps families') motivation, awareness, and willingness to report events they deem suspicious. Influences on health professionals' familiarity with and experience of these reporting systems are further questions about which little is known.

According to the WHO, '[s]uspicion alone is sufficient grounds for reporting, and the primary reporter is not expected to assess the causality that is implied' (WHO, 2016, p. 39). In theory, all AEFIs that worry patients, families, or professionals should be notified. Adverse events involving hospitalization or death, or associated with new vaccines, or which may have been caused by immunization errors, have to be given special attention. So do significant events of unexplained cause occurring within 30 days after vaccination and 'events causing significant parental or community concern' (WHO, 2016, p. 39). In many settings the primary reporter submits a report to the competent authority, which is generally a local public health authority, via internet, post, or phone.

Reporting forms vary slightly between countries, but all forms include demographic questions, questions about the type of vaccine, a space for the clinical history, descriptions of symptoms and signs, and categorization of the level of seriousness. Patients' and healthcare professionals' reports are coded according to a standard MedDRA (Medical Dictionary for Regulatory Activities) terminology, individually assessed by trained assessors and stored in the same database, to be analyzed. Usually, a general notification confirming the successful submission is sent to the reporter, with no further interaction between the agency and the reporter taking place.

Pharmacovigilance professionals analyze the data using statistical and analytical tools to detect potential rare events, to assess clusters of reports, and to detect safety signals for further evaluation (Rudolph et al., 2022). When a number of reports flag a potential issue, i.e. the number of reports about a specific symptom/disease/condition is more than the number of reports expected, this is called a 'signal'. For instance, in the case of COVID-19 vaccines, Vaccine Induced Thrombosis and Thrombocytopenia (VITT) following some adenoviral vectored vaccines, and myocarditis following mRNA vaccines, became 'signals'.

Following signal detection, a thorough evaluation process determines its clinical significance and its potential cause. This entails a detailed examination of available evidence, including the strength of the association, consistency of reports, biological plausibility, and the temporal relationship between drug/vaccine use and the adverse event. The final step is assessment of the likelihood that a given drug or vaccine actually caused the specific adverse event. If so, certain steps follow.

The case of myocarditis following mRNA COVID-19 vaccination is illustrative. The first signal of myocarditis following Comirnaty (Pfizer) was captured in Israel, which introduced it very early on. The Ministry of Health, as well as the EMA and FDA, then conducted investigations to confirm the potential link with the Pfizer vaccine. It was soon established that the benefits of using mRNA COVID-19 vaccines outweighed any risks in all populations, including adolescents and young adults, but that the Emergency Use Authorization (EUA) had to be modified to include information on the rare adverse event. The CDC created educational materials for both patients and healthcare providers about the potential risk of myocarditis, offering guidance to clinicians on recognizing concerning symptoms to ensure timely diagnosis and effective management (Gargano, 2021; CDC, 2023).

Despite the extension of pharmacovigilance systems to much of the world, estimates suggest that up to 95% of adverse reactions go unreported (Clothier et al., 2014). For decades, reporting through passive surveillance systems has typically been limited to healthcare professionals (HCPs), including (in some cases) pharmacists and nurses. However, their overall sensitivity is often low, and under-reporting has been acknowledged as a significant limitation. National agencies in the US, Australia, Scandinavian countries, and the Netherlands therefore raised the possibility of permitting direct reporting by patients and consumers. This question has been a matter of debate for two or three decades (van Grootheest et al., 2003). Would a 'lay reporter' (van Groothest et al., 2003, p. 214) be capable of providing good quality reports, or would they overload the system with information of little value? As summarized by van Grootheest et al. (2003, p. 214), 'Is a lay reporter capable of providing a clear and objective description of the adverse effects and can he or she supply the relevant clinical information necessary for an adequate evaluation of the report?' A number of studies exploring the quality and efficacy of lay reporting in the EU and beyond (van Hunsel et al., 2012, 2019; Inácio et al., 2017), suggest that patient-generated reports are as informative as, and qualitatively similar to, those from HCPs. Since 2004, LAREB, the Dutch drug reactions center, 'has accepted that ADRs [adverse drug reactions] reported by patients are of equal value to reports from healthcare professionals' (de Langen et al., 2008, p. 6), and found that patient reporting strengthens passive surveillance.

Patient involvement varies between Western European countries. For example, in the Netherlands (van Hunsel et al., 2019) and Denmark, the national pharmacovigilance centers started to include reports directly filed by consumers and patients in 2003, in Italy patient involvement started the following year, in the UK in 2005, and in Norway in 2013. In the EU, a pharmacovigilance reform of 2012 solidified and broadened patient participation as reporters, establishing the legal right for citizens to report adverse events directly to the competent authorities (Steurbaut & Hanssens, 2014). This commitment extends to the inclusion of patient representatives in the PRAC at the EMA.

During the COVID-19 pandemic, the EMA organized a public stakeholders' meeting about the development, evaluation, approval, and safety monitoring of COVID-19 vaccines in the EU (EMA, 2020). While this was an opportunity for the public to share their concerns and interests, it was not clear if (and if so, how) this feedback played any role in decision-making regarding COVID-19 vaccine regulation and surveillance. Moreover, during the pandemic, the first reports of menstrual irregularities following mRNA vaccines, which were coming from patients, were received with suspicion by the medical community. In response to the increasing number of social media posts describing menstrual disorders that, according to the reporters, were potentially related to vaccination, doctors and public health professionals worldwide rushed to reassure people, emphasizing that there were 'no data' and any link between the COVID-19 vaccine and menstrual irregularities was biologically implausible (Villarreal, 2021; Mezza, 2025). In addition to a lack of evidence linking the symptoms to the vaccine, public health authorities were concerned that this possible association could fuel vaccine hesitancy (Male, 2021; Edelman et al., 2022).

3.4 Social sciences and pharmacovigilance

A quick search of Web of Science in July 2024 shows that since the term 'vaccine hesitancy' was introduced, it has attracted the attention of researchers from many scientific disciplines. Of the nearly 2,800 articles published since 2010, roughly 360 can be considered 'social science' (including health policy and services, management, and economics). Pharmacovigilance has attracted nothing like the same attention. If we search Web of Science again, using 'vaccine' and 'regulation' as title search, our harvest is a mere 118 titles, of which only 10 or 12 are roughly 'social science'. Repeating the exercise with 'vaccine' as title and 'pharmacovigilance' as a 'topic' term yields 426 publications, of which 15–20 could be classified as 'social science'. The contrast between social scientists' attention to vaccine hesitancy and the limited attention paid to pharmacovigilance is striking. Attention for pharmacovigilance and for drug and vaccine regulation more generally has largely been limited to its regulatory component. Regulation involves a complex interplay between market forces and scientific expertise (Abraham & Lewis, 2014).

Studies by Carpenter (2004) showed a significant decrease in FDA approval times for new drugs, often involving reliance on less data and on surrogate measures. Reduced pre-marketing restrictions, facilitating faster drug approvals, are justified by the supposed strengthening of post-marketing checks. However, concerns remain about the ability of pharmacovigilance to compensate fully for reduced pre-market checks. To be sure, the rapid development and approval of COVID-19 vaccines demonstrated the potential benefits of accelerated approval pathways during a pandemic, and Dhanda et al. (2022) suggest that populations may be more willing to accept pre-marketing uncertainties in a public health crisis. Nevertheless, as Wardell's (1983) observations show, this trend towards faster approvals predates the pandemic by many years. Indeed, Davis and Abraham (2011) argue that changes in US regulations, like accelerated approval for cancer medications, might be a form of deregulation driven by the pharmaceutical industry, rather than a reaction to patient advocacy following the AIDS crisis.

Danish scholars are among the few who have examined how pharmacovigilance evidence is produced. Analyzing the Danish reporting system, they point to the difficulty in identifying and reporting adverse reactions, highlighting a lack of readily available knowledge among doctors, patients, and regulatory staff, and the system's inability to capture and process patients' tacit knowledge:

> Most doctors and patients find it difficult to determine whether an observation is an adverse reaction or not and therefore whether it should be reported ... Thus it is not possible for the authorities to control the process, because a great deal of tacit knowledge is presumably ignored or overlooked by patients or doctors or regulatory staff in the national agencies.
>
> *(Agaard et al., 2007, p. 1306)*

Analysing three specific cases, including oral contraceptives, Letigen, and Rofecoxib, Aagaard et al. (2007) question whether available pharmacovigilance data, which excludes tacit knowledge – in the sense the term was used by Nonaka and Takeuchi (1995) – provides an adequate basis for regulatory decisions.

The work of Lee et al. (2023) on sex disparities in adverse drug events (ADEs) focuses on how pharmacovigilance evidence is produced, including using gender as an axis of analysis. By analyzing reports from the US FDA Adverse Event Reporting System (FAERS), the authors demonstrate how gender norms and behaviors affect the reporting, perception, and seriousness attributed to ADEs. While much of the existing pharmacovigilance literature focuses on biological explanations for sex disparities in ADEs, Lee et al.'s (2023) study offers the 'Gender Hypothesis', positing that these disparities are also significantly influenced by social factors such as healthcare utilization patterns, clinical biases, gendered experiences of adverse events, and upstream social determinants of health.

Many critical questions remain un- or underexplored in the literature that specifically examines post-authorization surveillance systems. How does (vaccine) pharmacovigilance work in practice? Does it differ significantly from one country to another? Why has its growth and increasing methodological sophistication had so little influence on the extent of vaccine hesitancy? Are people aware that they can directly report their vaccine-related concerns and experiences? And if they do submit a report, what feedback would they like to receive? Where such questions have been addressed, it is by pharmacovigilance professionals themselves, not by social scientists. Since the results of these studies are written for and read by fellow professionals, they have had no influence on the disconnect between the field and civil society.

Our overview indicates the scope for more critical social scientific explorations. Public awareness of adverse events reporting systems is very low. In the UK, for instance, in 2011 only 8.5% of patients were aware of the possibility of reporting (Avery et al., 2011). In South Korea, less than 15% were aware of the national passive surveillance system, and even fewer respondents had direct reporting experience (Kim et al., 2020). Ideas about how patients could best be involved vary widely. For instance, while regulators and pharmaceutical groups focused on the involvement of patients in the design of educational and communication materials, patients' organizations mentioned full circle feedback, face-to-face communication, and developing trust as key activities. These discrepancies reveal that professionals might give priority to activities that are not considered meaningful by patients themselves (van Hoof et al., 2022).

Research conducted in the Netherlands showed that patients want to receive follow-up information about their reports, as well as additional information about the potential adverse reactions notified (van Hunsel et al., 2012, 2019). These studies, which to our knowledge constitute the only research about what patients want from pharmacovigilance, were conducted for drug adverse reactions in general, with no specific focus on immunization. Because of the complex social, cultural, and political dimensions of vaccination, it merits not only a specialized focus within the field of pharmacovigilance itself but also more attention from the social sciences.

3.5 Questions for the social sciences

Why has the growth in scale and sophistication of professional pharmacovigilance had so little effect on trust in vaccines? Could it be otherwise? By unpacking the power dynamics at play, and by exploring the ways in which pharmacovigilance evidence is produced, the social sciences can help provide answers to these important questions. We propose that a pharmacovigilance system more closely integrated with civil society could serve as a platform for dialogue and collaboration between public health institutions and communities, helping to bridge the growing divide and foster mutual trust.

3.5.1 Transparency, Public Awareness, and Trust

A 'well-functioning pharmacovigilance system, where patients are actively included, helps to increase the trust that the general public has in drugs' (van Hunsel et al., 2019, p. 479) and, we would add, in vaccines. Enhancing public awareness of these mechanisms must be the first step. How this should best be done, and the optimal structure and administrative location of a pharmacovigilance institution in a particular state, are questions in need of study.

The EU regulatory framework promotes patient-centered pharmacovigilance, but this seems to be more successful regarding drugs than vaccines. Given that pharmacovigilance professionals have tended to question patients' ability to describe their own experiences of vaccination, preferring 'objective descriptions' (van Grootheest et al., 2003, p. 214), and that the public is scarcely aware of reporting mechanisms, one might question professional commitment to promoting public engagement in vaccine pharmacovigilance.

Paradoxically, vaccine hesitancy seems to play a role in this professional hesitancy. A pharmacovigilance professional, presenting a platform to address knowledge gaps about AEFIs and 'the best way to immunize individuals' (INSIS, no date), expressed this concern. Answering a question from the audience about patient organizations' involvement in the platform, they said that there was a conversation on the topic, but that 'there was hesitancy, because of vaccine hesitancy' (ISoP, 2022).

According to Chinchilla et al. (2021, p. 188) a shift towards a patient-oriented pharmacovigilance has taken place, but 'a cultural shift where regulators understand patients' needs and the implementation of a series of regulatory improvements' is needed. Are the barriers to a more open and transparent pharmacovigilance essentially cultural? Does resistance reflect an attempt to protect professional authority and jurisdiction?

3.5.2 Re-negotiating Power

Orozco (2012) argues that the dominant narrative surrounding pharmacovigilance presents a picture of unified actors working towards a shared goal – patient safety. This narrative, however, overlooks the inherent tensions between stakeholders with conflicting interests. Pharmacovigilance itself falls under the broader umbrella of pharmaceutical regulation, a field described by Wiktorowicz (2003, p. 627) as an 'oligopolistic structure dominated by multinational, economically powerful companies'. Scholars like Wiktorowicz (2003), Abraham and Lewis (1999), Demortain (2015), and Coca et al. (2022) have highlighted the power imbalances between the pharmaceutical industry and regulatory agencies. Lack of resources within regulatory bodies (Wiktorowicz, 2003) and, in some cases, relationships 'too close for comfort' (Lexchin, 1990, p. 1257), can compromise the neutrality of these agencies. This raises crucial questions. Whose interests have shaped the current system, protocols, and practices of vaccine pharmacovigilance, and with what implications for vaccine safety? What spaces for negotiation are currently available for public participation, and what additional spaces should be sought? These questions point towards the urgency of addressing power imbalances and fostering greater public involvement in vaccine pharmacovigilance. But then, who constitutes the 'public' that should be negotiating for space and participation?

3.5.3 What Public?

In the case of medicines, patients' organizations and patients' representatives have become credible interlocutors for regulatory agencies and pharmaceutical companies. There are successful experiences of patient organization involvement in drug development, research, and regulatory process (Perfetto et al., 2015). But what of vaccines, which target varied groups of healthy individuals? How, if at all, is civil society represented in vaccine development, monitoring, and regulation? Who or what might legitimately represent it? How might civil society be involved in the research, design, development, approval, and surveillance of vaccines? At present, lay involvement in vaccine pharmacovigilance is largely limited to providing specific chunks of data through multiple-choice forms, in an extractive approach to patients and consumers' experiences and knowledge. However, as pointed out by some pharmacovigilance professionals (Chinchilla et al., 2021), patient involvement in pharmacovigilance could and should go beyond opening the reporting systems up to direct users' input.

3.5.4 What Evidence?

Vaccine pharmacovigilance plays a critical role in safeguarding public health by generating evidence and knowledge about vaccine safety. How is evidence defined and deemed legitimate within pharmacovigilance, and by whom? What counts as valid knowledge in safety assessments, and how do these definitions influence the understanding of vaccine risks and benefits? How are narratives in lay reports interpreted and analyzed by pharmacovigilance professionals?

In practice, there is an overwhelming emphasis on what is observable and quantifiable, analyzed through a statistical lens. Orozco (2012, p. 43) argues that this 'biomedical and statistical approach' prioritizes the interests of the pharmaceutical industry by emphasizing individual biological and medical issues, neglecting the social context of health. This prioritizes the participation of industry and the state, while marginalizing the contributions of other social actors (Orozco, 2012).

What is the effect of increasing reliance on large, aggregated data sets? Rare events should become more visible, but are there others (perhaps occurring only in a small population) which are potentially minimized or even rendered invisible? The case of menstrual disorders following COVID-19 vaccination exemplifies the challenges inherent in reliance on a specific kind of evidence. Initial reluctance to acknowledge this potential side effect stemmed from perceived biological implausibility, despite widespread reports and patient experiences. This resistance was eventually refuted by the European Medicines Agency (EMA, 2022), even if the evidence about the link was considered 'weak' because it was coming from patients (Mezza, 2025). We argue that a pluralist approach to knowledge production could help foster stronger links with civil society. However, a critical examination is equally important. We must actively question what experiences and events are rendered invisible by the current focus on individual biological and medical issues within pharmacovigilance (Orozco, 2012). Further investigation is needed to understand how potential structural biases accumulate at each level of evidence production within the system. The dominance of the biomedical paradigm leads to the marginalization not only of subjective experiences, but potentially also of any culturally or socially specific event.

3.5.5 Inequalities and 'Intersectionalities'

This chapter has focused on how pharmacovigilance systems work in Europe and the US, highlighting increased harmonization and institutional interconnectedness. Standards, protocols, and forms flow from those institutions, based in industrialized Western countries, to national agencies worldwide. How is pharmacovigilance done in the 'scientific periphery'? Adverse reactions to COVID-19 vaccines were largely identified in Israel, Europe, and the US, and so for the vaccines authorized in those areas. However, in much of the Global South, people were offered other vaccines, for which no new signal was analyzed following commercialization. Interrogating the pharmacovigilance system and the evidence produced by it through a decolonial lens would provide insights into the power geometries at play in flows of information between national agencies and transnational institutions. A flood of information from one quarter, but a mere trickle from another. What are the implications of this imbalance for (perceptions of) vaccine safety?

Intra-national inequalities in what is reported, and what remains unseen or undiagnosed, also need to be better understood. That people with similar symptoms but different sex, gender, race, ethnicity, and class, among others, may receive different diagnoses and treatments has been shown over and again. What do healthcare providers see? Who reports on their symptoms and anxieties? In other words, how do socio-economic inequalities influence what is known of vaccine safety and efficacy? While significant research has concentrated on ethnic biological differences, particularly variations in drug-metabolizing enzymes that influence drug efficacy and toxicity (Bjornsson et al., 2003), there remains a critical gap in exploring how the socio-cultural construct of race shapes and impacts these data. Phase III clinical trials have been privileged sites to observe how race, ethnicity, and geographical position are performed in health (McCarthy, 1994; Petryna et al., 2007; Prasad et al., 2022). By exploring how intersectional identities are performed in vaccine safety, and with which implications, we can address knowledge gaps, structural exclusions, and invisibilities in pharmacovigilance practice, evidence, and policy.

Additionally, this approach fosters advancements in social science's ontological and epistemological inquiries into how scientific knowledge produces bodies and subjectivities. Surveillance, particularly in its biopolitical forms, operates as a mechanism for governing populations by normalizing specific health, behavioral, and social standards (Foucault, 1977; Rose, 2001; Monahan & Wall 2007). Ontologically, pharmacovigilance operates as a system that categorizes and defines bodies according to their responses to drugs and vaccines, thereby influencing societal understandings of health, risk, and vulnerability. Questions arise about what constitutes an 'adverse reaction' and how these definitions shape the boundaries of normal and pathological bodies. For example, how does pharmacovigilance reinforce or challenge biomedical norms about which bodies are seen as 'typical' or 'atypical'? Additionally, how do these practices reify categories such as race, gender, and age, potentially embedding systemic biases into the very frameworks used to monitor health outcomes?

Epistemologically, pharmacovigilance privileges specific types of knowledge – quantifiable, clinical data – while often marginalizing other forms, such as patient narratives, experiential knowledge, or alternative medical paradigms. This raises questions about whose voices are included in pharmacovigilance processes and whose are excluded. For instance, how does the emphasis on standardized metrics and reporting systems obscure localized, culturally specific understandings of health and adverse effects? Furthermore, how do power dynamics between regulatory bodies, pharmaceutical companies, and patients influence what counts as legitimate knowledge in pharmacovigilance systems?

By addressing these questions, we can critically analyze how pharmacovigilance shapes not only the monitoring of drug safety but also broader societal norms and practices around health. This perspective invites a rethinking of pharmacovigilance as not merely a technical process but as an active site of knowledge production that constructs particular forms of subjectivity and embodiment, with implications for equity and inclusivity in global health systems.

3.6 Conclusions

This chapter has examined the historical and practical foundations of pharmacovigilance, exploring its structure, evidence production, and current limitations. We highlighted the disconnect between current pharmacovigilance practices and public trust in vaccines. Bridging this gap is not only a pressing public health challenge but also a significant opportunity for social science research.

While social science has delved deeply into vaccination and vaccine hesitancy, pharmacovigilance itself remains largely unexplored. Unpacking the inner workings of pharmacovigilance, the power dynamics at play, and the nature of evidence production – its strengths and limitations – is where social science can offer invaluable insights. By illuminating these aspects, social scientists can contribute to a more transparent and participatory pharmacovigilance system, ultimately fostering public confidence in vaccines. At present, however, few national (or international) agencies are willing to open their practices to external scrutiny. The extent to which restrictions on access might pose barriers to the implementation of our proposed research agenda remains to be seen. We believe our agenda offers both practical benefits and theoretical opportunities. By studying pharmacovigilance, social scientists can refine our understanding of trust, power, and risk perception. In addition, these questions contribute to insights into the social construction of scientific knowledge, colonial dynamics in scientific collaboration and medicine regulation, and expressions of gender, race, and ethnicity in scientific knowledge.

Note

1. https://www.grandviewresearch.com/industry-analysis/pharmacovigilance-industry

References

Aagaard, L., Søndergaard, B., Andersen, E., Kampmann, J.P. and Hansen, E.H., 2007. Creating knowledge about adverse drug reactions: A critical analysis of the Danish reporting system from 1968 to 2005. *Social Science & Medicine*, 65, pp. 1296–1309.

Abraham, J. and Lewis, G., 1999. Harmonising and competing for medicines regulation: How healthy are the European Union's systems of drug approval? *Social Science & Medicine*, 48(11), pp. 1655–1667.

Abraham, J. & Lewis, G., (2014). *Regulating Medicines in Europe: Competition, Expertise and Public Health*. Routledge.

AIFA, 2021. FAQ – Pharmacovigilance on COVID-19 vaccines. Available at: https://www.aifa.gov.it/en/vaccini-covid-19 [Accessed 11 June 2024].

Akbar, R., no date. Ten threats to global health in 2019. Available at: https://www.who.int/news-room/spotlight/ten-threats-to-global-health-in-2019 [Accessed 11 June 2024].

Avery, A.J., Anderson, C., Bond, C.M., Fortnum, H., Gifford, A., Hannaford, P.C., Hazell, L., Krska, J. et al., 2011. Evaluation of patient reporting of adverse drug reactions to the UK 'Yellow Card Scheme': Literature review, descriptive and qualitative analyses, and questionnaire surveys. *Health Technology Assessment*, 15(20), pp. 1–234. doi: 10.3310/hta15200.

Baber, N., 1994. International conference on harmonisation of technical requirements for registration of pharmaceuticals for human use (ICH). *British Journal of Clinical Pharmacology*, 37(5), pp. 401–404.

Bjornsson, T.D., Wagner, J.A., Donahue, S.R., Harper, D., Karim, A., Khouri, M.S., Murphy, W.R., Roman, K. et al., 2003. A review and assessment of potential sources of ethnic differences in drug responsiveness. *Journal of Clinical Pharmacology*, 43(9), pp. 943–967. https://doi.org/10.1177/0091270003256065.

Black, S.B., Law, B., Chen, R.T., Dekker, C.L., Sturkenboom, M., Huang, W.T., Gurwith, M., Poland, G., 2021. The critical role of background rates of possible adverse events in the assessment of COVID-19 vaccine safety. *Vaccine*, 39(19), pp. 2712–2718.

Blume, S., 2006. Anti-vaccination movements and their interpretations. *Social Science & Medicine*, 62, pp. 628–642.

Carpenter, D.P., 2004. The political economy of FDA drug review: Processing, politics, and lessons for policy. *Health Affairs*, 23(1), pp. 52–63.

CDC, 2023. *Clinical Considerations: Myocarditis and Pericarditis after Receipt of COVID-19 Vaccines Among Adolescents and Young Adults*. Available at: https://www.cdc.gov/vaccines/covid-19/clinical-considerations/myocarditis.html#print [Accessed 15 January 2025].

Chinchilla, K., Matos, C., Hall, V. and van Hunsel, F., 2021. Patient organizations' barriers in pharmacovigilance and strategies to stimulate their participation. *Drug Safety*, 44, pp. 181–191.

Clothier, H.J., Selvaraj, G., Easton, M.L., Lewis, G., Crawford, N.W. and Buttery, J.P., 2014. Consumer reporting of adverse events following immunization. *Human Vaccines & Immunotherapeutics*, 10(12), pp. 3726–3730.

Coca, J.R., Coca-Asensio, R. and Bueno, G.E., 2022. Socio-historical analysis of the social importance of pharmacovigilance. *Frontiers in Sociology*, 7, p. 974090.

Davis, C. and Abraham, J., 2011. Desperately seeking cancer drugs: Explaining the emergence and outcomes of accelerated pharmaceutical regulation. *Sociology of Health & Illness*, 33(5), pp. 731–747.

de Langen, J., van Hunsel, F., Passier, A., de Jong-van den Berg, L. and van Grootheest, K., 2008. Adverse drug reaction reporting by patients in the Netherlands: Three years of experience. *Drug Safety*, 31(6), pp. 515–524. doi: 10.2165/00002018-200831060-00006.

Demortain, D., 2015. The tools of globalization: Ways of regulating and the structure of the international regime for pharmaceuticals. *Review of International Political Economy*, 22(6), pp. 1249–1275.

Dhanda, S., Osborne, V., Lynn, E. and Shakir, S., 2022. Postmarketing studies: Can they provide a safety net for COVID-19 vaccines in the UK? *BMJ Evidence-Based Medicine*, 27(1), pp. 1–6.

Edelman, A., Boniface, E.R., Benhar, E., Han, L., Matteson, K.A., Favaro, C., Pearson, J.T., Darney, B.G., 2022. Association between menstrual cycle length and coronavirus disease 2019 (COVID-19) vaccination: A US cohort. *Obstetrics and Gynecology*, 139(4), pp. 481–489.

EMA, 2020. Public stakeholder meeting: Development and authorisation of safe and effective COVID-19 vaccines in the EU. Available at: https://www.ema.europa.eu/en/events/public-stakeholder-meeting-development-authorisation-safe-effective-covid-19-vaccines-eu [Accessed 11 June 2024].

EMA, 2021. Pharmacovigilance Risk Assessment Committee. Available at: https://www.ema.europa.eu/en/documents/other/prac-rules-procedure_en.pdf [Accessed 11 June 2024].

EMA, 2022. Meeting highlights from the Pharmacovigilance Risk Assessment Committee (PRAC) 24–27 October 2022. Available at: https://www.ema.europa.eu/en/news/meeting-highlights-pharmacovigilance-risk-assessment-committee-prac-24-27-october-2022 [Accessed 20 June 2024].

EMA, 2024. Pharmacovigilance: Overview. Available at: https://www.ema.europa.eu/en/human-regulatory-overview/pharmacovigilance-overview [Accessed 15 January 2025].

Foucault, M., 1977. *Discipline and Punish: The Birth of the Prison*. Pantheon Books.

Gargano, J.W., 2021. Use of mRNA COVID-19 vaccine after reports of myocarditis among vaccine recipients: Update from the Advisory Committee on Immunization Practices—United States, June 2021. *MMWR. Morbidity and Mortality Weekly Report*, 70.

HRSA, no date. About the National Vaccine Injury Compensation Program. Available at: https://www.hrsa.gov/vaccine-compensation/about#:~:text=The%20National%20Childhood%20Vaccine%20Injury,be%20injured%20by%20certain%20vaccines [Accessed 11 June 2024].

Inácio, P., Cavaco, A. and Airaksinen, M., 2017. The value of patient reporting to the pharmacovigilance system: A systematic review. *British Journal of Clinical Pharmacology*, 83(2), pp. 227–246.

INSIS, no date. About. Available at: https://insisvaccine.org/about [Accessed 20 June 2024].

ISoP, 2019. ESoP/ISoP History. https://isoponline.org/about-isop/esop-isop-history/

ISoP, 2022. A new era of pharmacovigilance: Challenges and opportunities. *Conference*, 20–23 September 2022.

Jeong, N.Y., Lee, H.I., Kim, M.J., Kim, H.J. and Choi, N.K., 2021. An introduction of the Accelerated Development of Vaccine Benefit-risk Collaboration in Europe (ADVANCE) project. *Journal of Health Informatics and Statistics*, 46(4), pp. 369–377.

Jethwa, H., Wong, R., & Abraham, S. (2021). Covid-19 vaccine trials: Ethnic diversity and immunogenicity. *Vaccine*, 39(27), pp. 3541–3543.

Kim, S., Yu, Y., You, M., Jeong H. Y. and Lee, E., 2020. A cross-sectional survey of knowledge, attitude, and willingness to engage in spontaneous reporting of adverse drug reactions by Korean consumers. *BMC Public Health*, 20, n. 1527. doi: 10.1186/s12889-020-09635-z.

Lee, K.M., Rushovich, T., Gompers, A., Boulicault, M., Worthington, S., Lockhart, J.W. and Richardson, S.S., 2023. A gender hypothesis of sex disparities in adverse drug events. *Social Science & Medicine*, 339, n. 116385. https://doi.org/10.1016/j.socscimed.2023.116385.

Lexchin, J., 1990. Drug makers and drug regulators: Too close for comfort. A study of the Canadian situation. *Social Science & Medicine*, 31(11), pp. 1257–1263.

Male, V., 2021. Menstrual changes after COVID-19 vaccination. *BMJ*, 374, n. 2211.

McBride, W.G., 1961. Thalidomide and congenital abnormalities. *The Lancet*, 278(7176), p. 1284.

McCarthy, C.R., 1994. Historical background of clinical trials involving women and minorities. *Academic Medicine*, 69(9), pp. 695–698.

Meade, T.W., 1975. Subacute myelo-optic neuropathy and clioquinol: An epidemiological case-history for diagnosis. *British Journal of Preventive and Social Medicine*, 29(3), pp. 157–169. doi: 10.1136/jech.29.3.157.

Mezza, M., 2025. Entangled evidence: Epistemic injustice, and systemic neglect in the assessment of menstrual disorders following COVID-19 vaccines. *Critical Public Health*, 35(1). doi: 10.1080/09581596.2024.2446763.

Monahan, T. and Wall, T., 2007. Somatic surveillance: Corporeal control through information networks. *Surveillance & Society*, 4(3), pp. 154–173.

Nonaka, I. and Takeuchi, H., 1995. *The Knowledge-Creating Company: How Japanese Companies Create the Dynamics of Innovation*. Oxford University Press.

Orozco, J.G., 2012. *De la farmacovigilancia al monitoreo crítico de los medicamentos. El proceso de registro de medicamentos en Colombia 2006*. Ph.D. Thesis. Universidad Nacional de Colombia.

Perfetto, E.M., Burke, L., Oehrlein, E.M. and Epstein, R.S., 2015. Patient-focused drug development. *Medical Care*, 53(1). Available at: https://doi.org/10.1097/mlr.0000000000000273.

Petryna, A., 2007. Clinical trials offshored: On private sector science and public health. *BioSocieties*, 2, pp. 21–40.

Potts, J., Genov, G., Segec, A., Raine, J., Straus, S. and Arlett, P., 2020. Improving the safety of medicines in the European Union: From signals to action. *Clinical Pharmacology & Therapeutics*, 107(3), pp. 521–529.

Prasad, S., Shahid, A., Co, E.L.F., Khatri, G., Cheema, H.A., Rocha, I.C.N., Bardhan, M. and Hasan, M.M., 2022. Vaccine apartheid: The separation of the world's poorest and most vulnerable and the birth of Omicron. *Therapeutic Advances in Vaccines and Immunotherapy*, 10, n. 25151355221107975.

Rose, N., 2001. The politics of life itself. *Theory, Culture & Society*, 18(6), pp. 1–30.

Rudolph, A., Mitchell, J., Barrett, J., Sköld, H., Taavola, H., Erlanson, N., Melgarejo-Gonzalez, C., Yue, Q.Y., 2022. Global safety monitoring of COVID-19 vaccines: How pharmacovigilance rose to the challenge. *Therapeutic Advances in Drug Safety*, 13, n. 20420986221118972.

Ruiz, J.B. and Bell, R.A., 2022. Parental COVID-19 vaccine hesitancy in the United States. *Public Health Reports*, 137(6), pp. 1162–1169. https://doi.org/10.1177/00333549221114346.

Sienkiewicz, K., Burzyńska, M., Rydlewska-Liszkowska, I., Sienkiewicz, J. and Gaszyńska, E., 2022. The importance of direct patient reporting of adverse drug reactions in the safety monitoring process. *International Journal of Environmental Research and Public Health*, 19(1), p. 413. doi: 10.3390/ijerph19010413.

Steurbaut, S. and Hanssens, Y., 2014. Pharmacovigilance: Empowering healthcare professionals and patients. *International Journal of Clinical Pharmacy*, 36(4), pp. 859–862.

Strom, B.L., 2012. What is pharmacoepidmeiology? In: Strom B.L., Kimmel, S.E. and Hennessy, S. (eds), *Pharmacoepidemiology*. Wiley & Sons, Ltd., pp. 1–22

van Grootheest, A.C. and van Puijenbroek, E.P., 2002. Pharmacovigilance in the Netherlands. In: Mann, R. and Andrews, E. (eds.), *Pharmacovigilance*. Wiley, pp. 309–315.

Van Grootheest, K., de Graaf, L. and de Jong-van den Berg, L.T., 2003. Consumer adverse drug reaction reporting: A new step in pharmacovigilance? *Drug Safety*, 26, pp. 211–217.

van Hoof, M., Chinchilla, K., Härmark, L., Matos, C., Inácio, P. and van Hunsel, F., 2022. Factors contributing to best practices for patient involvement in pharmacovigilance in Europe: A stakeholder analysis. *Drug Safety*, 45(10), pp. 1083–1098.

van Hunsel, F., Härmark, L., Pal, S., Olsson, S. and van Grootheest, K., 2012. Experiences with adverse drug reaction reporting by patients: An 11-country survey. *Drug Safety*, 35(1), pp. 45–60.

van Hunsel, F., Härmark, L. and Rolfes, L., 2019. Fifteen years of patient reporting – what have we learned and where are we heading to? *Expert Opinion on Drug Safety*, 18(6), pp. 477–484.

Veurink, M., Koster, M. and de Jong-van den Berg, L.T.W., 2005. The history of DES, lessons to be learned. *Pharmacy World and Science*, 27, pp. 139–143.

Villarreal, A., 2021. 'No data' linking Covid vaccines to menstrual changes, US experts say. *The Guardian*. Available at: https://www.theguardian.com/world/2021/apr/23/covid-vaccines-periods-menstruation-changes-data-experts [Accessed 11 June 2024].

Wardell, W. M. (1983). Introduction: Science and government in drug development, regulatory assessment, and postmarketing surveillance. In W. M. Wardell & G. P. Velo (eds), *Drug Development, Regulatory Assessment, and Postmarketing Surveillance*. Springer, pp. 1–12.

WHO, 2016. Immunization safety surveillance: Guidelines for immunization programme managers on surveillance of adverse events following immunization. Available at: https://iris.who.int/handle/10665/208262 [Accessed 11 June 2024].

WHO, 2022. The WHO programme for international drug monitoring. Available at: https://www.who.int/teams/regulation-prequalification/regulation-and-safety/pharmacovigilance/networks/pidm [Accessed 11 June 2024].

Wiktorowicz, M.E., 2003. Emergent patterns in the regulation of pharmaceuticals: Institutions and interests in the United States, Canada, Britain, and France. *Journal of Health Politics, Policy and Law*, 28(4), pp. 615–658.

4 Rethinking pharmaceutical innovation

Andrew Bartlett and Paul Martin

4.1 Introduction

While the twentieth century saw major advances in the development of pharmaceuticals, there are widespread concerns that the pace of innovation has slowed in the twenty-first century (Gaudillière, 2021), and at the same time the industry-reported costs of developing new drugs have reached astronomical levels (Wouters et al., 2020). These are core elements of a longstanding 'productivity crisis' (Pammolli et al., 2011), understood as being the product of multiple, inter-related scientific, clinical, and organisational problems. The 'low hanging fruit' has already been harvested and after a period of time what was the industry's intellectual property becomes public property. This results in a situation in which 'an ever-improving back catalogue of approved medicines increases the complexity of the development process for new drugs, and raises the evidential hurdles for approval, adoption and reimbursement' (Scannell et al., 2012, p. 193). At the same time, the completion of the Human Genome Project led to material developments in biotechnology – expanding the capabilities of the laboratory – and to *promises* of new medical developments, such as personalised medicine (Sturdy, 2017). In addition to this, the imperatives of late capitalism in the bioeconomy (Birch, 2017; Birch and Muniesa, 2020) have resulted in greater financialisation of the industry with an emphasis on maximising profits and shareholder value. Conti et al. (2008, p. 2), writing about biotechnology, argued that the high cost of development coupled with the risk posed by high failure rates – failure that can arise at the scientific, clinical, regulatory, or market level – are 'forces [that] push biotechnology research and development (R&D) into areas that meet specific investment criteria'. In navigating this landscape, the pharmaceutical industry has moved its focus towards personalised medicine (Tutton, 2016) and high-priced speciality drugs (Hayford, 2024), resulting in concerns about equitable access and sustainability. Nowhere are the effects of this nexus of technical and financial change more pronounced than in the case of the unmet medical needs of those with rare diseases, making the development of so-called 'orphan drugs' a prime site for sociological examination of the reorganisation of pharmaceutical innovation.

Social scientists have the privilege of both examining the world as it is and taking an active part in outlining new possibilities for how it might be different through the collective imagining of futures. 'Sociotechnical imaginaries' are 'collectively held, institutionally stabilised, and publicly performed visions of desirable futures, animated by shared understandings of forms of social life and social order attainable through, and supportive of, advances in science and technology' (Jasanoff, 2015, p. 4). Imaginaries are powerful in shaping how we understand the world and provide guidance for action, and in the response to sociotechnical change we can unpack the ways in which futures are constituted. In this chapter, we chart an emerging imaginary – and new sociality – of pharmaceutical innovation and supply designed to better serve public health (e.g., Duggal and Faulkner, 2020). These spaces, and their promise of a more responsive and responsible way of developing new medicines, are rich sites for social science research and intervention. Here, we sketch out a research agenda to explore this new imaginary, and the socialities by which it is both generated and constituted.

4.2 Failure, crises, and social innovation

There are two main axes of market failure that are particularly relevant to public health and therefore to this chapter. Despite the limitations of the 'market failure' concept, it is a usefully broad concept, especially as it is deployed by actors and stakeholders in pharmaceutical innovation. First, the high prices of many new medicines are causing major patient access issues worldwide. This is particularly true of drugs for rare diseases, where the median price of a new US orphan drug (2017–21) was $219,000, and oncology, where >95% of new US cancer drugs launched in 2023 had prices >$100,000 (IQVIA, 2024). This is also true of a series of complex cell and gene therapies for small patient populations, designated as Advanced Therapy Medicinal Products (ATMPs) in Europe, launched with prices in excess of £1,000,000 (Phares et al., 2024). Critically, a significant number of these have been withdrawn by manufacturers from the market due to commercial unsustainability, indicating difficulties finding viable business models (Srivastava and Foster, 2023). In some cases, non-profit organisations have stepped in to take over the development or manufacture of these products (e.g., San Raffaele Hospital, Fondazione Telethon) (Fondazione Telethon, 2023). The second form of market failure is seen in the lack of new products in several areas, not just in terms of drugs for rare diseases, but also new antibiotics to address antimicrobial resistance (AMR) and, notably, treatments for neglected tropical diseases (NTDs). Though this chapter focuses on social innovation in response to the unmet medical needs of people with rare diseases, developments mostly taking place in the more economically developed countries in the Global North, there are strong parallels between this and the challenges to developing, producing, and ensuring equitable distribution of drugs for NTDs, many of which are relatively common diseases mostly affecting people in less economically developed countries in the Global South.

Consequently, there has been a debate about the extent to which the existing innovation model is 'broken' and how to address its failure to meet key areas of medical need and broader public health objectives (e.g., Fleming, 2021; Sun et al., 2022). The established policy response to a lack of investment in some areas has been to incentivise industry, most notably through the enactment of orphan drug incentives for rare diseases. In addition, policy has also sought to speed up the development process by introducing a series of expedited approval pathways in the US and EU that grant market authorisation at an earlier stage and on the basis of more limited evidence. While these incentives have been successful in producing new drugs, a by-product of these incentives and attendant property protections is that the resulting drugs are often very expensive (Althobaiti et al., 2023). In this chapter we want to distinguish between initiatives to solve this problem by way of fixes to the existing innovation model – such as by making changes to the regulatory, intellectual property, and reimbursement environment in which the pharmaceutical industry operates – and initiatives to solve this problem by developing novel forms of collaboration, partnership, and organisation that exist outside and alongside – and in many cases include as one of a wider cast of actors – the existing pharmaceutical industry.

Of the first kind are, for example, proposals by Stiglitz and Jayadev (2010), who identified the tension between policy attempts to encourage innovation – such as extending intellectual property rights – and policy attempts to cut medical costs and extend the benefits of medical innovation to a higher number of people. They proposed four policies to address the problems facing the development of medicine for the public good: prize funds to encourage research on rare diseases, value-based pricing, public funding of clinical trials, and the development of 'research commons' for frontier technologies. These are not novel forms of social organisation in themselves, although changing the overarching social structures underlying pharmaceutical development may well allow new combinations of actors into these spaces. However, Conti et al. wrote that the 'tendency to rely on public policy to help guide the for-profit industry to undertake socially valuable R&D that does not meet investment criteria' had proven to be of mixed effectiveness (2008, p. 194); even with subsequent developments, more profound social innovation is perhaps required. A particularly radical (both organisationally and self-consciously politically) example of the second kind is the Open Insulin Project (Gallegos et al., 2018), which developed protocols for the manufacture of insulin that would take insulin supply out of the hands of the commercial pharmaceutical industry. The potential for pharmaceutical innovation and production to be removed from the constraints of the profit nexus has been discussed for much of the twenty-first centuryt (e.g., Hale et al., 2005; Conti et al., 2008).

None of this should be taken to deny the importance of commercial pharmaceutical and biotechnology companies in bringing new medicines and therapies to market and clinic. However, the absences that are the result of 'market failure' open up the space to develop new forms of public-private partnership that have the potential to move the emphasis in the development and distribution of medicines away from commercial interests and towards addressing public health needs. There has been social innovation in the face of these 'crises', and social scientists should also never let a crisis – a site of sociological inquiry at which the taken-for-granted is disrupted – go to waste.

There has been some social science work on these changes in the social organisation of innovation. This includes the Trans-Atlantic Platform-funded international research project on 'Social Pharmaceutical Innovation' led by Conor Douglas of York University, which organised the Global Conference for Advancing Social Pharmaceutical Innovation in Utrecht in March 2023 (Douglas et al., 2022). The project was established to investigate the growing number of initiatives exploring non-traditional models of drug innovation in many countries. The social, economic, and political conditions in which these alternative innovation models proliferate also have to be understood, specifically the systemic challenges, changes, and crises within the pharmaceutical sector. These are being examined in the Wellcome Trust-funded 'Orphanisation' project led by Paul Martin at the University of Sheffield (iHuman, 2024). In July 2024, these two projects convened an international workshop in Amsterdam to discuss these issues. Drawing participants from academia, clinical research, industry, and patient activism, the workshop addressed the obstacles to new forms of pharmaceutical innovation, particularly questions of late-stage clinical development, regulation, reimbursement, and investment. This chapter is intended to offer an outline of the broad terrain that is to be explored and to present a selection of speculative questions with which social researchers might wrestle.

4.3 Social innovation in pharmaceutical innovation

In recent years, as noted, there have been a growing number of initiatives aimed at developing and manufacturing new medicines outside the dominant commercial model. These initiatives have been driven by and have drawn in actors from the academic and non-profit sectors. These social innovations include university-based drug development programmes – with product development partnerships (PDPs) being seen as a way to 'keep costs down through collaboration' (Maxmen, 2016, p. 388) – and hospital-based manufacturing (Kleinhout-Vliek et al., 2024). They also include patient groups working in close collaboration with clinicians to collect data, including 'Real World Evidence', that can be used in drug design and regulatory spaces. Jonker et al. (2024, p. 5) write that 'Patient engagement is becoming increasingly important in drug repurposing initiatives, and patients can be the drivers of the drug repurposing process, as they can bring together the parties and funds for successful drug repurposing projects'. Importantly, they write that both SYMPATHIC and REMEDi4ALL – two European organising 'platforms' for drug repurposing – are developing training programmes to enable patients to act as 'drivers' of drug repurposing and to 'optimise' the process. Examples of this are the DevelopAKUre consortium (Rudebeck et al., 2021; Ranganath and Sireau, 2023) and the Canadian Fabry Disease Initiative. In the case of the Canadian Fabry Disease Initiative, a patient group lobbied for access to enzyme replacement therapy (provided by Genzyme, a commercial biotechnology company), which resulted in a clinician-led research protocol that allowed Fabry patients to receive the medicine as part of a study of the efficacy and cost effectiveness – a 'coverage-with-evidence' risk sharing agreement (RSA) (Douglas and Grunebaum, 2024).

Charities taking a driving role in drug discovery, manufacture, and access can also be understood as a form of social innovation, bringing new actors with novel capacities for fundraising, patient engagement and recruitment, political and regulatory lobbying, etc. into the mix. Patient groups and charities also bring their particular value systems and 'goal orientations' to drug development, as do new forms of commercial or semi-commercial drug development led by for-profit SMEs and public benefit companies (B corporations), established with the formal goal of reducing the cost of developing new medicines and increasing access. Some of these initiatives draw on new technologies such as artificial intelligence/machine learning (AI/ML) or strategies such as drug repurposing (e.g., HealX). However, little policy attention has been paid to both the growth of these new forms of organisations outside or orthogonal to the traditional pharmaceutical sector and how they could be better supported to benefit public health. In particular, there has yet to be a substantial discussion of the broader institutional and policy ecosystem needed for this purpose. Social science researchers, with a capacity to generate evidence and insight of the local and particular as well as the global and general, are well placed to contribute to and inform these discussions.

A number of these initiatives have been collectively described as forms of the aforementioned 'social pharmaceutical innovation' (SPIN). Douglas et al. (2022, p. 4) define SPINs as:

> collaborative processes, programs, policies, procedures and/or designs involving diverse sets of actors that break with conventional pharmaceutical innovation practices for the production of safe, effective, and accessible interventions that address unmet societal needs of rare disease patients that are not primarily market driven.

The 'constitution' of SPINs is key here, in two senses of the word; in being composed of 'diverse sets of actors', and in having as their explicit goal ends that are 'not primarily market driven'. Importantly, for social scientists, these are *social* innovations; new ways of organising collectively to produce knowledge, medicine, public goods, and commodities.

We can briefly sketch a selection of illustrative examples of the range of alternative innovation models and the organisations supporting them, demonstrating the diversity of these initiatives. These examples lean on national and international initiatives, but many others operate at a regional or local level. Within the broad scope of alternative innovation models there are a range of different aims and objectives; some initiatives seek to develop more efficient processes to create a greater number of lower-cost medicines for ultra-rare diseases – for example by the repurposing of existing drugs, a method that is the focus of REMEDi4ALL; others are working on manufacturing advanced therapies in the public sector – for example BioCanRx, 'a network of scientists, clinicians, cancer stakeholders, academic institutions, NGOs and industry partners' and 'a leader in the translation, manufacture and adoption of cancer immunotherapies' (BioCanRx, 2024); while a number of projects seek to create new drugs for NTDs – for example the Drugs for Neglected Diseases initiative (DNDi) – or to tackle antimicrobial resistance – for example the Global Antibiotic Research & Development Partnership (GARDP). These are all social innovations in the form of new, overarching collaborations that serve as platforms for projects to tackle particular diseases, to develop and bring to the clinic particular drugs. The Canadian Fabry Disease Initiative is an example of the way in which novel forms of social organisation have been used to provide access to a drug for an unmet need (Douglas and Grunebaum, 2024).

4.3.1 REMEDi4ALL

REMEDi4ALL is a consortium of 24 international organisations funded through the EU Horizon programme, which seeks to develop a 'standardised platform' and a 'more favourable regulatory environment' for drug repurposing, as well as building a drug repurposing community (REMEDi4ALL, 2024a). It is led by EATRIS, the European infrastructure for translational medicine, which provides access to research expertise and resources to both academia and industry (EATRIS, 2024), pointing to the complex interconnection of governmental, non-profit, academic, and commercial organisations in these spaces. REMEDi4ALL offers a 'concierge' service to those engaged in drug repurposing, and they claim that patients are 'the heart of research', arguing that 'the best treatments are those made by and with the people who use them' (REMEDi4ALL, 2004b). Donald Lo, of EATRIS, has been quoted as saying that the 'best case scenario [for REMEDi4ALL] would be to improve also the collaboration between the academic and the non-profit and commercial sectors' (REMEDi4ALL, 2023).

4.3.2 Canadian Fabry Disease Initiative

The Canadian Fabry Disease Initiative involved cooperation between patients, clinicians, and industry, resulting in an RSA, an innovative reimbursement approach. Enzyme replacement therapy (ERT) had not been approved for Fabry disease on the basis of expense and the poor quality of evidence. Fabry disease patients, however, politically organised (supported by Genzyme, one of the manufacturers of ERT) and campaigned for access. However, the initiative itself was clinician-led, not patient-led; the clinicians produced a research protocol that would allow Fabry patients to receive ERT as part of a study of efficacy and cost effectiveness – a 'coverage-with-evidence' RSA (Douglas and Grunebaum, 2024).

4.3.3 Drugs for Neglected Diseases Initiative (DNDi)

DNDi concentrates on the 'most neglected diseases'. DNDi advocates an 'open and collaborative approach to R&D – driven by patient needs, not profits' (DNDi, 2024). Projects involve both repurposing and novel drug development. Funded by an array of governments, NGOs, and philanthropic organisations, it 'maintains a policy of not relying on any individual donor for more than 25 percent of its budget' (Lezaun and Montgomery, 2015). Light (2020, p. 1) argues that DNDi is a 'working, successful model of a non-profit, virtual collaborative that researches, tests, gains approval, manufactures, and distributes clinically superior medicines at low cost and for wide access, thus reducing health care disparities'. While it is non-profit and orientated towards access and addressing health inequalities, it cooperates with the pharmaceutical industry; for example, when developing a treatment for sleeping sickness, DNDi partnered with Sanofi, which took responsibility 'for the manufacturing, supply, registration, and distribution' of the drug (DNDi, 2020).

4.4 A new mixed economy of pharmaceutical innovation?

While the concept of a 'mixed economy' describes a system in which there is a role for both private companies and the state in economic life, the term '*new* mixed economy' has been used to mark the distinctiveness of those sectors in which there is a significant role for 'third sector' actors – charities, 'social enterprises', non-governmental organisations, and not-for-profit organisations. This is particularly the case in the economies of services such as housing or social care (Byrne et al., 2006). Giddens (1998, pp. 99–100) argued that while the old mixed economy involved the subordination of the market to the state in the pursuit of public good, 'The new mixed economy looks instead for a synergy between public and private sectors, utilizing the dynamism of markets but with the public interest in mind'. To this end, this involved policy enthusiasm for the provision of public goods by public-private partnerships, private finance initiatives, and the reorganisation of public services in ways that envisaged the user as a 'customer'.

We borrow this concept to help us to understand the potential for these new forms of social organisation to alter the economy of pharmaceutical innovation. The notion of a new mixed economy *of innovation* captures what we see as the most sociologically and politically significant aspect of the response to 'market failure' in pharmaceutical innovation – the entry of new actors *as actors* into the pharmaceutical innovation system that are neither (purely) government agencies nor private commercially-orientated corporations. This concept helps capture the broader environment constituted by a diverse and heterogeneous group of initiatives operating at different levels, researching, producing, and delivering medicines. While the idea of a 'new' mixed economy is intended to capture the role of 'third sector' organisations in addition to the state/private dichotomy conventionally implied by 'mixed economy', it is inseparable from neoliberal 'reform' – privatisation – of public services. In this context, it should be noted that while the development of 'new' mixed economies in many sectors has involved the penetration of private, commercial interests into what had previously been public sectors, the case of a new mixed economy of innovation involves the incorporation of non-commercial interests into what had been a largely private sector.

Any confusion here is likely the result of the multiple meanings of 'public' and 'private'. Weintraub (1997, p. 3) warns us that this is a dichotomy which contains multiple meanings, a 'complex family' of paired oppositions, and that we should be careful when using these terms to ensure that we do not 'generate confusion (or absurdity) when their categories are casually or unreflectively blended'. In our case, this confusion arises from the different meanings of public in what Weintraub calls 'the liberal-economistic model' and 'the republican-virtue approach'. In both of these understandings, 'public' is used to delineate the limits of the political, but where in the former the public-political is embodied by the state, in the latter it is used to describe the 'world of discussion, debate, deliberation, collective decision making, and action in concert' (Weintraub, 1997, p. 11). In the case of a new mixed economy of pharmaceutical innovation, both of these are at play; patient groups, charities, social interest corporations, etc. are taken to be agents of the 'public' interest; they are a key part of what makes these forms of pharmaceutical innovation 'social'. This is a 'new' public sector for an age of entrenched neoliberalism, in which the solution to market failure must be found by bringing new actors within the totalising conceptual space of the market.

At this point, it is worth reflecting on how the social organisation of innovation in pharmaceuticals has been understood in order to cast the contemporary challenges and changes in this system into sharp relief. Historically, both public policy and industry have stressed a division of labour in the production of pharmaceutical knowledge, a 'mixed economy' involving the public and private sectors. Crudely, this is characterised as the public sector providing funding and other resources for basic research into understanding disease processes and characterising potential drug targets. Much of this work takes place in universities and research institutes, many of which, if not strictly 'public', operate on a non-commercial basis. This knowledge is then transferred to companies, either through the 'commons' of the scientific literature or increasingly through the commercial transfer of some kind of property rights, where it is used in the development of new medicines; the knowledge is transformed into commodities. This is, of course, only a crude characterisation; large companies have also funded a great deal of research and development, including fundamental studies of disease mechanisms and drug targets, and universities are increasingly concerned with the commercialisation and commodification of knowledge themselves. Nevertheless, as a consequence of this perceived division of responsibilities, capabilities, and capacities, the public sector has traditionally not been involved in the material development and distribution of medicines other than at a small, local scale in hospitals or in particular disease areas, such as vaccines for infectious diseases (e.g., Blume and Baylac-Paouly, 2021).

However, science, technology, and innovation scholars have challenged this description and stressed the shortcomings of this 'linear model' as well as studying different, 'non-linear' models. First, knowledge production and translation is a complex process of exchange between the laboratory, clinic, industry, and academia (da Silva et al., 2021). Second, the structure of the pharmaceutical sector has changed in critical ways since the 1980s, in terms of a vertical disintegration in the organisation of R&D following the growth in biotechnology. Increasingly, biotechnology SMEs are the main source of new medicines (Schuhmacher et al., 2023). Large integrated drug companies now focus on late-stage product development, regulatory approval, and marketing, with a high proportion of R&D outsourced to smaller firms (PPD, 2022). As a consequence, a greater range of commercial actors are now involved in the production of pharmaceutical knowledge. Third, there has been a shifting boundary between the public and private sectors in several crucial areas – in part due to technological and scientific changes such as the advent of cell and gene therapies. Here, the public sector plays a key role in creating the resources and technical infrastructures needed to support the development of novel therapeutics, often in close collaboration with private companies. Taken together, these changes represent a fundamental shift in how medicines are discovered and developed and foreshadow the move to much more open and networked forms of innovation involving a diversity of actors. This has resulted in value chains and innovation systems becoming more distributed.

It is in this changing context that the entry of alternative innovation initiatives must be placed and understood. These also build on a long history of non-profit involvement in the development of new medicines in areas such as NTDs (Rotondoa et al., 2016). It will be critical to delineate the ways in which there can be the space for a new mixed economy alongside the dominant regime of pharmaceutical innovation based on large (multinational) pharmaceutical companies. This calls for a new social contract between the pharmaceutical industry, government, and society, in which the different contributions of each stakeholder are more clearly recognised, and the interdependencies between them are made more explicit. In doing this, the dominant conceptual model of innovation within policy circles needs to be rethought to take these systemic changes into account. However, it must be stressed that these new initiatives are not a direct threat to either established pharmaceutical companies or to more recently established biotech and biopharmaceutical firms. Public and non-profit drug development initiatives of the kinds described here are unlikely to match the scale or complexity of the work done by the innovative pharmaceutical and biotechnology industries, and their work should continue to be fully supported. At the same time, it should also be recognised that the existing system of developing new medicines is not fully addressing many public health needs.

Weintraub wrote that 'many discussions take for granted that distinguishing "public" from "private" is equivalent to establishing the boundary of the political' (1997, p. 2). And we see that here, at least in the soft form, the introduction of 'public' interests is understood as considered, deliberate intervention in the market; making the domain of private interests subject to public concern and scrutiny. Note that these interventions do not seek to do away with 'medicine as commodity', only to shape this necessary, given fact into ends that better meet the public interest. Paraphrasing Weintraub, we know that debates about how to divide the social world of pharmaceutical innovation between public and private are not an 'innocent analytic exercise' because the normative aspects are viscerally foregrounded.

4.5 Re/placing the pharmaceutical industry

None of these efforts to address 'market failure' envisage the solution being outside the market entirely. Faith in the power of the state – the public sector – alone to accomplish complex, large-scale, innovative projects has faded since the 1970s. More than that, even the successes of state-led innovation tend to be, in fact, examples of the success of the mixed economy. 'Moonshot' is a popular metaphor, shorthand for a large-scale project that would launch a new field of science and technology. But NASA was always a success of the military-industrial complex, with leading roles to play for aerospace companies and countless contractors and consultants. Even if there were to be an equivalent of a 'moonshot' in pharmaceutical innovation, it would take place in the context of a landscape in which much of the capacity to develop, manufacture, secure regulatory approval for, and distribute drugs lies in the hands of the private sector, in which pharmaceuticals, regardless of the particularities of the social organisation of innovation, are licensed for entry to the 'market', not the 'commons'.

Furthermore, before considering the relationship between alternative innovation models and pharmaceutical companies, it must be noted that the latter category is highly differentiated. Whilst dominated by a relatively small number of huge, integrated, multinational companies (often called 'Big Pharma'), many medium-sized and smaller firms conduct research and development or provide manufacturing and other services. Most notably, these include the huge number of research-intensive biotechnology firms. Within the biotech sector, there is a range of companies and various business models. Many mimic the traditional pharmaceutical approach to drug discovery, while others are creating new technologies that may transform the discovery and development process, including the use of AI/ML. Both pharmaceutical and biotech companies are supported by a wide range of service providers, including contract research organisations (CROs), bioinformatics firms, companies specialising in safety testing, reagent and equipment manufacturers, etc. It must be stressed that it is very difficult for hospitals or charities to succeed in bringing a new therapy to market without the active involvement, expertise, and capacity of at least some of these companies.

Given this, the prime questions are not whether these new forms of organising innovation involve commercial actors but those examining the particular contours of these collaborations, questions that are all to some degree variations on 'how do the different actors involved exercise power?' The interests and goals of the various actors – commercial actors large and small, regulators, healthcare systems, clinicians, charities, academics, patient groups, etc. are not identical and neither is the power which they can bring to bear. The answers to this question – which will be variable – will help us to unpack what is the 'social' of SPINs; including, but not limited to, the way in which the goals, interests, and goods are contested and produced. A number of the alternative innovation models/SPINs involve close working relationships with private companies that supply essential expertise, resources, and services. It should also be stressed that this is not a simple one-way relationship. Companies also not only benefit from knowledge created in the academic and public sectors – as per the conventional model of innovation – but these new forms of collaboration allow the industry greater access to other resources essential to developing and bringing to market new drugs. For example, the support and participation of patient organisations brings with it access to trial subjects, clinical data, and 'Real World Evidence', as well as the political weight of patients, their families, and their stories. It is against this backdrop that major industry players are patrons and supporters of umbrella groups such as Beacon for Rare Disease. The industry may also benefit significantly from the long-term growth of alternative innovation models as they can help the characterisation of new molecular targets, provide proof-of-principle demonstrations for new compounds and therapeutic modalities, and support the co-development of complex advanced therapies that require much greater participation from clinicians and the public sector in providing essential infrastructure. Alternative models can therefore help determine what is required for successful innovation in emerging technology areas, further reducing business risk. This could enable more sustainable commercial and economic models in return for transparent and equitable benefit sharing.

Though it is possible for non-commercial actors to exercise control over much of the drug development 'pipeline' – Jarosławski and Toumi (2019) present Généthon as an example of a rare organisation that has brought 'in-house' the marketing authorisation, manufacturing, and distribution aspects of drug development and supply that most non-profits outsource – it is clear that most alternative models of innovation will involve some kind of relationship with the pharmaceutical industry. Questions can be asked as to how these collaborations that incorporate commercial interests will protect their commitment to addressing unmet medical needs and public health problems. However, some posit more radical solutions; these incorporate actors who represent 'social' interests into pharmaceutical innovation and seek a more radical break with the commercial interests and market logic. An example of this is Public Pharma for Europe, which explicitly positions itself as antagonistic to 'Big Pharma'. They point critically at many of the existing attempts to encourage the industry to meet public health needs as using public resources to 'de-risk' private interests. This, then, is a more radical sociotechnical imaginary; one in which there is a 'pharmaceutical commons' in which innovation is directed, conducted, and publicly owned, one in which commercial companies would still be involved, but not as monopolists of knowledge. By its very nature, the sociality that generates and is constituted by this imaginary is not itself involved in pharmaceutical innovation; it is a political campaign to transform pharmaceutical innovation (Public Pharma for Europe, 2024). The idea of a 'pharmaceutical commons' is gaining ground, even if sometimes the term is used to offer a measure of political acceptability to examples that are geared towards the production of private property; 'a new pharmaceutical "commons" is posited as a holding bay for inventions of questionable value prior to their enclosure at an unspecified point in the future' (Lezaun and Montgomery, 2015, p. 16). In this future, pharmaceutical knowledge will be held in common often under the auspices of 'open innovation' where basic science and early stage discoveries are accessible to all researchers. However, this is only until such a point as valuable portions that may form the basis for commercial products can be carved out as private property in the form of patents that grant private monopolies, enclosed behind the fences of the global intellectual property regime.

4.6 Obstacles to social innovation in pharmaceutical innovation

Challenges in developing new medicines cover a spectrum of scientific, technical, clinical, business, economic, and regulatory fields. Instead of providing a comprehensive inventory of these challenges, the focus here is on identifying the main systemic obstacles facing alternative innovation initiatives. Drawing on research in the academic field of science, technology, and innovation studies provides the conceptual tools and empirical evidence to help identify critical issues and possible solutions. Alternative drug innovation models will depend on changing a number of the key economic, commercial, legal, and institutional arrangements within the existing drug innovation system. This will require social, organisational, and institutional innovation, including new legal and regulatory measures, original contract forms and (dispersed) methods of ownership, novel forms of financing and reimbursement, and potentially new types of data and pioneering ways of collecting them – such as the involvement of patient groups in determining clinical end points (Deal et al., 2017) and the collection of 'Real World Data' (Liu et al., 2022) – which brings with it questions as to how such data will be incorporated into existing systems of regulatory and reimbursement decision-making.

One of the most relevant ideas within this literature is understanding innovation as a complex sociotechnical process of bringing together different actors, artefacts, forms of knowledge, resources, organisations, and practices within network structures (Geels, 2004). The term 'sociotechnical' is used to blur the division between technology and society. In this framework technology is shaped by and in turn shapes society; these two domains cannot be easily separated. All innovation is a fundamentally collaborative process that requires both scientific and technical expertise as well as work in social and economic domains. It is not just in the laboratory that there are processes of experimentation, failure, and collective learning. Each of the alternative initiatives to address the unmet medical needs of rare disease patients mentioned above faces challenges heavily influenced by their local context; there is no simple solution for many of the problems they face. However, many of these obstacles have common characteristics related to the structure of the current innovation system. It can be argued that the most significant challenges faced by these new forms of pharmaceutical innovation, pioneered in response to the challenge of rare diseases, are in the late-stage clinical and product development processes. Certainly, with much social science work on the transition of knowledge from the lab to the clinic (Martin et al., 2008), these later stages represent particularly fruitful sites for future research.

The existing literature identifies several issues. While novel forms of pharmaceutical innovation are an attempt to surmount or sidestep some of the obstacles to rare disease drug development in a profit-driven industry, they face both some of the familiar problems of research on rare diseases – such as small population size – as well as challenges specific to their novel modes of social organisation. Jarosławski et al. (2018) identified two main challenges non-profit pharmaceutical innovators face. First, they often lack the expertise and resources to obtain market access (a challenge identified as a problem by many authors, e.g., Davies et al., 2017) or to manufacture, market, and distribute their drug. Second, they are not often sustainable – a commitment to sell their drug at a low price in order to maximise access means that funding for any future ventures has to come from a new round of donations. Jarosławski et al. (2018) also identified four examples of approaches that non-profit pharmaceutical developers have used to surmount these challenges and bring new drugs to the patient: DNDi, which outsourced production and distribution; Généthon, which built capacity to carry these tasks 'in-house'; Janssen R&D Ireland, which used market competition to manufacture and distribute their drug at a low price, granting non-exclusive licences to several generic companies; and finally, the formal collaboration between DNDi and the pharmaceutical multinational Sanofi.

Drug repurposing as a particular strategy has also prompted discussion of obstacles (e.g., Breckenridge and Jacob, 2019; Krishnamurthy et al., 2022; van der Pol et al., 2023), which include questions of funding and reimbursement – to which forms of organisation such as public-private partnerships are often touted as a solution – intellectual property barriers, the application and protections afforded by 'orphan' status, and the 'regulatory burden' of market access. Kleinhout-Vliek et al. (2024), in their research on novel reimbursement routes for eculizumab and grant-funded, hospital-based manufacturing of CAR-T cell therapy, identified a determinedly 'social' problem, that these new forms of social organisation often lack 'legitimacy'. Their novelty, existing across multiple institutional domains, means that other actors may fail to recognise these collaborations as legitimate, or may opt to not recognise the collaborations if they are seen as disruptive.

There are initiatives attempting to mitigate some of these barriers in different ways. For example, the conscious pursuit of goal alignment across different actors and the mobilisation of professional expertise may overcome the lack of legitimacy (Kleinhout-Vliek et al., 2024). Concerns that academics lack the expertise to navigate the regulatory paths from laboratory to patient access have led to initiatives to correct this deficit, such as the Dutch Medicine for Society platform publishing a 'roadmap' (Rosenberg et al., 2023).

4.7 Unhappy is the land in need of heroes

Many current alternative innovation models rely heavily on project and philanthropic funding and/or the heroic work of highly motivated individuals. Whilst this might have been essential to the early development of the field, it is not sustainable over the long run. Instead, there is a need to build a 'circular economy' in which alternative innovation models can generate a surplus that is recycled back into supporting further efforts to develop new medicines. This would require the construction of a new innovation ecosystem and appropriate financial arrangements, as the constitution of many individual instances of new forms of pharmaceutical innovation militate *against* sustainability (Jarosławski et al., 2018). How can a model for innovation be sustainable when it is constituted with the goal of developing a medicine for one disease, a product that will have a necessarily limited 'customer' base? What surplus can be generated when one of the crises being addressed is access and affordability?

It is likely that for alternative innovation systems to succeed they will by necessity develop structures which mimic many of the key functions performed by the mainstream model. This may include elements already existing in the current system, but will also require creating novel policies, organisations, and institutions. Whilst this can be achieved in a highly distributed manner, involving many different groups, organisations, and stakeholders, a critical factor for success will be coordinating these activities, organising investment and generating recurrent income, holding drug licences, and making strategic investment decisions. This will involve a form of market intermediation with brokerage between the public and non-profit sectors and the private sector. One way of achieving this would be the creation of independent non-profit organisations to carry out these core activities. Several of these already exist in different countries with a subset of these functions but in specific areas such as rare diseases (e.g., LifeArc, Remedi4All, Eatris, etc.).

Such bodies could coordinate vital parts of the broader ecosystem, build infrastructure, provide training and advice, liaise with regulators and payers, etc., perhaps acting as a kind of 'boundary organization' (Guston, 2001). Crucially, such a market intermediary must become self-financing, a process which would involve the coordination of public and philanthropic funds and resources. This raises many questions about the scope, remit, and governance of such intermediaries and their relationship to market and non-market actors. Would it be possible for such an organisation (or a tightly coordinated network) to act as an honest broker focused on producing social benefits, actively addressing some of the most critical systemic barriers identified in this chapter, whilst at the same time providing tangible benefits to the private sector (e.g., by 'derisking' projects)?

Any social science programme that seeks to understand these new forms of pharmaceutical innovation cannot neglect the emergence of a policy framework that can promote – or inhibit – the development of a 'new mixed economy'. This includes paying close attention to the way in which policy (and policy-makers and -framers) understand the changing relationships and boundaries between the pharmaceutical industry, academia, the non-profit sector, and government. In some cases, the state will play an active role in supporting alternative innovation models that address areas of unmet medical need. For example, DNDi is partially funded by several governments, and BioCanRx receives funding from the Canadian federal government. There will also develop an 'ecosystem' of support organisations, networks, and platforms that act as market intermediaries, as described above, prompting questions as to how *these* social innovations are constituted vis-à-vis the interests and goals of the various actors. There will also be the development of novel incentives for private investment that go beyond traditional forms of patents and IP protection, leading to questions as to the ways in which these might 're-privatise' alternative drug development initiatives (Lezaun and Montgomery, 2015). And, of course, central to any reshaping of pharmaceutical innovation is the response of the pharmaceutical industry; in what ways will the industry grasp the new *commercial* opportunities to support and facilitate alternative innovation initiatives?

We might end this section on a few cautionary notes. Ferpozzi (2023) examined PDPs through the critical lens of Science, Technology, and Society studies. They argued that:

> private actors that join PDPs can respond to increasing demands for corporate responsibility, enhance their public image, and contribute funds and critical expertise to relegated health issues; partnerships also allow private actors to exert greater influence on the global and international regulatory scene and, because of this, gain privileged access to unconquered markets and untapped scientific resources in developing countries.
>
> *(Ferpozzi, 2023, p. 614)*

Quoting Martens (2003), Ferpozzi reminds us that 'the term "partnership" is eminently political and not just stylistic: it "implicitly downgrades the role of governments and intergovernmental organizations and upgrades the (political) status of private actors" such as transnational corporations' (2023, p. 614). They note that PDPs are intended to not only correct for market failure but also public health failures, and in doing so they carve out greater space for the operation of private interests.

Similarly, Lezaun and Montgomery (2015, p. 21) warned that:

> the new pharmaceutical 'commons' crafted by the PDPs rests on the expectation of future enclosures, whether they are in the guise of property rights and marketing opportunities attached to new medicines against NTDs [and rare diseases], or result from an expanded ability to extract profit from drugs for unrelated diseases in 'emerging markets'.

In imagining a new way of making medicines that better serves public health and decentres the profit motive, social scientists must remain reflexive and critical if they are to avoid reproducing the existing innovation system and the social relations embedded in it (Martin, 2022). We must ask ourselves, whose interests are at play in these new social spaces?

That there is a 'crisis', that people have come to see the existing business model of pharmaceutical innovation and access to medicine as being 'broken', suggests that there is the possibility for significant social change. The market, as it is currently constituted, *does* leave medical needs unmet; whether this is in the context of rare diseases in richer countries, or in that of common, but neglected diseases in poorer countries. Recognition of this by governments, academics and clinicians, non-profit organisations, and patients themselves – as agents, not just subjects – promises the potential for innovation in new forms of social organisation, a setting ripe for social science research; not just new imaginaries and socialities to explore, but also a setting in which the social researcher can contribute to change.

4.8 Opportunities for social research

As described in this chapter, new models of pharmaceutical innovation are rich sites for social research. With the application of a sociological imagination combined with the multiplicity of theoretical, methodological, and political perspectives, there are countless possibilities, so we will only offer a selection here.

At the lowest level of resolution, the particular social, economic, and political conditions in which these alternative innovation models proliferate could be a fruitful research area. Comparative studies – taking a 'bird's eye view' of, say, the US, the UK, and the EU – would help us understand the types of models produced and sustained within different economic, healthcare, and regulatory systems.

At a slightly higher level of resolution, social researchers could explore the contribution of the new models of innovation to 'public health', a programme which might not be limited to raw measures of, say, quality-adjusted life years (QALYs), but also the contestation over the way in which 'public health' is understood. A research programme addressing these questions would also bring patients, and patient organisations, into the frame *as actors*, through the way in which their perspectives and demands shape the generation of knowledge. For example, Project HERCULES, which involved a consortium of actors – including patient groups – involved with Duchenne muscular dystrophy research, produced new measures of health states validated by patients and their carers which can be used in the development and assessment of new therapies (Broomfield et al., 2024).

Tightening the focus further, we can begin to reveal the particular textures and contours of these new forms of organisation, often involving novel collaborations. As suggested in the chapter, there are many questions at this level that are variations on 'how do the different actors involved exercise power?' At this level, the differences and tensions between the goal orientation and normative systems of the variety of participants are made most patent. While the relationship between for-profit and non-profit actors may be the most immediately eye-catching, and obviously warrants significant attention, social researchers should not neglect the exploration of the contestation between patient groups, academics, academic institutions, charities and philanthropic funders, and the various arms of the state. These actors have different goals, measures of success, modes of accountability, etc.

References

Althobaiti, H., Seoane-Vazquez, E., Brown, L.M., Fleming, M.L. and Rodriguez-Monguio, R. (2023) 'Disentangling the cost of orphan drugs marketed in the United States'. *Healthcare*, 11(4), n. 558. https://doi.org/10.3390/healthcare11040558

BioCanRx (2024) 'About BioCanRx'. https://biocanrx.com/about/about-biocanrx

Birch, K. (2017) 'Rethinking value in the bio-economy: finance, assetization, and the management of value'. *Science, Technology, & Human Values*, 42(3), pp. 460–490.

Birch, K. and Muniesa, F. (eds.) (2020) *Assetization: Turning Things into Assets in Technoscientific Capitalism*. Cambridge, MA: MIT Press.

Blume, S. and Baylac-Paouly, B. (eds.) (2021) *Immunization and States: The Politics of Making Vaccines*. Chicago, IL: Routledge.

Breckenridge, A. and Jacob, R. (2019) 'Overcoming the legal and regulatory barriers to drug repurposing'. *Nature Reviews Drug Discovery*, 18(1), pp. 1–2.

Broomfield, J., Hill, M., Chandler, F., Crowther, M.J., Godfrey, J., Guglieri, M., Hastie, J., Larkindale, J., Mumby-Croft, J., Reuben, E., Woodcock, F. and Abrams, K.R. (2024)

'Developing a natural history model for Duchenne muscular dystrophy'. *PharmacoEconomics Open*, 8, pp. 79–89.

Byrne, P., Adamson, D. and Bromiley, R. (2006) *Towards a 'New Mixed Economy'. An Exploration of the Relationship Between Social Enterprise and Private Sector Micro and Small to Medium Enterprises (SMEs) in Wales*. Cardiff: Llywodraeth Cymru / Welsh Government. https://www.gov.wales/sites/default/files/statistics-and-research/2019-07/070424-towards-new-mixed-economy-en.pdf

Conti, R.M., Meltzer, D.O. and Ratain, M.J. (2008) 'Nonprofit biomedical companies'. *Clinical Pharmacology & Therapeutics*, 84(2), pp. 194–197.

da Silva, R.G.L., Chammas, R. and Novaes, H.M.D. (2021) 'Rethinking approaches of science, technology, and innovation in healthcare during the COVID-19 pandemic: the challenge of translating knowledge infrastructures to public needs'. *Health Research Policy and Systems*, 19, n. 104. https://doi.org/10.1186/s12961-021-00760-8

Davies, E.H., Fulton, E., Brook, D. and Hughes, D.A. (2017) 'Affordable orphan drugs: a role for not-for-profit organizations'. *British Journal of Clinical Pharmacology*, 83(7), pp. 1595–1601.

Deal, L.S., Goldsmith, J.C., Martin, S., Barbier, A.J., Roberds, S.L. and Schubert, D.H. (2017) 'Patient voice in rare disease drug development and endpoints'. *Therapeutic Innovation & Regulatory Science*, 51(2), pp. 257–263.

DNDi (2020) 'Innovative single-dose oral sleeping sickness treatment to be co-developed by Sanofi and DNDi partnership'. https://dndi.org/press-releases/2020/innovative-single-dose-oral-sleeping-sickness-treatment-to-be-co-developed-by-sanofi-and-dndi/

DNDi (2024) 'Who we are'. https://dndi.org/about/who-we-are/

Douglas, C.M.W., Aith, F., Boon, W., de Neiva Borba, M., Doganova, L., Grunebaum, S., Hagendijk, R., Lynd, L., Mallard, A., Mohamed, F.A., Moors, E., Oliveira, C.C., Paterson, F., Scanga, V., Soares, J., Rabeharisoa, V. and Kleinhout-Vliek, T. (2022) 'Social pharmaceutical innovation and alternative forms of research, development and deployment for drugs for rare diseases'. *Orphanet Journal of Rare Diseases*, 17, n. 344. https://doi.org/10.1186/s13023-022-02476-6

Douglas, C.M. and Grunebaum, S. (2024) 'Lessons learned from the Canadian Fabry Disease Initiative for future risk-sharing and managed access agreements for pharmaceutical and advanced therapies in Canada'. *Health Policy*, 143, n. 105044. https://doi.org/10.1016/j.healthpol.2024.105044

Duggal, S. and Faulkner, A. (2020) 'Promissory and protective imaginaries of regenerative medicine: expectations work and scenario maintenance of disease research charities in the United Kingdom'. *Public Understanding of Science*, 29(4), pp. 392–407.

EATRIS (2024) 'About EATRIS'. https://eatris.eu/about/

Ferpozzi, H. (2023) 'Public-private partnerships and the landscape of neglected tropical disease research: the shifting logic and spaces of knowledge production'. *Minerva*, 61, pp. 607–629.

Fleming, S. (2021) 'A new perspective on how to fix pharma's broken business model', *Forbes*, 27 January 2021. https://www.forbes.com/sites/stanfleming/2021/01/27/fixing-the-broken-business-model-that-threatens-pharmas-future/

Fondazione Telethon (2023) 'Fondazione Telethon announces commitment to make gene therapy for Wiskott-Aldrich syndrome available to patients'. https://www.telethon.it/en/stories-and-news/news/from-telethon-foundation/fondazione-telethon-announces-commitment-to-make-gene-therapy-for-wiskott-aldrich-syndrome-available-to-patients/

Gallegos, J.E., Boyer, C., Pauwels, E., Kaplan, W.A. and Peccoud, J. (2018) 'The Open Insulin Project: a case study for "biohacked" medicines'. *Trends in Biotechnology*, 36(12), pp. 1211–1218.

Gaudillière, J.P. (2021) 'Pharmaceutical innovation and its crisis: drug markets, screening, and the dialectics of value'. *BioSocieties*, 16, pp. 411–432.

Geels, F. (2004) 'From sectoral systems of innovation to socio-technical systems: insights about dynamics and change from sociology and institutional theory'. *Research Policy*, 33(6–7), pp. 897–920.

Giddens, A. (1998) *The Third Way: The Renewal of Social Democracy*. Cambridge: Polity Press.

Guston, D.H. (2001) 'Boundary organizations in environmental policy and science: an introduction'. *Science, Technology, & Human Values*, 26(4), pp. 399–408.

Hale, V.G., Woo, K. and Lipton, H.L. (2005) 'Oxymoron no more: the potential of nonprofit drug companies to deliver on the promise of medicines for the developing world'. *Health Affairs*, 24(4), pp. 1057–1063.

Hayford, T.B. (2024) 'Role of specialty drugs in rising drug prices for Medicare Part D'. *JAMA Health Forum*, 5(5), e241188. https://doi.org/10.1001/jamahealthforum.2024.1188

iHuman (2024) 'The orphanisation project'. https://www.sheffield.ac.uk/ihuman/our-work/biosocial-humans/orphanisation-home

IQVIA (2024) *The Use of Medicines in the U.S.* https://www.iqvia.com/insights/the-iqvia-institute/reports-and-publications/reports/the-use-of-medicines-in-the-us-2024

Jarosławski, S. and Toumi, M. (2019) 'Non-profit drug research and development: the case study of Genethon'. *Journal of Market Access & Health Policy*, 7(1), n. 1545514. https://doi.org/10.1080/20016689.2018.1545514

Jarosławski, S., Toumi, M., Auquier, P. and Dussart, C. (2018) 'Non-profit drug research and development at a crossroads'. *Pharmaceutical Research*, 35, n. 52. https://doi.org/10.1007/s11095-018-2351-3

Jasanoff, S. (2015) 'Future imperfect: science, technology, and the imaginations of modernity', in Jasanoff, S. and Kim, S. (eds.), *Dreamscapes of Modernity: Sociotechnical Imaginaries and the Fabrication of Power*. Chicago, IL: University of Chicago Press, pp. 1–29.

Jonker, A.H., O'Connor, D., Cavaller-Bellaubi, M., Fetro, C., Gogou, M., 't Hoen, P.A.C., de Kort, M., Stone, H., Valentine, N. and Pasmooij, A.M.G. (2024) 'Drug repurposing for rare: progress and opportunities for the rare disease community'. *Frontiers in Medicine*, 11, n. 1352803. https://doi.org/10.3389/fmed.2024.1352803

Kleinhout-Vliek, T.H., Boon, W.P.C., Hagendijk, R.P., Hoekman, J. and Moors, E.H.M. (2024) 'Together for the greater goods: legitimising social innovation in the pharmaceutical field'. *Innovation: The European Journal of Social Science Research*, 37(1), pp. 60–84.

Krishnamurthy, N., Grimshaw, A.A., Axson, S.A., Choe, S.H. and Miller, J.E. (2022) 'Drug repurposing: a systematic review on root causes, barriers and facilitators'. *BMC Health Services Research*, 22, n. 970. https://doi.org/10.1186/s12913-022-08272-z

Lezaun, J. and Montgomery, C.M. (2015) 'The pharmaceutical commons: sharing and exclusion in global health drug development'. *Science, Technology, & Human Values*, 40(1), pp. 3–29.

Light, D.W. (2020) 'Addressing health care disparities: a radical perspective and proposal'. *Frontiers in Sociology*, 5, n. 29. https://doi.org/10.3389/fsoc.2020.00029

Liu, J., Barrett, J.S., Leonardi, E.T., Lee, L., Roychoudhury, S., Chen, Y. and Trifillis, P. (2022) 'Natural history and real-world data in rare diseases: applications, limitations, and future perspectives'. *The Journal of Clinical Pharmacology*, 62, pp. S38–S55.

Martens, J. (2003) 'The future of multilateralism after Monterrey and Johannesburg'. Berlin: Friedrich Ebert Stiftung, Dialogue on Globalization Occasional Paper No. 10.

Martin, P.A. (2022) 'The challenge of institutionalised complicity: researching the pharmaceutical industry in the era of impact and engagement'. *Sociology of Health & Illness*, 44, pp. 158–178.

Martin, P.A., Brown, N. and Kraft, A. (2008) 'From bedside to bench? Communities of promise, translational research and the making of blood stem cells'. *Science as Culture*, 17(1), pp. 29–41.

Maxmen, A. (2016) 'Busting the billion-dollar myth: how to slash the cost of drug development'. *Nature*, 536(7617), pp. 388–390.

Pammolli, F., Magazzini, L. and Riccaboni, M. (2011) 'The productivity crisis in pharmaceutical R&D'. *Nature Reviews Drug Discovery*, 10, pp. 428–438.

Phares, S., Trusheim, M., Emond, S.K. and Pearson, S.D. (2024) *Managing the Challenges of Paying for Gene Therapy: Strategies for Market Action and Policy Reform*. Boston, MA: Institute for Clinical and Economic Review. https://icer.org/wp-content/uploads/2024/04/Managing-the-Challenges-of-Paying-for-Gene-Therapy-_-ICER-NEWDIGS-White-Paper-2024_final.pdf

PPD (2022) *Trends in Pharmaceutical Research and Development Report: The State of the Drug Development Industry*. Waltham, MA: Thermo Fisher Scientific. https://www.ppd.com/wp-content/uploads/2022/09/PPD_Trends_in_Pharmaceutical_Research_and_Development_Report_d02-1.pdf

Public Pharma for Europe (2024) 'Conference Programme Public Pharma for Europe – Brussels March 2024'. Public Pharma for Europe. https://publicpharmaeurope.taplink.ws/

Ranganath, L.R. and Sireau, N. (2023) 'Clinical development innovation in rare diseases: overcoming barriers to successful delivery of a randomised clinical trial in alkaptonuria—a mini-review'. *Orphanet Journal of Rare Diseases*, 18, n. 1.

REMEDi4ALL (2023) 'REMEDi4ALL's first workshop for funders on innovating drug repurposing'. https://remedi4all.org/remedi4alls-first-workshop-for-funders-on-innovating-drug-repurposing/

REMEDi4ALL (2024a) 'Remedi4All platform'. https://remedi4all.org/about

REMEDi4ALL (2024b) 'Remedi4All patients homepage'. https://remedi4all.org/remedi4all-homepage-patients/

Rosenberg, N., van den Berg, S., Stolwijk, N.N., Jacobs, B.A.W., Post, H.C., Pasmooij, A.M.G., de Visser, S.J. and Hollak, C.E.M. (2023) 'Access to medicines for rare diseases: a European regulatory roadmap for academia'. *Frontiers in Pharmacology*, 14, n. 1142351. https://doi.org/10.3389/fphar.2023.1142351

Rotondoa, L.A., Harrison, W., Bush, S., Hopkins, A.D. and Koporce, K. (2016) 'The Neglected Tropical Disease Non-governmental Development Organization Network (NNN): The value and future of a global network aiming to control and eliminate NTDs'. *International Health*, 8(Suppl 1), pp. i4–i6.

Rudebeck, M., Scott, C., Rhodes, N.P., van Kan, C., Olsson, B., Al-sbou, M., Hall, A.K., Sireau, N. and Ranganath, L.R. (2021) 'Clinical development innovation in rare diseases: lessons learned and best practices from the DevelopAKUre consortium'. *Orphanet Journal of Rare Diseases*, 16, n. 510. https://doi.org/10.1186/s13023-021-02137-0

Scannell, J., Blanckley, A., Boldon, H. and Warrington, B. (2012) 'Diagnosing the decline in pharmaceutical R&D efficiency'. *Nature Reviews Drug Discovery*, 11, pp. 191–200.

Schuhmacher, A., Hinder, M., Dodel, A., Gassmann, O. and Hartl, D. (2023) 'Investigating the origins of recent pharmaceutical innovation'. *Nature Reviews Drug Discovery*, 22, pp. 781–782.

Srivastava, S. and Foster, J.C. (2023) 'The new economics of cell and gene therapy'. https://www.cellandgene.com/doc/the-new-economics-of-cell-and-gene-therapy-0001

Stiglitz, J.E. and Jayadev, A. (2010) 'Medicine for tomorrow: some alternative proposals to promote socially beneficial research and development in pharmaceuticals'. *Journal of Generic Medicines*, 7(3), pp. 217–226.

Sturdy, S. (2017). 'Personalised medicine and the economy of biotechnological promise'. *The New Bioethics*, 23(1), pp. 30–37.

Sun, D., Gao, W., Hu, H. and Zhou, S. (2022) 'Why 90% of clinical drug development fails and how to improve it?' *Acta Pharmaceutica Sinica B.*, 12(7), pp. 3049–3062.

Tutton, R. (2016). *Genomics and the Reimagining of Personalized Medicine*. London: Routledge.

van der Pol, K.H., Aljofan, M., Blin, O., Cornel, J.H., Rongen, G.A., Woestelandt, A.-G. and Spedding, M. (2023) 'Drug repurposing of generic drugs: challenges and the potential role for government'. *Applied Health Economics and Health Policy*, 21, pp. 831–840.

Weintraub, J. (1997) 'The theory and politics of the public/private distinction', in Weintraub, J. and Kumar, K. (eds.), *Public and Private in Thought and Practice: Perspectives on a Grand Dichotomy*. Chicago, IL: University of Chicago Press, pp.1–42.

Wouters, O.J., McKee, M. and Luyten, J. (2020) 'Estimated research and development investment needed to bring a new medicine to market, 2009–2018'. *JAMA*, 323(9), pp. 844–853.

5 Towards digital mental health? Entwining expectations, novelty, and value

Martyn Pickersgill and Jorge Crespo Suarez

5.1 Introduction[1]

Within psychiatry and psychology, digital artefacts and infrastructures have been presented as imperative. These are very varied and include text messaging, websites, blogs, social media, and chatbots (Mohr et al., 2017; Torous et al., 2021). Therapeutic interactions enabled by videoconferencing (i.e., telepsychiatry) and computer-based interventions like online cognitive behavioural therapy (CBT) platforms are widely advocated. This includes through programmes such as the National Health Service's (NHS) England 'Talking Therapies' initiative, which has influenced discourse on the provision of psychological care at an international scale (Pickersgill, 2019a).

Further, commonly and sometimes enthusiastically used smartphone applications (i.e., apps) have proliferated (Flore, 2023). These leverage algorithms and artificial intelligence (AI) to offer various mental health-orientated services, such as self-help, mood tracking and monitoring, and various self-guided or assisted interventions. Entwining various notions of neurobiological, psychological, and social experience, these apps - alongside chatbots accessed through web browsers - often promise to help individuals live with or recover from feelings and experiences associated with psychiatric disorders.

Digital interventions have been argued to have "recast the spatiality and temporality of healthcare" (Trnka, 2016, p. 248). They are sometimes framed as desirable precisely because of their distinctiveness from the praxis of conventional mental healthcare, and indeed through their elision of input from actual clinicians. Increasingly, digital tools and technologies are employed not only as interventions for mental ill-health, but are also on occasion positioned as a means of generating new kinds of information about patients and pathologies per se.

In this chapter, we contextualise and historicise some of these developments, charting innovation and discussion about telepsychiatry, mobile health (also known as 'mHealth' or 'm-health'), and what has more recently been called digital psychiatry or digital mental health. We argue that these have been partly constituted through the implicit and explicit extolment of various professional values and concerns in expectational statements about them, which interact with and propel characterisations of novelty.

5.2 Value, expectations, and novelty in biomedicine

To analyse the emergence of digital mental health, we engage with the sociologies of value, expectations, and novelty. Professional values and concerns, and the value that professionals place in particular discourses and practices, are well known to constitute the terrain of biomedicine (Freidson, 1970). So, too, does the economic value attributed to biological substances and processes (Birch and Tyfield, 2013). Through widespread instantiation across a range of registers (e.g., public-facing documents and intra-professional conversations), values and that which is valued articulate and reciprocally constitute each other (Dussauge et al., 2015). Articulations of value might exert disciplining effects on actual practices (Lamont, 2012), with value consequently having an ambiguous existence as promise and actuality. Values also morph as the technologies to which they are associated traverse epistemic contexts and agendas. Take, for instance, the long-established value for healthcare that is associated with genetic technologies: this has been reconstituted in terms of its potential to enhance the learning of children and young people as these techniques interact with the educational sciences (Williamson et al., 2024).

The rhetoric and instantiation of value can be strategically and more spontaneously deployed to support various professional endeavours (Birch and Tyfield, 2013). This is particularly evident when the canonical biomedical value, the value of life itself, is used to justify continued symbolic and material investment in technological processes that are yet to demonstrate clinical worth. Paul Martin and colleagues (2008) provide a striking example of this through a case study of private umbilical cord blood stem cell banking. Martin et al. demonstrated how a market emerged, underpinned by visions of cord blood as having *potential* therapeutic applications for assorted life-limiting or threatening disorders that a newborn baby might one day experience. Accordingly, the biomedical value of extending life – or at least, limiting severe suffering – has played a key role in powering a promissory bioeconomy (Martin et al., 2008). More generally, diverse forms of therapeutic promise (Rubin, 2008, p. 13) have been constituted via various kinds of biomaterials, configuring these as promissory substrates (Brown et al., 2006, p. 330) to which hopes and capital – i.e., symbolic and economic values – are associated.

Professional projects that might involve the strategic deployment of biomedical value and values to justify their necessity include practices of what – following Hacking (2004) – has been termed "performative nominalism" (Pickersgill, 2019b). In other words, the act of naming and the ongoing utterance of names are central to the consolidation of ontologies and the economic and symbolic infrastructures that give life to these. This concept also underscores the role of agency in generating notions of novelty and value: co-emergence can be intentionally fostered by agents who reflexively reconfigure their identities in the process (Galasso et al., 2024). Practices reminiscent of performative nominalism come from a variety of fields; sociologists of biomedical ethics, for instance, have demonstrated how ethical commentary shapes technoscientific development and thus the need for bioethicists (Conrad and De Vries, 2011; Hedgecoe and Martin, 2003).

Such insights emerge from wider work on the sociologies of expectations and novelty, which undergird much of the analysis presented here (Borup et al., 2006; Brown, 2003; Pickersgill, 2021; Webster, 2002). In the case of biomedicine, the promise of new health technologies involves mobilising "a range of claims about their future therapeutic impact" (Webster, 2002, p. 443). This includes psychiatry, where investments in neuroscience, for instance, are predicated in part upon the promise that these will enhance clinical practice – aligning with social promises in various domains (Pickersgill, 2023). Novelty is reflective and constitutive of high expectations; it is usefully regarded as a social accomplishment rather than quintessential to a technology, idea, or practice (Pickersgill, 2019c; Webster, 2002). In what follows, we draw on the inter-relating sociologies of value, expectations, and novelty to unpack the development and operations of digital mental health.

5.3 Psychiatry and technology

> What greater scourge could befall psychiatry than becoming impersonal – which means losing sight of the persona of the patient? The great technological advances that have taken place in medicine within the last three-quarter century raise this threat – the loss of the personal relationship with the patient. The whole tradition is based on healing and caring for the sick as persons, through constant personal contact between the doctor and the patient.
>
> *(Bartemeier, 1952, p. 1)*

These comments come from Leo H. Bartemeier's 1952 Presidential Address to the American Psychiatric Association (APA). In it, he sounded caution at the rise of techn(olog)ical approaches to clinical practice and underscored the therapeutic import of interpersonal relationships. Bartemeier's anxieties orientate us to how psychiatrists have long engaged with multiple technologies – including electroencephalography (EEG), positron emission tomography (PET), and magnetic resonance imaging (MRI). In the mid-twentieth century US, psychiatrists like Bartemeier commonly emphasised psychoanalysis; at the same time, interventions into neurological structure and function to treat mental ill-health were widely employed. Most controversially, these included electroconvulsive therapy (ECT) and lobotomy. Sadowsky (2006, p. 22) has illuminated how receptive many psychoanalysts were to ECT, underscoring "the extent of eclecticism in American psychiatry". For lobotomy, Raz (2008, p. 387) demonstrated that "psychosurgical discourse adopted key concepts from psychoanalytical discourse" and vice versa. Hence, technical apparatuses within psychiatry can be understood to help direct practitioner attention, while also becoming enfolded within existing theoretical and operational regimes that embed particular ontologies and values.

"Telepsychiatry" is a more contemporary instantiation of a (partial) psychiatric embrace of an external technological innovation, namely, telemedicine. This was defined in the first editorial of the *Telemedicine Journal* as: "the delivery of care to patients anywhere in the world by combining communications technology with medical expertise" (Goldberg, 1995). For decades now, clinicians and policymakers have advocated telemedicine explicitly in terms of two kinds of value: as a means of containing healthcare costs, and of enhancing access (Greene, 2022). In the UK, for instance, early policy announcements emphasised "the novelty and potential of telemedicine systems in a rhetoric that stresses the technology's place in a paradigm shift in the conceptualization and organization of British health care" (May et al., 2001, p. 1890). It was in part through such discourse, and via journals, research groups, professional associations, and conferences that bore the name 'telemedicine', that the field was constituted. This can be regarded as a form of performative nominalism: the coining of "telemedicine" and the badging of activities as such contributed to galvanising hopes and resources in ways that facilitated its consolidation.

Telepsychiatry is defined by organisations like the APA as "any synchronous or asynchronous consultation with a patient or other practitioner by regular telephone, text, or videoconferencing" (2021, p. 1), and the Royal Australian & New Zealand College of Psychiatrists (RANZCP) as "a consultation between a patient and a psychiatrist conducted via videoconference or by telephone" (RANZCP, 2023). Specific uses of telepsychiatry include medication management, as well as direct therapy (APA, 2021; see, similarly, RANZCP, 2023). We can see, then, that this mode of technical practice straightforwardly contains a range of professional ontologies – from the overtly neurobiological to the explicitly psychosocial.

In the twenty-first century, the use of telepsychiatry has greatly expanded, with its instantiation purported to have "revealed opportunities to increase access to and continuity of psychiatric care" (APA, 2021, p. 1), and to promote "health equity by increasing access to care" (ibid). Accordingly, it is deemed "a critical component of the mental health delivery system" (ibid). Similarly, the New Zealand Telehealth Forum – funded by the New Zealand Ministry of Health – emphasises the importance of telehealth for "remote patients" and clinicians in rural facilities (NZ Telehealth, 2024).

Research and practice initiatives around telepsychiatry in various nations have been configured with recourse to the value of access. With moral and clinical value overtly imbricated in this style of thought, epistemic endeavour has been orientated towards generating results that can be narrated through the value of access. Intervention trials are a case in point, with these commonly noting the utility of the technology in terms of enhancing admission into therapy for those who might otherwise be excluded from care (e.g., Kessler et al., 2009; O'Reilly et al., 2007). The impetus for the deployment of telepsychiatry was extended with the COVID-19 pandemic, where a range of countries used this in light of social distancing requirements. This shift has significantly extended outwards the imperative of access to care via telepsychiatry from a "traditional" locus of rurality (e.g., Cano et al., 2021; Javed et al., 2020).

Clinicians, though, have often been presented as resistant to telepsychiatry due to assumed deleterious effects on the relationship between doctor and patient deemed central to therapeutic engagement and success. As May et al. (2001) have shown, such matters have inflected the reception of telepsychiatry – and telemedicine more generally (May et al., 2003) – for decades now. Responses from policymakers and those with a stake in technological innovation to perceived practitioner reticence are not always sympathetic. Clinicians are often castigated for not only valuing the "wrong" thing (i.e., a particular therapeutic relationship versus access per se), but also for inaccurately characterising that upon which value judgements rest (i.e., that telepsychiatry does not "really" trouble therapeutic relationships). Of course, such castigations themselves embed certain imaginaries of psyche and social context. Still, and despite what many might see as the success of telepsychiatry during the COVID-19 pandemic, the technological shaping of inter-subjective action constitutive of telepsychiatric practice remains an object of clinical concern.

In sum, the praxis of telepsychiatry directs attention to two potentially conflicting values: access to care "versus" the quality of the clinical encounter. On the one hand, and most importantly within promissory discourse, telepsychiatry might be valued as a novel means to increase access to therapy. Even half a century ago, access had been – in the words of APA Medical Director Walter Barton – "a concern of the APA for a long time" (Barton, 1971, p. 522). Today, the value of enhancing access continues to be (co-)constituted through a range of (inter)national policy and clinical debates (Pickersgill, 2026). On the other hand, telepsychiatry is sometimes judged to have the potential to undercut a positive doctor-patient relationship understood by many therapists as holding considerable clinical (and personal) value. Its importance is an enduring trope within biomedicine; as Allan Tasman put it during an APA Presidential Address, it is of "central importance" to psychiatry (Tasman, 2000, p. 1762). The value of this relationship is also underscored by a wide-ranging literature describing various purported challenges to it, including industrial, economic, and political impacts on healthcare systems.

5.4 "Mobilising" psychiatry

In the previous section, we saw how telepsychiatry has been a major focus for psychiatric praxis concerning interweaving information and communication technologies into clinical practice. It represents a striking example of how critical biomedical values intersect, and configure field-building and the negotiation and reception of novelty. It is not the only illustration that could be advanced: online, often largely self-directed, therapy is another.

Interactive and self-guided psychological therapy – particularly CBT, delivered via online platforms, apps, or computer software without real-time therapist interaction

– has been a topic of international advocacy and debate. Numerous articles on this subject have been published in a range of journals focused on different national psy-communities. Evaluation studies of such modalities for CBT are also increasing, and evidence is being provided regarding the values of "acceptability" and "cost effectiveness" compared to other options. In the UK, for instance, online therapy portals like Beating the Blues have been rolled out across the NHS. They are endorsed by bodies such as the National Institute for Health and Care Excellence (NICE) in England and the Scottish Intercollegiate Guidelines Network (SIGN). In much the same way as in-person CBT is delivered through NHS Talking Therapies, web-based CBT is, in some senses, ontologically agnostic: it is focused on 'solutions' rather than necessarily 'causes'. Still, despite its high dose of pragmatism, this vision of the psyche might enfold particular neurobiological notions, given the (US) psychiatric origins of much of the theory and research styles informing contemporary CBT (Pickersgill, 2019b).

Online therapies, where users navigate through pre-set text, audio, video, animation, and exercises, tend to be associated with the treatment of so-called "mild to moderate" instantiations of common conditions like depression, and deployed through psychological and primary care services. As well as pre-set content, other chatbot tools are more interactive – such as Woebot, a "fully automated conversational agent" (Fitzpatrick et al., 2017). Considerations of telepsychiatric approaches as avenues for treatment vary more widely across a range of conditions, including those like schizophrenia – a contested and biomedically coded term – for which psychiatrists often take clinical responsibility (e.g., Henson et al., 2020). In recent years, telepsychiatry has become frequently operationalised through mobile phones, and web-based psychological therapies – once accessed largely through desktop computers – have also been "mobilised" as smartphone apps. Next, we explore how apps are being promoted through the diverse field of mHealth.

5.5 Promoting mobile health

mHealth is a key facet of the matrix of illness, optimisation, and technology. As Williams et al. (2015, p. 1045) have discussed, through mobile digital technologies "patients, proto-patients and the wider public may now track their bodies, share their data, participate in online discussion and support groups, and use the information they gather to improve or optimise their health". Institutions like the APA (undated) contribute to constructing mHealth as a novel and important development, asserting that the "expanding use of mobile health (mHealth) technologies is unprecedented in the history of medicine". Its value is seemingly evidenced in the "growing patient, clinical, government, and payer interest in the potential of mHealth technologies for psychiatric clinical care". To this end, the APA convened a working group to interrogate mobile phone apps that purport to promote wellbeing and treat mental ill-health. This subsequently developed an evaluation model for psychiatrists to use when ascertaining whether an app might afford value for a given patient – to help users and clinicians rate apps and "make the best choice for clinically meaningful app use" (Lagan et al., 2020, p. 7).

Deploying digital mental health can entail varying forms of responsibilisation. In telepsychiatry, the onus initially seems to lie with the clinician to cultivate new skills and care practices (although patients are expected to learn how to operate relevant technologies and software). With apps and chatbots, the responsibility lies more obviously with the user. This connects with established, broader values of "patient empowerment" which over the last decade or more have become embroiled with digital mental health (e.g., WHO, 2013, p. 14). At the same time, apps can also "passively" collect data from people's use of their phones, to generate clinically actionable psyknowledge about mood and an assumed "mental state" (De La Fabián, 2024). This, in turn, requires different interpretative work from clinicians when such data is passed to them.

Implementation of mHealth in the UK has for years been supported by a strong policy push towards innovation (Mental Health Taskforce, 2016, p. 38; National Information Board, 2014), one which increasingly also foregrounds AI (DSIT et al., 2023). Until December 2021, NHS Digital provided an online app library where patients were encouraged to discover digital resources to manage and enhance their health. Following the merger of NHS Digital with NHS England, "a new way of recommending apps" was implemented (NHS, 2023). People were then suggested to create an account and use the NHS App to access services and recommendations. Yet, in the NHS App's "Terms of Use", a disclaimer stated that the "NHS App and services within it are not a substitute for seeking medical advice. Always follow any medical advice given by your healthcare professionals" (NHS, 2024). Clinical expertise thus remains valued, even as some (potential) patients are encouraged to contribute to their care in isolation from mental health practitioners.

Epistemic and financial investment in research has come from funders like the Wellcome Trust and the UK National Institute for Health Research (NIHR); for example, MindTech: "a national centre focussing on the development, adoption and evaluation of new technologies for mental healthcare and dementia" (see: http://www.mindtech.org.uk). In the US, the National Institute of Mental Health (NIMH) also actively sought to configure the value of mHealth, including through expectational statements. It was, for instance, explicitly flagged within the agency's Strategic Plan for Research, with digital technologies, such as "mobile devices, information systems, artificial intelligence", posited as holding value for addressing ongoing problems around access to healthcare (NIMH, 2023a).

Like telepsychiatry before it, mHealth is thus presented as a technological fix to issues of healthcare policy, planning, and delivery. Nevertheless, the value of direct clinical care remains inscribed into the NIMH's Strategic Goals, with the institution still making it clear that digital tools "may not replace a mental health professional" (NIMH, 2023b). Still, mobile technologies could give "the public, health care providers, and researchers new ways to access help, monitor progress, and increase understanding of mental wellbeing" (ibid) – conjuring expectations of novelty and import. As for specific uses, mobile apps are widely framed as having value in being able to monitor symptoms and track individual "progress", and purportedly facilitate large-scale, personalised, and context-specific data collection. Apparently, "Digital Health tools have the potential to truly improve our understanding of mental illness, to track the course of illnesses, and to provide as-needed mental health care" (ibid). Accordingly, they are promised to enhance the understanding of mental health trends, triggers, and interventions in everyday life. Presented as a novel offering to increase knowledge production, digital technologies for mental health through their data collection and processing potential could shape wider mental research agendas.

Within funder discourses like those of the US NIMH, the entangling of the actual and the expectational re-creates enthusiasm and underscores the novelty of digital approaches to mental health. These organisations are also folding digital mental health into the highly financed regimes of "global health", with specific funding for research in what the World Bank terms "low and middle income countries" (LMICs). The NIMH Center for Global Mental Health Research has a "Digital Global Mental Health Program", aiming "to substantially improve mental health outcomes in LMICs through innovative digital mental health technologies that improve the detection, assessment, prevention, and treatment of mental illnesses, and that improve the delivery, management, and scalability of mental health care" (NIMH, 2024). The programme fosters research across diverse domains to advance digital mental health technologies. Key priorities include developing and testing tools to enhance screening, diagnosis, treatment adherence, and the management of ill-health (ibid). One focus is on leveraging emerging technologies, such as AI and machine learning, to improve health outcomes. The programme also emphasises efforts to optimise data capture, real-time assessment, and predictive analytics for "at-risk" populations, as well as strategies to boost engagement with digital tools.

Another way to track the evolution and increasing visibility of mHealth is through the statements made about it by the psychiatrist and former NIMH Director Thomas Insel (in post 2002–2015). Once cautious about the use of technological interventions in mental health (Shoham and Insel, 2011), Insel (2018) became an ever more vocal advocate of (mobile) digital techniques in psychiatric settings. When, during a 2013 *Boston Globe* interview, he was queried about the future of psychotherapy, Insel described how it "might be that what we call 'psychotherapy' is a mobile app that you download and is crafted for your specific cognitive domain" (Koven, 2013). A year later, *Psychology Today* asked Insel "What's a clinical innovation you're excited about?"; he responded: "Web-based and mobile CBT" (Nemko, 2014).

In 2015, Insel left the NIMH to work for Alphabet – a technology-driven American conglomerate with a broad range of subsidiary companies (most notably Google) – on device-orientated approaches to mental health. In a discussion with *Fortune* magazine, he accounted for this interest in technology as relating to wider shifts in understandings of psychopathology: where once disorders like depression were seen as "just a chemical imbalance", now they can be considered "problems with how neural circuits are communicating" – an issue that "we may be able to modulate with devices" (Sukel, 2015). Clearly, ostensibly psychological modalities can easily contain highly neurological ontologies.

Insel subsequently had various private sector and policy roles, more recently co-founding Humanest Care, which provides mHealth services to individuals and organisations, and Vanna Health, which offers services to people living with "serious mental illness" – with a "member-facing digital platform [...] available as an option" (see: www.vanna.health). Subsequently, Insel (2022, 2023) has gestured to an array of social, chemical, and technological solutions as offering the best way forward for people experiencing mental ill-health. In this respect, he seems to resonate with much mainstream opinion within a number of countries that have celebrated and entwined digital mental health within wider approaches to care and ontologies of psychopathology.

Despite the lauding of digital mental health, concerns have nevertheless also been raised about the security and commodification of the data that technologies might harness, given their commonly commercial origins (Erikainen et al., 2019; Lupton, 2014). This includes mental health apps (Egher, 2022), with one professional news piece, for instance, addressing the problem explicitly and bluntly: "Many app developers may be selling patient data for profit" (Torous et al., 2016a). What clinicians, patients, and developers value about digital mental health might thus be very different. In a review of opportunities and challenges associated with apps, psychiatrists Marley and Farooq (2015) also highlighted concerns about the clinical accuracy of information presented and the (lack of a) role of medical expertise in the development of some software – as well as overt risk to patients using apps partly as a consequence of errors and omissions. Discussions about the hazards of mHealth proliferating within psychiatric discourse underscore the increasingly everyday nature of mobile digital technologies for mental health. They also cast light on the responsibility many clinicians feel regarding the need to better understand the risks and benefits associated with technology when negotiating patients' own questions and concerns.

In part as a response to clinical concerns, mental health apps have come under increasing regulatory scrutiny (e.g., Zagorski, 2023). This includes interrogation of what, in fact, they are; are they, for instance, medical devices – and, if so, should they be regulated in ways congruent with other technologies that are perceived as such? As then UK Minister for Mental Health, Caroline Jackson, noted in 2022: "Digital mental health tools can be incredibly useful to help build resilience and prevent problems worsening, but it's crucial these are regulated properly" (MHRA, 2022). Such regulatory anxieties appear to have intensified within healthcare over the last decade or more, with the proliferation of devices with uses that further blur the lines between health, wellness, and recreation (Faulkner, 2017; Lievevrouw et al., 2022). In the case of mental health apps, processes of potential ontological respecification (Woolgar and Neyland, 2013) themselves produce notions of novelty. Expectational regulatory discourse also affirms the value of apps, with the (costly) attention paid to them implicitly and sometimes explicitly legitimised via their perceived significance.

Through disseminating and defining the concept of mHealth, and generating ethical discourse around its instantiations, professional associations, funders, and governments contribute to reifying mHealth as an object of novelty and fascination. Within the concerns of physicians, the disclaimers of NHS websites, and the tacit and overt endorsement of mental health apps by health-related organisations, we can see at least two assemblages of value (beyond the enhancement of access) playing a role in this performative nominalism. For one, there is the therapeutic, political, and economic value of encouraging self-care (e.g., WHO, 2013). Public health in a range of countries commonly emphasises care of the self to stave off pathology and optimise present health, with clinicians and societies framing self-care as a means of empowering patients and cutting healthcare costs. In recent years, digital technologies – including apps – have featured prominently within discourses of patient self-care (Henwood and Marent, 2019; Petrakaki et al., 2018).

Second, there is the moral, personal, and professional value of clinical responsibility. When, for instance, the apps recommended by the NHS carry with them a disclaimer that they are not a substitute for clinical consultation, we can see how the ultimate responsibility for addressing mental ill-health is often formally apportioned to a healthcare professional, even if in practice rather more diverse mediations of responsibility play out. While articulations of clinical responsibility are necessarily demarcations of power and expertise, they are also configured as virtuous in legalistic healthcare contexts where responsibility is inscribed in hard and soft law. Hence, the formal holding of clinical responsibility and the performance of being a responsible clinician (in a broader sense) mutually reinforce and blur the lines between descriptive and normative dimensions of responsibility. Through reminders to patients and professionals that mobile technologies should not be substituted for clinical inputs or through reassurances that clinicians have oversight of a process entailing digital mental health technologies, the value – and, indeed, virtue – of responsibility comes to legitimise endeavours to innovate the development and implementation of digital devices.

5.6 Consolidating the digital in mental health

2017 saw the publication of The World Psychiatric Association-Lancet Psychiatry Commission on the Future of Psychiatry: a report "intended to stimulate thought, debate, and the change necessary for psychiatry to fulfil its potential as an innovative, effective, and inclusive medical specialty in the 21st century" (Bhugra et al., 2017, p. 776). An accompanying editorial highlighted "the apparently relentless progress of digital technology", which has "the potential to render physical distance irrelevant to some areas of psychiatric practice" (*The Lancet Psychiatry*, 2017, p. 733). This, seemingly, created a new "challenge" to psychiatry "to use such innovations to enhance, rather than replace, the humane and humanistic aspects of practice" (ibid). Similar comments about progress and risks were made in the report's Executive Summary:

> Digital technology might offer psychiatry the potential for radical change in terms of service delivery and the development of new treatments. However, it also carries the risk of commercialised, unproven treatments entering the medical marketplace with detrimental effect. Novel research methods, transparency standards, clinical evidence, and care delivery

> models must be created in collaboration with a wide range of stakeholders. Psychiatrists need to remain up to date and educated in the evolving digital world.
>
> *(Bhugra et al., 2017, p. 775)*

The Commission comprised six key sections, one of which was a segment specifically on "digital psychiatry". This level of attention to the role of digital technology within mental health research and practice indicated a wider and sustained growth in prominence that, as we have seen, has been constituted through policy positioning, funding drivers, and researcher commentaries. What comprises "digital psychiatry" in the Commission, as elsewhere today, is wide-ranging. It encompasses digital devices such as smartphones, wearable sensors, augmented reality glasses, virtual reality headsets, and smartwatches, along with their animative technological infrastructures like algorithms, machine learning, and AI. Smartphones were given primary prominence by the Commission, with smartphone apps juxtaposed with more futuristic possibilities such as augmented reality glasses. These were judged to be just "entering the mental health space" (Bhugra et al., 2017, p. 799), albeit in somewhat undefined ways which continue to lack sharpness and granularity. Through talk of apps and more advanced technologies that "are already projected to change health care" (ibid), digital psychiatry was presented as moving "beyond traditional telepsychiatry" (ibid, p. 798) – with such novelty hence requiring focused attention and debate.

The Commission and subsequent writings reviewing the state of digital psychiatry, or digital mental health more generally, point to the apparent inevitability of clinical integration. One recurrent figure within contemporary writings on technology and mental health is US psychiatrist John Torous. Director of the Digital Psychiatry Division at the Beth Israel Deaconess Medical Center (Boston, USA) and a co-author of the WPA-Lancet Psychiatry Commission, Torous can be regarded as having worked for some years now to actively constitute a dedicated field of digital psychiatry, in part through the documentation of its possibilities. This includes articles examining the ethical hurdles associated with using digital technologies and providing provisional roadmaps for navigating these (e.g., Torous et al., 2021; Torous and Nebeker, 2017). Through raising (and sometimes resolving) ethical issues, Torous and others contribute to performing the novelty and value of digital innovation in psychiatric praxis. "Digital psychiatry", then, and "digital mental health" more generally, appear not so much as relatively bounded sites of sociotechnical practice, but rather as manifest through expectational discourse about the rise of digital technologies and their epistemic and clinical ramifications (cf. Brown, 2003; Hedgecoe and Martin, 2003).

According to the WPA-Lancet Psychiatry Commission report, the "digital psychiatry revolution has arrived" (Bhugra et al., 2017, p. 798). Aside from apps to treat mental disorders, the report also highlighted the increasingly discussed possibility of enrolling these as sources of data for research into the nature of psychopathology. As clinical psychologist Dror Ben-Zeev wrote in the first column of an ongoing series in *Psychiatric Services* on technology and mental health: "Advancements in Web, mobile, sensor, and informatics technology can do more than serve as tools to enhance existing models of care. Novel technologies can help us better understand the very nature of mental illness" (2017, p. 107). With similar optimism, the NIMH (2023b) has described on one of their public-facing pages how "receiving widescale information from many people at the same time can increase researchers' understanding of mental health and help them develop better interventions". As indicated in the previous section, the NIMH – as with other funders – is now actively supporting work in this area.

The direct data that people themselves enter into apps is widely considered to have considerable value, with new industry-academic partnerships emerging to capitalise on this potential. For example, the website of the mental health social networking app TalkLife bills itself as working "[t]ogether with researchers at Harvard University, Massachusetts Institute of Technology and Microsoft Research" to "have developed unique classifiers to better understand and predict self-harm" (TalkLife, 2024). Apparently: "Our world first platforms use this machine learning and human in the loop computing to be able to offer users assistance and services, specific to their individual circumstances, in real time". The Commission also noted the importance of passive data obtained via some of the additional features of smartphones (like GPS) (Bhugra et al., 2017). Other articles and commentaries have similarly flagged this, with sleep- and activity-tracking highlighted as means of generating new temporally fine-grained insights into psychopathology as experienced in everyday life (e.g., Marzano et al., 2015; Mendes et al., 2022).

Threading through all these commentaries is another biomedical value: the augmentation of the insights, learning, and understanding of psychiatrists and other mental health professionals and the expansion of the biomedical evidence base upon which this is commonly regarded as resting. According to Torous et al. (2016b), "Smartphone sensors and phone usage patterns, when coupled with appropriate statistical learning tools, are able to capture various social and behavioural manifestations of illnesses, in naturalistic settings, as lived and experienced by patients" (p. 1). In essence, technologies might contribute to this so-called "digital phenotyping" (Birk et al., 2021; Birk and Samuel, 2020), imparting new means of researching mental ill-health – and hence of knowing individual patients. Accordingly, perceptions of the very nature of psychopathology could also be transformed, while longstanding processes of medicalisation and neuropsychologisation could be reenergised (De La Fabián et al., 2023).

5.7 Looking back, looking forward

Innovations in digital mental health research, promotion, and treatment have generated excitement internationally (e.g., Rojas et al., 2019; Torous et al., 2021) – with one corollary of this being concern and disquiet. In this chapter, we have sought to historicise and enrich contextual understandings of these digital developments. We have seen how contemporary uses and future possibilities are connected in ways that imply psychotechnical novelty and the value and the inevitability of further innovation.

Through discussions of scenarios emerging from commentaries on digital mental health, some organisations and individuals adopt roles as "mediators of hope" (Martin et al., 2008, p. 127) about the prospects of technologies for patient benefit. Indeed, some even act as what we call "inoculators of certainty" (Crespo Suarez and Pickersgill, in press) concerning the psychiatric body politic and the positive role of digital technologies. In so doing, they contribute to a "discourse of inevitability" (Leonardi, 2008; Pickersgill, 2019a, 2026) about the imbrication of mental health praxis and technological artefacts that help to realise futures for understanding and treating mental ill-health that entwine not only psyche and society but also the neurobiological.

Among such mediators, agencies like the NIMH have the economic capacity to materialise a selection of the innovations they anticipate and the discourses they promote. Strategies of field-building consequently occur with and through leveraging value and values, or concrete investment and change. These appear to be playing out with a view to realising and further propelling such expenditure and innovation. Some of these strategies can be characterised as practices of performative nominalism. In this regard, purported members of ostensibly new fields act, in effect, to talk these into existence. Through mirroring such rhetoric, funders and governments themselves contribute actively to this consolidation.

As the sociology of expectations reminds us, promissory statements are vitally important to the constitution of biomedical endeavours and the generation of bio(medical) value(s) (Rubin, 2008; Tyfield and Birch, 2013) – including within the domain of digital health (Erikainen et al., 2019; Geiger and Gross, 2017). Indeed, when uttered so often, they can make alternative futures hard to imagine and the roads that might take psychiatry there challenging if not impossible to traverse – contributing to a form of path dependency. Within expectational statements, the implicit and explicit extolment of biomedical value and values plays an important legitimising function. Emphases of different values about the technological mediation of mental health care have shifted over time as the attention of psychiatry has ranged around various modalities. To date, the moral, clinical, and economic value of enhancing access to treatment has been key to propelling technological innovation in mental health – as, more recently, has the encouragement of self-care.

Today, mobile technologies are also being folded into regimes of mental health data collection, constituted through the value of the enhancement of clinical wisdom. In particular, service-orientated research is being conducted and urged to ascertain the potential for information gleaned from mobile phones (including via apps and activity monitoring functions) to assist with clinical decision-making. This work has been argued to have the potential to reshape therapeutic encounters, whereby the epistemic salience of patient testimony regarding their subjective experience is dissipated as objectivity is delegated to devices. Investigations are also emerging into how digital technologies might provide insights into the nature – especially the temporalities – of symptoms like low mood (Malhi et al., 2017; Merikangas et al., 2019). Research in this vein resonates with broader epistemological shifts in psychiatry into the analysis of symptoms and (often neurobiological) mechanisms of psychopathology, which have rendered problematic the existence of established nosological categories like schizophrenia.

Imbricating with all of this is another biomedical value: maintaining a positive doctor-patient relationship. It is striking how much the editorial accompanying the aforementioned WPA-Lancet Psychiatry Commission report, for instance, which advanced concerns about the "challenge" of innovation for "humane and humanistic aspects of practice" (*The Lancet Psychiatry*, 2017, p. 733), echoes the worries of psychiatrists in decades past. In particular, Leo Bartemeier's anxieties about the "threat" of technology to the psychiatrists' "personal relationship with the patient", set out almost 75 years ago in his APA Presidential Address, continue to resonate.

5.8 Conclusion

While digital mental health has been much vaunted, uncertainties remain concerning how readily and in what ways mental health professionals will accommodate digital technology in their practice and how patients and publics will respond to and reconfigure emergent strategies of research and care (Meadows and Hine, 2024). This is even as the direction of travel towards more, rather than less, digitisation is being encouraged through multiple discourses and direct enjoinments. Nevertheless, psychiatric practice is nothing if not eclectic and pragmatic. Further, as we have seen, technologically facilitated psychiatry may contain multiple and intersecting biological, psychological, and social ontologies of subjective distress. This enables, to an extent, the elision of customary debates within the mental health professions about how an emerging therapeutic modality could intensify or counter one particular ontological commitment or another – which might positively impact adoption.

Consequently, it does not feel unreasonable to anticipate a greater instantiation of digital technology within mental health than the aforementioned concerns might suggest. That said, we are of course mindful of contributing ourselves to the aforementioned expectational discourse of inevitability in digital mental health. Regardless, the normative dimensions of (any) digital instantiations within psychiatric praxis will certainly continue to require sociological scrutiny. Collectively, the processes characterised in this chapter underscore the need for ongoing, indeed revitalised, research on mental health, technology, and society. Potential areas of exploration include the impact on patient agency and autonomy; the shifting dynamics of dominance and marginalisation of different actors, institutions, and discourses; the normativities and implications of datafication; and the reconfiguring of professional, patient, and psychopathological ontologies.

Acknowledgements

We want to thank Alex Faulkner and the reviewers for insightful comments on an earlier version of this chapter. We are also grateful to the Wellcome Trust for supporting this research [209519/Z/17/Z; 106612/Z/14/Z; 094205/Z/10/Z]. Work undertaken through additional grants funded by the Wellcome Trust [223615/Z/21/Z], the UK Medical Research Council [MR/S035818/1; MC_PC_MR/R01910X/1], the UK Economic and Social Research Council [ES/S013873/1], the UK Arts and Humanities Research Council [AH/W011417/1], and National Agency for Research and Development of Chile (ANID) [72210001] has further informed our thinking, and we likewise acknowledge their support.

Note

1. This chapter develops from and extends arguments made within the following texts: Pickersgill, M. (2019a). Digitising psychiatry? Sociotechnical expectations, performative nominalism and biomedical virtue in (digital) psychiatric praxis. *Sociology of Health & Illness*, *41*(1), 16–30; Crespo Suarez, J., & Pickersgill, M. (in press). De la telepsiquiatría a la salud mental digital: realizando expectativas, novedad y virtud en psiquiatría. In De La Fabián, R., Jiménez, A., & Pizarro, F. (Eds.), *¿Somos Sujetos Digitales? Tecno-Promesas, Saberes Psi y la Digitalización de la Vida Cotidiana*. Santiago: RIL Editores.

References

American Psychiatric Association [APA]. (2021). Position statement on telemedicine in psychiatry. https://www.psychiatry.org/getattachment/a9405e26-3a69-4e9d-95b6-5df9568fb443/Position-Telemedicine-in-Psychiatry.pdf

American Psychiatric Association [APA]. (undated). App advisor. https://www.psychiatry.org/psychiatrists/practice/mental-health-apps

Bartemeier, L. H. (1952). Presidential address. *American Journal of Psychiatry*, *109*(1), 5–7.

Barton, W. E. (1971). Report of the medical director. *American Journal of Psychiatry*, *128*(4), 522–524.

Ben-Zeev, D. (2017). Technology in mental health: Creating new knowledge and inventing the future of services. *Psychiatric Services*, *68*(2), 107–108.

Bhugra, D., Tasman, A., Pathare, S., Priebe, S., Smith, S., Torous, J., Arbuckle, M. R., Langford, A., et al. (2017). The WPA-Lancet Psychiatry commission on the future of psychiatry. *The Lancet Psychiatry*, *4*(10), 775–818.

Birch, K., & Tyfield, D. (2013). Theorizing the bioeconomy. *Science, Technology, & Human Values*, 38(3), 299–327.

Birk, R., Lavis, A., Lucivero, F., & Samuel, G. (2021). For what it's worth: Unearthing the values embedded in digital phenotyping for mental health. *Big Data & Society*, *8*(2), 20539517211047319. https://doi.org/10.1177/20539517211047319

Birk, R., & Samuel, G. (2020). Can digital data diagnose mental health problems? A sociological exploration of 'digital phenotyping'. *Sociology of Health & Illness*, *42*(8), 1873–1887.

Borup, M., Brown, N., Konrad, K., & Van Lente, H. (2006). The sociology of expectations in science and technology. *Technology Analysis & Strategic Management*, *18*(3–4), 285–298.

Brown, N. (2003). Hope against hype: Accountability in biopasts, presents and futures. *Science Studies*, *16*(2), 3–21.

Brown, N., Kraft, A., & Martin, P. (2006). The promissory pasts of blood stem cells. *BioSocieties*, *1*(3), 329–348.

Cano, J. F., González-Díaz, J. M., Vallejo-Silva, A., Alzate-García, M., & Córdoba-Rojas, R. N. (2021). El rol del psiquiatra colombiano en medio de la pandemia de COVID-19. *Revista Colombiana de Psiquiatría*, *50*(3), 184–188.

Conrad, E. C., & De Vries, R. (2011). Field of dreams: A social history of neuroethics. In Pickersgill, M., Keulen, I. V., & Rothman, B. K. (Eds.), *Sociological Reflections on the Neurosciences*. Bingley: Emerald, pp. 299–324.

Crespo Suarez, J., & Pickersgill, M. (in press). De la telepsiquiatría a la salud mental digital: Realizando expectativas, novedad y virtud en psiquiatría. In De La Fabián, R., Jiménez, A., & Pizarro, F. (Eds.), *¿Somos Sujetos Digitales? Tecno-Promesas, Saberes Psi y la Digitalización de la Vida Cotidiana*. Santiago: RIL Editores.

De La Fabián, R. (2024). Digital therapeutic cultures and their new regime of psychological truth. *Sociological Research Online*, *29*(2), 299–315.

De La Fabián, R., Jiménez-Molina, Á., & Pizarro Obaid, F. (2023). A critical analysis of digital phenotyping and the neuro-digital complex in psychiatry. *Big Data & Society*, *10*(1), 20539517221149097. https://doi.org/10.1177/20539517221149097

Department for Science, Innovation and Technology [DSIT], Department of Health and Social Care [DHSC], The Rt Hon Michelle Donelan, The Rt Hon Steve Barclay MP, and The Rt Hon Rishi Sunak MP. (2023). New £100 million fund to capitalise on AI's game-changing potential in life sciences and healthcare. 29 October 2023. https://www.gov.uk/government/news/new-100-million-fund-to-capitalise-on-ais-game-changing-potential-in-life-sciences-and-healthcare

Dussauge, I., Helgesson, C.-F., & Lee, F. (Eds.) (2015) *Value Practices in the Life Sciences & Medicine*. Oxford: Oxford University Press.

Egher, C. (2022). *Digital Healthcare and Expertise: Mental Health and New Knowledge Practices*. London: Palgrave.

Erikainen, S., Pickersgill, M., Cunningham-Burley, S., & Chan, S. (2019). Patienthood and participation in the digital era. *Digital Health*, 23(5), 2055207619845546. https://doi.org/10.1177/2055207619845546

Faulkner, A. (2017). Blood informatics: negotiating the regulation and usership of personal devices for medical care and recreational self-monitoring. In Lynch, R., & Farrington, C. (Eds.), *Quantified Lives and Vital Data: Exploring Health and Technology through Personal Medical Devices*. London: Palgrave, pp. 203–228.

Fitzpatrick, K., Darcy, A., & Vierhile, M. (2017). Delivering cognitive behavior therapy to young adults with symptoms of depression and anxiety using a fully automated conversational agent (Woebot): A randomized controlled trial. *JMIR Mental Health*, *4*(2), e19. https://doi.org/10.2196/mental.7785

Flore, J. (2023). *The Artefacts of Digital Mental Health*. London: Palgrave.

Freidson, E. (1970). *Profession of Medicine: A Study of the Sociology of Applied Knowledge*. New York: Harper & Row.

Galasso, I., Erikainen, S., Pickersgill, M., & Testa, G. (2024). "Different names for the same thing"? Novelty, expectations, and performative nominalism in personalized and precision medicine. *Social Theory & Health*, *22*(2), 139–155.

Geiger, S., & Gross, N. (2017). Does hype create irreversibilities? Affective circulation and market investments in digital health. *Marketing Theory*, *17*(4), 435–454.

Goldberg, M. (1995). Telemedicine Journal: a new journal for a new age. *Telemedicine Journal*, *1*(1), 1–2. https://doi.org/10.1089/tmj.1.1995.1.1

Greene, J. A. (2022). *The Doctor Who Wasn't There: Technology, History, and the Limits of Telehealth*. Chicago: Chicago UP.

Hacking, I. (2004). *Historical Ontology*. Cambridge, MA: Harvard University Press.

Hedgecoe, A., & Martin, P. (2003). The drugs don't work: Expectations and the shaping of pharmacogenetics. *Social Studies of Science*, *33*(3), 327–364.

Henson, P., Barnett, I., Keshavan, M., & Torous, J. (2020). Towards clinically actionable digital phenotyping targets in schizophrenia. *npj Schizophrenia*, *6*(1), 13. https://doi.org/10.1038/s41537-020-0100-1

Henwood, F., & Marent, B. (2019). Understanding digital health: Productive tensions at the intersection of sociology of health and science and technology studies. *Sociology of Health & Illness*, *41*(S1), 1–15.

Insel, T. (2018). Digital phenotyping: A global tool for psychiatry. *World Psychiatry*, *17*(3), 276–277.

Insel, T. (2022). *Healing: Our Path from Mental Illness to Mental Health*. New York: Penguin.

Insel, T. (2023). Digital mental health care: Five lessons from Act 1 and a preview of Acts 2–5. *npj Digital Medicine*, *6*(1), 9. https://doi.org/10.1038/s41746-023-00760-8

Javed, A., Mohandas, E., & De Sousa, A. (2020). The interface of psychiatry and Covid-19: Challenges for management of psychiatric patients. *Pakistan Journal of Medical Sciences*, *36*(5), 1133–1136.

Kessler, D., Lewis, G., Kaur, S., Wiles, N., King, M., Weich, S., Sharp, D., Araya, R., et al. (2009). Therapist-delivered internet psychotherapy for depression in primary care: A randomised controlled trial. *The Lancet*, *374*(9690), 628–634.

Koven, S. (2013). Taking a new approach to psychiatric research. 16 December 2013. https://www.bostonglobe.com/lifestyle/health-wellness/2013/12/16/with-thomas-insel-director-national-institute-mental-health/nZ9Qjw88QmJtXWNQft1CFN/story.html

Lagan, S., Aquino, P., Emerson, M. R., Fortuna, K., Walker, R., & Torous, J. (2020). Actionable health app evaluation: Translating expert frameworks into objective metrics. *npj Digital Medicine*, 3(1), 100. https://doi.org/10.1038/s41746-020-00312-4

Lamont, M. (2012). Toward a comparative sociology of valuation and evaluation. *Annual Review of Sociology*, *38*, 201–222.

Leonardi, P. (2008). Indeterminacy and the discourse of inevitability in international technology management. *The Academy of Management Review*, *33*(4), 975–984.

Lievevrouw, E., Marelli, L., & Van Hoyweghen, I. (2022). The FDA's standard-making process for medical digital health technologies: Co-producing technological and organizational innovation. *BioSocieties*, *17*(3), 549–576.

Lupton, D. (2014). Critical perspectives on digital health technologies. *Sociology Compass*, *8*(12), 1344–1359.

Malhi, G. S., Hamilton, A., Morris, G., Mannie, Z., Das, P., & Outhred, T. (2017). The promise of digital mood tracking technologies: Are we heading on the right track? *Evidence Based Mental Health*, *20*(4), 102–107. https://doi.org/10.1136/eb-2017-102757

Marley, J., & Farooq, S. (2015). Mobile telephone apps in mental health practice: Uses, opportunities and challenges. *BJPsych Bulletin*, *39*(6), 288–290.

Martin, P., Brown, N., & Turner, A. (2008). Capitalizing hope: The commercial development of umbilical cord blood stem cell banking. *New Genetics and Society*, *27*(2), 127–143. https://doi.org/10.1080/14636770802077074

Marzano, L., Bardill, A., Fields, B., Herd, K., Veale, D., Grey, N., & Moran, P. (2015). The application of mHealth to mental health: Opportunities and challenges. *The Lancet Psychiatry*, *2*(10), 942–948.

May, C., Gask, L., Atkinson, T., Ellis, N., Mair, F., & Esmail, A. (2001). Resisting and promoting new technologies in clinical practice: The case of telepsychiatry. *Social Science & Medicine*, *52*(12), 1889–1901.

May, C., Harrison, R., Finch, T., MacFarlane, A., Mair, F., & Wallace, P. (2003). Understanding the normalization of telemedicine services through qualitative valuation. *Journal of the American Medical Informatics Association: JAMIA*, *10*(6), 596–604.

Meadows, R., & Hine, C. (2024). Entanglements of technologies, agency and selfhood: Exploring the complexity in attitudes toward mental health chatbots. *Culture, Medicine, and Psychiatry*, *48*(4), 840–857.

Mendes, J., Moura, I., Van de Ven, P., Viana, D., Silva, F., Coutinho, L., Teixeira, S., Rodrigues, J., et al. (2022). Sensing apps and public data sets for digital phenotyping of mental health:

Systematic review. *Journal of Medical Internet Research*, *24*(2), e28735. https://doi.org/10.2196/28735

Mental Health Taskforce. (2016). *The Five Year Forward View for Mental Health: A Report from the Independent Mental Health Taskforce to the NHS in England*. https://www.england.nhs.uk/wp-content/uploads/2016/02/Mental-Health-Taskforce-FYFV-final.pdf

Merikangas, K. R., Swendsen, J., Hickie, I. B., Cui, L., Shou, H., Merikangas, A. K., Zhang, J., Lamers, F., et al. (2019). Real-time mobile monitoring of the dynamic associations among motor activity, energy, mood, and sleep in adults with bipolar disorder. *JAMA Psychiatry*, *76*(2), 190–198.

MHRA. (2022). Press Release: Mental health funding of £1.8m welcomed by MHRA and NICE to explore regulation of digital mental health tools. 10 October 2022. https://www.gov.uk/government/news/mental-health-funding-of-18m-welcomed-by-mhra-and-nice-to-explore-regulation-of-digital-mental-health-tools#:~:text=The%20Medicines%20and%20Healthcare%20products,regulating%20digital%20mental%20health%20tools

Mohr, D., Weingardt, K., Reddy, M., & Schueller, S. (2017). Three problems with current digital mental health research ... and three things we can do about them. *Psychiatric Services*, *68*(5), 427–429.

National Information Board. (2014). *Personalised Health and Care 2020: Using Data and Technology to Transform Outcomes for Patients and Citizens. A Framework for Action*. https://www.gov.uk/government/uploads/system/uploads/attachment_data/file/384650/NIB_Report.pdf

National Institutes of Mental Health [NIMH]. (2023a). *National Institute of Mental Health Strategic Plan For Research*. https://www.nimh.nih.gov/sites/default/files/documents/about/strategic-planning-reports/NIMH_Strategic_Plan_for_Research_2023_Update.pdf

National Institutes of Mental Health [NIMH]. (2023b). Technology and the future of mental health treatment. https://www.nimh.nih.gov/health/topics/technology-and-the-future-of-mental-health-treatment

National Institutes of Mental Health [NIMH]. (2024). Digital global mental health program. https://www.nimh.nih.gov/about/organization/cgmhr/digital-global-mental-health-program

Nemko, M. (2014). The present and future of treatment for depression. 30 September 2014. https://www.psychologytoday.com/intl/blog/how-do-life/201409/the-present-and-future-treatment-depression

NHS. (2023). NHS apps library. https://digital.nhs.uk/services/nhs-apps-library

NHS. (2024). NHS apps terms of use. Version 5.2, 25 November 2024. https://digital.nhs.uk/services/nhs-apps-library

NZ Telehealth. (2024). About Telehealth. https://www.telehealth.org.nz/health-provider/what-is-telehealth/

O'Reilly, R., Bishop, J., Maddox, K., Hutchinson, L., Fisman, M., & Takhar, J. (2007). Is telepsychiatry equivalent to face-to-face psychiatry? Results from a randomized controlled equivalence trial. *Psychiatry Services*, *58*(6), 836–843.

Petrakaki, D., Hilberg, E., & Waring, J. (2018). Between empowerment and self-discipline: Governing patients' conduct through technological self-care. *Social Science & Medicine*, *213*(9), 146–153.

Pickersgill, M. (2019a). Digitising psychiatry? Sociotechnical expectations, performative nominalism and biomedical virtue in (digital) psychiatric praxis. *Sociology of Health & Illness*, *41*(1), 16–30.

Pickersgill, M. (2019b). Access, accountability, and the proliferation of psychological therapy: On the introduction of the IAPT initiative and the transformation of mental healthcare. *Social Studies of Science*, *49*(4), 627–650.

Pickersgill, M. (2019c). Psychiatry and the sociology of novelty: Negotiating the US National Institute of Mental Health "Research Domain Criteria" (RDoC). *Science, Technology, & Human Values*, *44*(4), 612–633.

Pickersgill, M. (2021). Negotiating novelty: Constructing the novel within scientific accounts of epigenetics. *Sociology*, *55*(3), 600–618.

Pickersgill, M. (2023). Neuroscience, novelty, and the sociology of the brain. In Petersen, A. (Ed.), *Handbook on the Sociology of Health and Medicine*. Cheltenham: Edward Elgar Publishing, pp. 525–540.

Pickersgill, M. (2026). *Configuring Psychology: Access to Therapy and the Transformation of Psychological Care*. Cambridge: Cambridge University Press.

Raz, M. (2008). Between the ego and the icepick: Psychosurgery, psychoanalysis, and psychiatric discourse. *Bulletin of the History of Medicine*, *82*(2), 387–420.

Rojas, G., Martínez, V., Martínez, P., Franco, P., & Jiménez-Molina, Á. (2019). Improving mental health care in developing countries through digital technologies: A mini narrative review of the Chilean case. *Frontiers in Public Health*, *7*. https://doi.org/10.3389/fpubh.2019.00391

Rubin, B. (2008). Therapeutic promise in the discourse of human embryonic stem cell research. *Science as Culture*, *17*(1), 13–27.

Sadowsky, J. (2006). Beyond the metaphor of the pendulum: Electroconvulsive therapy, psychoanalysis, and the styles of American psychiatry. *Journal of the History of Medicine and Allied Sciences*, *61*(1), 1–25.

Shoham, V., & Insel, T. (2011). Rebooting for whom? Portfolios, technology, and personalized intervention. *Perspectives on Psychological Science*, *6*(5), 478–482.

Sukel, K. (2015). Google's NIH health hire: Smartphones can detect mental health breakdowns. 17 September 2015. http://fortune.com/2015/09/17/googles-nih-health-hire-smartphones-can-detect-mental-health-breakdowns/

TalkLife. (2024). What is TalkLife? https://www.talklife.com/about

Tasman, A. (2000). Presidential address: The doctor-patient relationship. *American Journal of Psychiatry*, *157*(11), 1762–1768.

The Lancet Psychiatry. (2017). Editorial: New wave. *The Lancet Psychiatry*, *4*(10), 733.

The Royal Australian & New Zealand College of Psychiatrists [RANZCP]. (2023). *Professional Practice Guideline 19. Telehealth in Psychiatry*. https://www.ranzcp.org/getmedia/2148dcf0-9fcd-4dc2-80bb-4bef2f44f2ca/ppg-19-telehealth-in-psychiatry-oct-2023-v2.pdf

Torous, J., Chan, S., & Luo, J. (2016a). Are your patients using 'digital supplements'? *Psychiatric News*, *51*(22). https://psychiatryonline.org/doi/10.1176/appi.pn.2016.11b16

Torous, J., Kiang, M., Lorme, J., & Onnela, J. (2016b). New tools for new research in psychiatry: A scalable and customizable platform to empower data driven smartphone research. *JMIR Mental Health*, *3*(2), e16. https://doi.org/10.2196/mental.5165

Torous, J., & Nebeker, C. (2017). Navigating ethics in the digital age: Introducing connected and open research ethics (CORE), a tool for researchers and institutional review boards. *Journal of Medical Internet Research*, *19*(2), e38. https://doi.org/10.2196/jmir.6793

Torous, J., Bucci, S., Bell, I. H., Kessing, L. V., Faurholt-Jepsen, M., Whelan, P., Carvalho, A. F., Keshavan, M., Linardon, J., & Firth, J. (2021). The growing field of digital psychiatry: Current evidence and the future of apps, social media, chatbots, and virtual reality. *World Psychiatry*, *20*(3), 318–335.

Trnka, S. (2016). Digital care: Agency and temporality in young people's use of health apps. *Engaging Science, Technology, and Society*, 2, 248–265. https://doi.org/10.17351/ests2016.119

Webster, A. (2002). Innovative health technologies and the social: Redefining health, medicine and the body. *Current Sociology*, *50*(3), 443–457.

Williams, S., Coveney, C., & Meadows, R. (2015). 'M-apping' sleep? Trends and transformations in the digital age. *Sociology of Health & Illness*, *37*(7), 1039–1054.

Williamson, B., Kotouza, D., Pickersgill, M., & Pykett, J. (2024). Infrastructuring educational genomics: Associations, architectures, and apparatuses. *Postdigital Science and Education*, *6*, 1143–1172. https://doi.org/10.1007/s42438-023-00451-3

Woolgar, S., & Neyland, D. (2013). *Mundane Governance: Ontology and Accountability*. Oxford: Oxford University Press.

World Health Organization [WHO]. (2013). *Mental Health Action Plan: 2013–2020*. http://apps.who.int/iris/bitstream/handle/10665/89966/9789241506021_eng.pdf;jsessionid=BA0F36F7931A83B9A956063E52793754?sequence=1

Zagorski, N. (2023). Digital mental health apps need more regulatory oversight. *Psychiatric News*, *58*(12). https://doi.org/10.1176/appi.pn.2023.12.11.35

6 Following technologies, understanding governance: A bio-moralities approach to emerging reproductive genetic technologies

Ingrid Metzler and Erik Aarden

6.1 Introduction[1]

Newly emerging biomedical technologies often spark debates about the meaning of core values that shape how communities coexist. Non-invasive prenatal testing (NIPT), which uses platforms to analyze fetal DNA fragments (of placental origin) circulating in pregnant women's blood, is a good example of this (Hui and Bianchi, 2017). The rise of this form of testing was frequently accompanied by debates, which centered on how this test could empower women and enhance their reproductive freedom (Ravitsky, 2017). In Belgium, public healthcare authorities made this test available to all pregnant women, fully reimbursing its cost, to increase their reproductive autonomy (Van Den Bogaert *et al.*, 2021). In Germany, the use of this test sparked debates that revealed conflicting views about the meaning of women's self-determination and the role public healthcare authorities should play in protecting their freedoms (Braun and Könninger, 2018; Raz *et al.*, 2022; Metzler, 2024). In Austria, concerns about unresolved ethical questions have kept the test primarily as a private service that women must pay for themselves (Metzler, 2020). In contrast, the Netherlands took unresolved questions and uncertainties as an impetus to conduct comprehensive studies aimed at generating a common ground that could help address these very concerns (van der Meij *et al.*, 2019). How can we understand and explain such differences? Why do similar concerns lead some countries to pursue public solutions, while others leave these issues to private markets? And what do notions such as 'autonomy' or 'freedom' come to mean in different situations?

In this chapter, we introduce the concept of 'bio-moralities' to address such questions. We argue that while bio-moralities can be found in many spaces, they can be particularly well studied in engagements with technological governance. In turn, distilling bio-moralities that sustain technological governance can help us better understand its contemporary configuration. We base our argument on reflections on social science research on technological governance in reproductive genetic testing (RGT), as this body of literature and our own attempts to contribute to it have inspired us to start developing this concept.

RGT involves biomedical technologies that generate information about genetic structures of prospective parents, IVF embryos, or fetuses, such as chromosome numbers or genetic variants associated with specific diseases. RGT can be categorized by testing stage: carrier testing examines genetic material of prospective parents, typically before pregnancy; preimplantation genetic testing (PGT) analyzes genetic material of IVF embryos before their transfer; and prenatal testing analyzes genetic structures from cell-free DNA in women's bloodstream or cells from amniotic fluid or placenta during pregnancy. RGT results inform reproductive choices, ranging from deciding not to have children (with a particular partner), using PGT to choose embryos, terminating pregnancies, or preparing for a child with special needs.

The emergence, expansion, and routinization of RGT have sparked debates about appropriate uses of biomedical technologies. RGT has enabled couples to have healthy children, turning 'chances' into 'choices' (Buchanan *et al.*, 2001), and increasing women's reproductive autonomy. While many welcomed this as progress, they also questioned how to oversee these technologies to achieve a 'reproductive autonomy worth having' (Johnston and Zacharias, 2017, p. 5). Others challenged the desirability of transforming natural contingencies into human choices, arguing that this could undermine the egalitarian relationships fundamental to liberal democracies (Habermas, 2001). Critics also problematized the consequences of RGT for unborn lives, individuals living with tested conditions (Kerr, 2009), and our understandings of human life and human nature in biological, social, and biosocial terms.

In more abstract terms, the debates surrounding the emergence, adoption, and governance of RGT technologies have intertwined with discussions about human life and, borrowing Hannah Arendt's (2019) term, 'the human condition.' These debates often addressed fundamental questions. Some were framed in biological and legal terms: when does human life and personhood begin (Jasanoff, 2011b; Hurlbut, 2017)? Others aligned with philosophical anthropology and political theories: what is human nature? What freedoms should individuals have to ensure collective flourishing? What role should biomedical technologies play in advancing these freedoms? Answers to these questions often extended beyond biology. In this chapter, we engage with combinations of moralities—or understandings of what humans *should* do—together with conceptions of human nature and the human condition. We refer to such combinations as bio-moralities.

As a working definition, bio-moralities encompass forms of normativity—such as ideas, visions, values, principles, and rationalities (which are often tied to practices, institutions, and technologies)—that are linked to conceptions of the human condition and that both sustain and are sustained by measures to protect human life, enhance human well-being, and do justice to the human condition. Bio-moralities thus encapsulate both biological and other (e.g., social, biographical) conceptions of human life. They appear in many contexts: commercial companies' promotional videos presenting visions of good life and responsible parenthood enabled by their technology; bioethicists' judgments on appropriate therapeutic uses of biomedical technologies based on particular conceptions of human life; or healthcare advocates' campaigns warning against unquestioned use of new biomedical technologies they see as threatening.

However, looking for competing bio-moralities is particularly valuable when engaging with technological governance. On the one hand, technological governance is grounded in specific bio-moralities, and thus in specific assumptions about human nature that justify developing, using, funding, restricting, or banning biomedical technologies. On the other hand, technological governance is also a site where bio-moralities are made durable and mobile, e.g., through the travels of technologies and the moralities traveling along with them. Following biomedical technologies, unpacking the measures that actors, experts, and authorities call for, take, or problematize, and asking systematically 'how do actors conceptualize human nature if these measures are appropriate to do justice to that nature,' can help us better understand technological governance and the distribution of responsibilities between actors involved in it.

In this chapter, we use a broad concept of governance drawing together elements from several scholars (Rose, 2006; Gottweis, 2008; Gottweis *et al.*, 2008; Laurent, 2022). We approach governance as the range of measures taken by formal and informal authorities to shape the actions of subjects and the flows of objects in specific spaces. The measures, the governing authorities' identities, and the boundaries of the spaces that authorities govern vary (Gottweis *et al.*, 2008). Measures can include uses of technologies, enforceable laws, soft regulations, public healthcare programs providing access to particular technologies, or nudges to incentivize certain actions. Authorities may be formal, legally entitled to make decisions for and on behalf of others, or informal—deriving their authority from the 'epistemic authority' tacitly attributed to national and international professional societies (Hurlbut, 2015), or from the 'infrastructural power' (Kelton *et al.*, 2022) of companies controlling technical devices constitutive of biomedical technologies.

The well-documented multitude of authorities involved in contemporary technological governance is one of the main reasons why we have commenced thinking about the concept of bio-moralities. Scholars have drawn attention to the 'sphere transgressions' (Sharon and Gellert, 2023) or the 'regulatory capture' (Saltelli *et al.*, 2022; Chomanski and Lauwaert, 2024) by big tech companies. Such insights have informed our understanding that we need concepts that are broad enough to capture the diversity of spaces, authorities, and measures in contemporary technological governance, while also helping us to better understand the ongoing redistribution of power and authority.

We base our argument on reflections on social science research on technological governance in RGT. Our engagement is necessarily selective. We discuss research on the governance of RGT in liberal democracies in Europe and the United States, neglecting research on RGT in other contexts. We engage with social science perspectives that describe, explain, or critique RGT governance, omitting more prescriptive contributions about how biomedical technologies should be governed. We focus on social science research that has shaped our reasoning, situating our thoughts on bio-moralities and acknowledging the concepts and insights we build upon. However, while we have begun to develop the concept primarily in conversation with literature on technological governance in RGT, we think that the concept holds potential for engagements with other biomedical technologies.

We begin by describing key aspects of 'new RGT' that emerged from the 1960s onward. We then examine two theoretical perspectives on RGT governance: one building on Foucault's concepts of biopower and governmentality to explore governance through technologies, and another analyzing governance of technologies through regulations and access policies. Subsequently, we discuss 'next generation RGT,' which has emerged since the turn of the century, and a third set of perspectives that has highlighted the involvement of informal authorities in the governance of newly emerging technologies. In our concluding reflections, we will draw together these perspectives and reflect on how the concept of bio-moralities seeks to combine them to inform future research on technological governance—in and beyond RGT.

6.2 Research perspectives on the governance of new reproductive genetic testing

6.2.1 The Emergence of New Reproductive Genetic Testing

The awareness that some conditions are passed from one generation to the next predates the rise of the 'new genetics' in the second half of the twentieth century. From the eighteenth century onward, physicians began to differentiate conditions caused by accidents from those produced by 'bad blood' (Löwy, 2018a, p. 40). In the early twentieth century, geneticists began ordering hereditary conditions into 'recessive' (caused by two pathogenic copies of a gene), 'dominant' (caused by one pathogenic copy of a gene), and 'sex-linked' (caused by a gene located on a sex chromosome). In eugenic programs, people deemed to have hereditary conditions were discouraged, and often also prohibited, from having children (Kevles, 1985).

This began to change in the 1960s when the emergence of technologies for RGT enabled couples deemed at risk of passing a condition to their children to have children without these conditions. In 1959, scientists linked inborn anomalies, such as Down syndrome, to variations in chromosome numbers, which they could now visualize with laboratory technologies (Löwy, 2018a). In the late 1960s, biomedical professionals developed 'amniocentesis,' which allowed them to sample fetal cells from the amniotic fluid of a pregnant woman (Rapp, 2000). The cells were cultured and analyzed in laboratories to detect an abnormal number of chromosomes or the presence of a pathogenic copy of a gene, which could be detected with then-available laboratory technologies. Some of these latter technologies were also used to identify (healthy) carriers of recessive genetic conditions in carrier screening programs (Antonarakis, 2019).

While RGT was initially uncommon, it became a more widespread practice in the 1980s and 1990s. New molecular-genetic technologies increased the number of detectable genetic conditions (Kerr, 2009). Moreover, RGT was combined with other technologies. In 1990, combining genetic testing with in vitro fertilization (IVF) through pre-implantation genetic testing expanded reproductive options for carriers of genetic conditions (Franklin and Roberts, 2006). Additionally, blood and ultrasound markers helped identify women at higher risk of carrying fetuses with common autosomal trisomies, making screening for these conditions a routine for many pregnant women (Kerr, 2009; Löwy, 2018b; Wahlberg and Gammeltoft, 2018).

The emergence and expansion of biomedical technologies used in RGT were accompanied by debates about their purpose, consequences, and oversight. These moral debates differed between contexts. They intensified with increased uses of these technologies, often peaking when RGT and IVF merged through PGT. Social sciences and humanities scholars also weighed in, alternating between advancing moral arguments and analyzing how moral positions emerged in relation to these technologies through critical or interpretive lenses.

Early scholarship questioned these new choices and freedoms by examining their consequences on women and their influence on understandings of human life. Barbara Katz Rothman (1993) showed how amniocentesis transformed women's experiences of pregnancies into 'tentative' ones. Rayna Rapp's (2000) study of amniocentesis in the United States showed how women who had this test not only made individual choices but also contributed to clarifying a contested issue as 'moral pioneers.' Others described how 'dangerous diagnostics,' to quote Nelkin and Tancredi (1994), threatened to reduce understandings of health and disease to genetic ones. This critique was also captured by the notion of 'geneticization' (Lippman, 1993; Hedgecoe, 1998), which served as a mainstream social science position on the consequences of genetic testing. While early social science engagements primarily formulated critiques of RGT, research soon moved to questions of how authorities responded to it.

6.2.2 Biomedical Technologies as Technologies of Governance

A first set of perspectives on governance built on Michel Foucault's (2003) work on biopolitics, biopower, and governmentality to analyze the governance of women, populations, and 'life itself' (Rose, 2001) through RGT. In these writings, RGT did not so much figure as an object overseen and governed by authorities, but as a technology that governed—e.g., by producing effects on individuals' and couples' actions, 'molecularizing' human life and leading to new forms of self-governance (Rose, 2001). In the introduction of a volume on 'Genetic Governance,' the editors Robin Bunton and Alan Petersen (2005, p. 1) wrote:

> While there remains extensive public debate about the rights and wrongs of such developments, there has been less concern for the detailed effects these envisaged changes will

> have on the ways we make decisions about our bodies and ourselves, our communities and environment; in short *on the ways in which we are governed.* (Italics added)

Scholars developing this perspective described the moralities—or, in the terms they tended to use: the 'rationalities'—tied to technologies, comparing new rationalities with previous eugenic ones (Lemke, 2005). They showed that, unlike previous top-down interventions on human reproduction, the new technologies worked through individualizing choices (Rose, 2001; Helén, 2004; Lupton, 2012).

Combinations between understandings of the human condition and uses of technology were already present in this research, focusing on how individuals governed themselves. For instance, Nikolas Rose described biomedical technologies used in RGT and other fields as giving rise to an 'ethopolitics'—'the politics of life itself and how it should be lived ' (Rose, 2001, p. 18). This concept was meant to capture the:

> ways in which the ethos of human existence, the sentiments, moral nature or guiding beliefs of persons, groups, or institutions – have come to provide the 'medium' within which the self-government of the autonomous individual can be connected up with the imperatives of good government.
>
> *(Rose, 2001, p. 18)*

Thus, these early writings introduced the combination between conceptions of human life and moralities, conceptualizing moralities in terms of rationalities tied to technologies. This first set of perspectives on governance sensitized us to the agency of technologies in the governance of human life, while neglecting the questions of who governs these technologies and how. These questions became central in a second set of perspectives on the governance of biomedical technologies, which localized moralities and thereby also pluralized technologies.

6.2.3 The Governance of Biomedical Technologies by State Authorities

The question of who governs RGT technologies was central in a second set of perspectives that 'brought the state back in' (Evans *et al.*, 1985) to discussions on RGT governance. This research contextualized biomedical technologies and moralities, locating them on a national scale.

Much of this research focused on PGT, the genetic testing of IVF embryos before their transfer, which was then largely known as preimplantation genetic diagnosis (PGD). Particularly during the peak of research on PGT governance around the turn of the millennium, this procedure sparked debates about the destruction of human life through unused embryos, the devaluation of lives of people with conditions that could now be 'prevented,' and concerns that PGT would enable the creation of 'designer babies.'

In their ethnographic study of PGT in the UK, Sarah Franklin and Celia Roberts (2006) argued that the complex social meaning of ethical and political questions surrounding PGD required analysis of regulation and governance. They emphasized that their descriptions of PGT were specific to the UK and its distinct regulatory approach, noting that 'some of the divergent patterns of PGD usage internationally suggest that PGD is always to some extent a nationally specific technology' (Franklin and Roberts, 2006, p. 130). Understanding the effects of technologies now also required engaging with their governance.

Social science scholars began examining how state authorities governed biomedical technologies, often focusing on the making of laws and regulations. Some research mapped out the actors and institutions involved in regulating PGT. Ivar Bleiklie and colleagues produced an overview of the governance of PGT in 13 countries, positioning them on a scale from restrictive to permissive regulation (Bleiklie *et al.*, 2003). They described how different moralities (in our terms) around a specific biomedical technology were constructed by describing how regulatory procedures, authorities, and institutions produced different regulations.

Other scholars compared the governance of biomedical technologies in a smaller number of countries, using concepts such as 'discourses,' 'political cultures,' or 'bioconstitutional imaginaries' to reveal and explain different moralities. For instance, Svea Luisa Herrmann (2009) compared the 'problematizations'—the constructions of problems that state authorities were expected to address—in her comparison of PGT and embryo research debates in the UK and in Germany and unpacked the different 'discourses' at work in the two countries. In an expansive comparative study of the governance of biotechnology in Germany, the UK, and the United States, Sheila Jasanoff (2005) explored national specificities with reference to the role of 'political culture.' She described how distinct institutional configurations, political norms, and public evaluations of (scientific) knowledge claims shaped both biomedical technologies and their governance. She reconstructed how new entities and technologies were coproduced with particular norms and rules for doing and regulating science.

Extending this work on the coproduction of forms of life and norms for life, Jasanoff and colleagues later developed the concept of 'bioconstitutionalism' (Jasanoff, 2011a; Hurlbut *et al.*, 2020). Jasanoff (2011a, p. 3) argued that:

> periods of significant change in the life sciences and technologies should be seen as constitutional or, more precisely, *bio*constitutional in their consequences. Revolutions in our understanding of what life is burrow so deep into the foundations of our social and political structures that they necessitate, in effect, a rethinking of law at a constitutional level.

Bioconstitutionalism builds on the understanding that definitions of what human life *is* and visions of what it *ought to be* are shaped by a 'constant, mutually constitutive interplay of biological and legal conceptions of life, the former focusing on life's definition and the latter on its entitlements' (Jasanoff, 2011a, p. 3). In a later formulation, Jasanoff and colleagues described bioconstitutionalism in terms of a mutually sustaining combination between descriptions of the human, 'that are at once and the same time biological and legal' (Hurlbut *et al.*, 2020, p. 983), and prescriptions of the 'state's responsibilities towards the lives in their care' (Hurlbut *et al.*, 2020, p. 981).

A further strand of research has analyzed governance through cross-national differences in access and funding of these technologies. Returning once more to the example of PGT, we examined how technological governance manifests in the practical organization, delivery, and provision of RGT (Aarden *et al.*, 2008, 2009). While maintaining focus on comparable national specificities, this work showed how distinct national approaches to governing PGT also included particular kinds of clinics where the procedure would be available, specific applications for the procedure, and specific legal, normative, and medical rationalities shaping for whom the procedure is available and paid for. These considerations expanded the meaning of governance from legal regulations to shaping uses of technologies by providing particular forms of RGT.

6.3 Next generation reproductive genetic testing

6.3.1 The Emergence of Next Generation Reproductive Genetic Testing

After the turn of the millennium and the completion of the Human Genome Project, new technological platforms like microarrays and next-generation sequencing platforms transformed RGT practices.

Firstly, new platforms expanded RGT's scope, shifting from a targeted search for specific variants in prospective parents', IVF embryos', or fetuses' genomes to more comprehensive screening for many 'variants,' i.e., differences in the DNA sequence compared to reference sequences (Hashiloni-Dolev *et al.*, 2019). Language changes reflect these technological transformations. 'T' (testing) or 'S' (screening) replaced 'D' (diagnosis) in acronyms like PG*D* (preimplantation genetic diagnosis) or PN*D* (prenatal diagnosis). These technological changes also affect bio-moralities, as the new technological possibilities also raise questions of what kinds of conditions should be tested for.

Secondly, as the new platforms have rendered genetic analysis less labor-intensive, they have also made it technically feasible to offer RGT to more individuals and couples than in the past (Rowe and Wright, 2020). This is most visible in the field of prenatal testing. Using new technological platforms to analyze short fragments of cell-free DNA shed from the placenta to a pregnant woman's bloodstream has made it thinkable to screen all pregnancies for conditions such as common autosomal trisomies with a test known as 'non-invasive prenatal testing' (NIPT) (Bianchi *et al.*, 2014; Hui and Bianchi, 2017), opening the question of whether such a general screening is also morally desirable.

Thirdly, new technologies have transformed the actors, experts, and authorities involved in RGT, with commercial actors playing a more prominent role than in the past, and testing practices traveling in new forms. At the risk of overstating differences between 'new RGT' and 'next generation RGT,' previous RGT practices typically operated as public healthcare programs targeted at specific risk groups. For instance, amniocentesis was offered to pregnant women over 35 (due to their statistically higher chance of carrying a fetus with a common autosomal trisomy). Carrier screening was provided to specific subgroups deemed to have a higher chance of unknowingly passing a recessive disorder to their children (Prainsack and Siegal, 2006; Beck and Niewöhner, 2009; Antonarakis, 2019). Such forms of RGT were often pioneered by biomedical professionals who convinced public healthcare authorities of the value of RGT, whether for public health or for advancing women's autonomy. They also involved building local infrastructures for counseling women and couples and processing samples.

In comparison, the forms—and associated spaces and flows—of next generation RGT are more diverse (Löwy, 2022). Next generation RGT can take the shape of public healthcare programs, where local biomedical professionals, public healthcare authorities, and laboratories play a key role; however, it can also take the shape of consumer services that rely on infrastructures distributed across geographical distances. In such cases, biomedical professionals counsel women and couples, take samples, and send them to laboratories located across large geographical distances (Metzler, 2020). Next generation RGT often travels as a consumer service, enabled by distributed infrastructures. This raises new questions about who governs these technologies and how.

6.3.2 Research Perspectives on the Governance of Next Generation RGT

When studying the governance of next generation RGT, scholars have continued to examine how national contexts shape technologies in relation to country-specific moralities.

Much of this research involved NIPT. Studies have shown that NIPT shapes are configured by cultures and regulations (Zeng *et al.*, 2016; Ravitsky *et al.*, 2021; Bowman-Smart *et al.*, 2022; Löwy, 2022; Raz *et al.*, 2022). Scholars have also documented variations in NIPT coverage. Ilana Löwy (2022) emphasized how preexisting structures influenced such decisions, noting that the rolling out of NIPT has diverged, 'depending, among other things, on whether countries already have state-sponsored screening for Down syndrome risk, or whether NIPT is delivered via market-based healthcare.' Other studies examined the moralities involved in cost coverage. Kathrin Braun and Sabine Könninger (2018) analyzed the controversy over cost coverage in Germany, scrutinizing whether public authorities 'realize' their responsibilities, e.g., by imposing effective restrictions on the use of NIPT. Following up on this work, we have engaged with the same controversy to distill competing 'bioconstitutional visions' at work in the debate—a liberal one and a societal (or, in retrospect, a communitarian) one (Metzler, 2024). While the former framed NIPT as a biomedical technology that could enable women to exercise their right to know, the latter framed NIPT as a selective technology that threatened human life on a societal scale. We argued that healthcare authorities sought to reconcile these competing visions when deciding to reimburse the costs for NIPT on an individual level.

6.3.3 Private Actors Shaping Soft Mechanisms of Governance

Some scholars have begun to specifically examine informal authorities' role in RGT governance, using conceptual lenses from research on 'regulatory governance' and 'regulation of diagnostics' (Hogarth *et al.*, 2022). Both bodies of scholarship have taken larger transformations as a starting point, drawing specific attention to the proliferation of 'regulatory authorities' situated at a distance from traditional state authorities in new constellations of governance (Majone, 1994). They have highlighted the simultaneous relocation and multiplication of governance with the notion of 'polycentric' regulatory actions (Hogarth *et al.*, 2022, p. 1), drawing attention to the many sites where biomedical tests are governed: sites where formal and informal authorities validate and evaluate testing technologies; sites where professional societies draft recommendations on whether and how tests ought to be used; and sites where formal and informal authorities make reimbursement decisions. They have also highlighted the diverse kinds of actors and authorities at work at these sites, underlining the salience of commercial actors.

Building upon this research perspective, Holloway and colleagues described the mechanisms governing the dissemination of NIPT in the United States, conceptualizing them as a diffuse and polycentric 'regulatory regime' shaped by a multitude of actors (Holloway *et al.*, 2021, p. 1). They discussed two sets of mechanisms governing the flows of NIPT within the American healthcare system: clinical practice guidelines and cost coverage systems. And they underlined the salience of 'private actors,' i.e., actors 'not tied to a public authority' (Holloway *et al.*, 2021, p. 4), in the production of knowledge and evidence shaping decisions at these sites.

Our own research on the emergence of NIPT in Austria has found a similar pattern. When trying to make sense of the rapid uptake of NIPT in private centers of prenatal testing in Austria, we also noted the importance of national and international professional societies, which worked as mediators between commercial companies envisioning and providing NIPT and biomedical professionals offering NIPT to pregnant women (Metzler, 2020). While we did not use the conceptual vocabulary of regulatory governance, we also concluded that the moralities shaping technologies were increasingly influenced by authorities situated at a distance from traditional public healthcare authorities.

6.4 Future research perspectives

Before examining how bio-moralities can inform future research on technological governance—both within and beyond RGT—we will summarize key insights from these three research perspectives and their contribution to our understanding of bio-moralities.

6.4.1 Looking Back

We discussed a first set of perspectives which discussed how biomedical technologies in RGT govern women, populations, and life. Drawing on Foucault's work, this research showed how biomedical technologies shape people's choices, their self-understandings, and 'the ways in which [they] are governed' (Bunton and Petersen, 2005, p. 1). Biomedical technologies acted as active agents that transformed understandings of human life, relations, and moralities.

While the first set of perspectives examined governance through how biomedical technologies governed people, two other perspectives focused on how various authorities governed these technologies. Both approaches situated technologies by examining how authorities shaped their uses, e.g., by stipulating provisions on their uses or by providing access to these technologies. However, these perspectives differed in how they conceptualized authorities.

A second set of perspectives examined moralities at the nation-state level, moving beyond universal rationalities to explore nation-specific moralities. These studies analyzed how public authorities shaped RGT through statutory regulations, infrastructure development, and funding. Using concepts like 'discourses,' 'political cultures,' or 'bioconstitutional imaginaries,' they illuminated variations between countries. The 'bioconstitutionalism' framework particularly influenced our understanding of bio-moralities by highlighting the mutually sustaining combination between conceptions of human nature and measures taken to do justice to that nature.

Findings from a third set of perspectives, focused on next generation RGT, explain why we retain the 'bio' while replacing 'constitutions' with 'moralities.' These perspectives underlined the importance of soft governance instruments like clinical practice guidelines in shaping uses and flows of newly emerging biomedical technologies, highlighting the agency of informal authorities, such as commercial companies or professional societies, operating both within and beyond the nation-state.

Commercial actors were less prominent in earlier research on RGT governance—most likely because they played a less significant role in the field. However, research that underlines their growing importance demands concepts and methods that can both capture and explain their current influence. Like bioconstitutionalism, the concept of bio-moralities examines how conceptions of human nature inform uses of biomedical technologies, and, vice versa, how uses of biomedical technologies inform conceptions of human nature. However, it remains more agnostic regarding which authorities are involved in this coproduction, which measures solidify understanding of the human conditions and related moralities, and their geographic scope. This approach transforms questions about authorities, their measures, and moral reach into empirical ones—creating an agenda for future research.

6.4.2 Looking Ahead

First, our proposal to develop the concept of bio-moralities builds on key questions from the bioconstitutionalism framework. It is valuable to examine explicit and implicit understandings of human nature that underpin the governance of biomedical technologies, as these conceptions define and limit what authorities can and should do. However, the metaphor of constitutionalism might lead scholars to focus only on formal lawmaking and to map moralities along national boundaries, potentially overstating differences between countries while missing variations and conflicts within them. In shifting to bio-moralities, we maintain focus on the coproduction between conceptions of human nature and measures taken to do justice to that nature, while expanding the analysis to examine multiple spaces, authorities, and forms of moralities. The concept of bio-moralities recognizes that we need concepts and methodologies attentive to the diverse authorities shaping our understanding of humanness—including civil society organizations, commercial actors, and national and transnational professional societies and expert groups.

One such methodology consists of following a specific biomedical technology across different spaces, unpacking and comparing these spaces, and exploring how these intersect and interact. Such spaces include: spaces where technologies are envisioned and designed (Hilgartner, 2015; Sharon, 2018); spaces where technologies are used in practice; and spaces where they are 'problematized' (Laurent, 2017, 2022), i.e., where these technologies become matters of concern, and actors assemble to assess and evaluate technologies, write soft guidelines or regulations, or decide on whether to provide them or cover costs for its uses (Aarden *et al.*, 2009; Holloway *et al.*, 2021). Such a methodology would recognize the broad variety of measures that authorities can take to seek to govern technologies. Such a methodology would examine the range of authorities involved in these spaces, distill their values, visions, and ideas from their articulation and practices, and ask: what is the authorities' conception of human nature, if the suggested measures are deemed appropriate to do justice to that nature? This methodology would build on pragmatist approaches (Laurent, 2017), temporally suspending our own moralities to understand the actors' reasoning and practices through their conception of the human condition, comparing these across spaces, and exploring their relationships. It would be specifically attentive to differences and conflicts, without, however, prematurely sidelining one perspective.

In proposing this technology-centered methodology to study governance, we do not argue that traditional sites of governance have become irrelevant; rather, we argue that their influence cannot be taken for granted. Technological governance increasingly emerges from former peripheries and transcends national boundaries. This requires a methodology that moves beyond predetermined centers of authority. By following biomedical technologies to where they are envisioned, used, and problematized, and by examining the bio-moralities operating in these contexts, we can better understand contemporary technological governance. The relationships between these spaces, their authorities, and their associated bio-moralities are empirical questions that vary across different biomedical technologies.

Second, future research should continue to examine the prominence of commercial actors and other non-state actors, such as civil society organizations and professional groups, in biomedical technology governance while also seeking to explain their prominence. Studies of RGT—and biomedical technologies more broadly—often emphasize commercial actors' power, sometimes viewing them as drivers of contemporary transformations. We suggest that analyzing technological governance through the lens of bio-moralities could provide a more relational understanding of these actors' significance, which would include, e.g., how professional organizations or NGOs align with and give legitimacy to commercial actors' claims to authority. This approach would not deny the well-documented power and agency of commercial actors in contemporary governance (Sharon, 2016; Prainsack, 2018; Birch and Muniesa, 2020); rather, it would treat their power not merely as the *cause* of contemporary transformations, but also as an *effect* of changes in the bio-moralities underlying biomedical technology governance. Such research would move beyond criticizing the current distribution and delegation of responsibilities. It would examine formal authorities' reasoning by asking: what conception of good human life underlies their vision that empowering commercial companies or pursuing deregulation will achieve that life? What vision of the human condition leads formal authorities to believe that empowering commercial companies or reducing regulations will benefit society? Examining the bio-moralities that sustain technology governance can help us explain not just *that* authority is being redistributed, but also *how* and *why* this redistribution is happening and gaining legitimacy.

Third, we also think that exploring biomedical governance through the lens of bio-moralities might help us develop a better understanding of the geographies of technological governance. In the previous sections, we argued that the three research perspectives we discussed located moralities at different levels. A first set of perspectives understood bio-moralities in terms of seemingly universal rationalities, a second set of perspectives located moralities on a national scale. The third perspective drew attention to informal authorities operating within countries, without, however, addressing the scope of their authority, which might be located below or above the level of nation-states. Moreover, when describing new RGT and next generation RGT, we observed that these two generations came with different shapes, spaces, and flows. Earlier, new RGT typically involved biomedical experts taking samples from patients for analysis in local and national laboratories. More recent next generation RGT often involves shipping samples to laboratories across large geographical distances. Thus, the geographies of technological infrastructures differ. We think that it is important to be attentive to such differences when engaging with technological governance, as it has consequences for how life can be governed through technologies and how bio-moralities become durable and mobile. This is another reason why following technologies and unpacking the bio-moralities that sustain their governance is valuable; it helps transform the often implicit geographies of technological governance into explicit research questions.

Note

1. This research was funded in part by the Austrian Science Fund (FWF) [grant DOI 10.55776/P37208]. For open access purposes, the authors have applied a CC BY public copyright license to any author accepted manuscript version arising from this submission. We would also like to acknowledge support by the Open Access Publishing Fund of the Karl Landsteiner University of Health Sciences, Krems, Austria.

References

Aarden, E., Hoyweghen, I.V., Horstman, K. and Vos, R. (2008) 'Learning from co-evolution of policy and technology. Different PGDs in the Netherlands, Germany and Britain', *Journal of Comparative Policy Analysis: Research and Practice*, 10(2), pp. 191–206. Available at: https://doi.org/10.1080/13876980802028131.

Aarden, E., Van Hoyweghen, I., Vos, R. and Horstman, K. (2009) 'Providing preimplantation genetic diagnosis in the United Kingdom, The Netherlands and Germany: a comparative in-depth analysis of health-care access', *Human Reproduction*, 24(7), pp. 1542–1547. Available at: https://doi.org/10.1093/humrep/dep054.

Antonarakis, S.E. (2019) 'Carrier screening for recessive disorders', *Nature Reviews Genetics*, 20(9), pp. 549–561. Available at: https://doi.org/10.1038/s41576-019-0134-2.

Arendt, H. (2019) *The Human Condition*. 2nd Edition. Enlarged Edition. Chicago: The University of Chicago Press.

Beck, S. and Niewöhner, J. (2009) 'Localising genetic testing and screening in Cyprus and Germany: contingencies, continuities, ordering effects and bio-cultural intimacy', in P. Atkinson, P. Glasner and M. Lock (eds), *The Handbook of Genetics and Society*. London and New York: Routledge, pp. 76–93.

Bianchi, D.W., Parker, R.L., Wentworth, J., Madankumar, R., Saffer, C., Das, A.F., Craig, J.A., Chudova, D.I. et al. (2014) 'DNA sequencing versus standard prenatal aneuploidy screening', *New England Journal of Medicine*, 370(9), pp. 799–808. Available at: https://doi.org/10.1056/NEJMoa1311037.

Birch, K. and Muniesa, F. (eds) (2020) *Assetization: Turning Things into Assets in Technoscientific Capitalism*. Cambridge, Mass: MIT Press.

Bleiklie, I.A., Goggin, M.L. and Rothmayr, C. (eds) (2003) *Comparative Biomedical Policy: Governing Assisted Reproductive Technologies*. 1st Edition. London and New York: Routledge.

Bowman-Smart, H., Wiesemann, C. and Horn, R. (2022) 'Non-invasive prenatal testing in Germany: a unique ethical and policy landscape', *European Journal of Human Genetics*, 31, pp. 1–6. Available at: https://doi.org/10.1038/s41431-022-01256-x.

Braun, K. and Könninger, S. (2018) 'Realizing responsibility. Institutional routines, critical intervention, and the "big" questions in the controversy over non-invasive prenatal testing in Germany', *New Genetics and Society*, 37(3), pp. 248–267. Available at: https://doi.org/10.1080/14636778.2018.1495555.

Buchanan, A., Brock, D.W., Daniels, N. and Wikler, D. (2001) *From Chance to Choice: Genetics and Justice*. Cambridge: Cambridge University Press.

Bunton, R. and Petersen, A. (2005) 'Genetics and governance. An introduction', in A. Petersen and R. Bunton (eds), *Genetic Governance: Health, Risk and Ethics in a Biotech Era*. 1st Edition. New York: Routledge, pp. 1–27.

Chomanski, B. and Lauwaert, L. (2024) 'Digital privacy and the law: the challenge of regulatory capture', *AI & SOCIETY* [Preprint]. Available at: https://doi.org/10.1007/s00146-024-02041-8.

Evans, P., Rueschemeyer, D. and Skocpol, T. (eds) (1985) *Bringing the State Back In*. Cambridge: Cambridge University Press.

Foucault, M. (2003) *'Society Must be Defended'. Lectures at the Collège de France, 1975–76*. New York: Picador.

Franklin, S. and Roberts, C. (2006) *Born and Made. An Ethnography of Preimplantation Genetic Diagnosis*. Princeton and Oxford: Princeton University Press.

Gottweis, H. (2008) 'Biobanks in action: new strategies in the governance of life', in H. Gottweis and A. Petersen (eds), *Biobanks: Governance in Comparative Perspective*. London and New York: Routledge, pp. 22–37.

Gottweis, H., Braun, K., Haila, Y., Hajer, M., Loeber, A., Metzler, I., Reynolds, L., Schultz, S. and Szerszynski, B. (2008) 'Participation and the new governance of life', *BioSocieties*, 3(3), pp. 265–286. Available at: https://doi.org/10.1017/S1745855208006194.

Habermas, J. (2001) *Die Zukunft der menschlichen Natur. Auf dem Weg zu einer liberalen Eugenik?* Frankfurt am Main: Suhrkamp.

Hashiloni-Dolev, Y., Nov-Klaiman, T. and Raz, A. (2019) 'Pandora's pregnancy: NIPT, CMA, and genome sequencing—A new era for prenatal genetic testing', *Prenatal Diagnosis*, 39(10), pp. 859–865. Available at: https://doi.org/10.1002/pd.5495.

Hedgecoe, A. (1998) 'Geneticization, medicalisation and polemics', *Medicine, Health Care, and Philosophy*, 1(3), pp. 235–243. Available at: https://doi.org/10.1023/a:1009969226655.

Helén, I. (2004) 'Technics over life: risk, ethics and the existential condition in high-tech antenatal care', *Economy and Society*, 33(1), pp. 28–51. Available at: https://doi.org/10.1080/0308514032000176720.

Herrmann, S.L. (2009) *Policy Debates on Reprogenetics. The Problematisation of New Research in Great Britain and Germany*. Frankfurt and New York: Campus.

Hilgartner, S. (2015) 'Capturing the imaginary: vanguards, visions and the synthetic biology revolution', in S. Hilgartner, C.A. Miller and R. Hagendijk (eds), *Science and Democracy. Making Knowledge and Making Power in the Biosciences and Beyond*. New York and London: Routledge, pp. 33–55.

Hogarth, S., Miller, F.A. and Sturdy, S. (2022) 'Multidisciplinary perspectives on the regulation of diagnostic technologies', *Social Science & Medicine*, 304, p. 115059. Available at: https://doi.org/10.1016/j.socscimed.2022.115059.

Holloway, K., Miller, F.A. and Simms, N. (2021) 'Industry, experts and the role of the "invisible college" in the dissemination of non-invasive prenatal testing in the US', *Social Science & Medicine*, 270, p. 113635. Available at: https://doi.org/10.1016/j.socscimed.2020.113635.

Hui, L. and Bianchi, D.W. (2017) 'Noninvasive prenatal DNA testing: the vanguard of genomic medicine', *Annual Review of Medicine*, 68(1), pp. 459–472. Available at: https://doi.org/10.1146/annurev-med-072115-033220.

Hurlbut, B. (2017) *Experiments in Democracy: Human Embryo Research and the Politics of Bioethics*. 1st Edition. New York: Columbia University Press.

Hurlbut, J.B. (2015) 'Remembering the future: science, law and the legacy of Asilomar', in S. Jasanoff and S.-H. Kim (eds), *Dreamscapes of Modernity: Sociotechnical Imaginaries and the Fabrication of Power*. Chicago and London: Chicago University Press, pp. 126–151. Available at: http://www.press.uchicago.edu/ucp/books/book/chicago/D/bo20836025.html (Accessed: 22 May 2015).

Hurlbut, J.B., Jasanoff, S. and Saha, K. (2020) 'Constitutionalism at the nexus of life and law', *Science, Technology, & Human Values*, 45(6), pp. 979–1000. Available at: https://doi.org/10.1177/0162243920921236.

Jasanoff, S. (2005) *Designs on Nature: Science and Democracy in Europe and the United States.* Princeton and Oxford: Princeton University Press.

Jasanoff, S. (2011a) 'Introduction: rewriting life, reframing rights', in S. Jasanoff (ed), *Reframing Rights. Bioconstitutionalism in the Genetic Age.* Cambridge, Mass: MIT Press, pp. 1–27.

Jasanoff, S. (2011b) 'Making the facts of life', in S. Jasanoff (ed), *Reframing Rights: Bioconstitutionalism in the Genetic Age.* Cambridge, Mass: MIT Press, pp. 59–83.

Johnston, J. and Zacharias, R.L. (2017) 'The future of reproductive autonomy', *The Hastings Center Report*, 47(Suppl 3), pp. S6–S11. Available at: https://doi.org/10.1002/hast.789.

Kelton, M., Sullivan, M., Rogers, Z., Bienvenue, E. and Troath, S. (2022) 'Virtual sovereignty? Private internet capital, digital platforms and infrastructural power in the United States', *International Affairs*, 98(6), pp. 1977–1999. Available at: https://doi.org/10.1093/ia/iiac226.

Kerr, A. (2009) 'Reproductive genetics: from choice to ambivalence and back again', in P. Atkinson, P. Glasner and M. Lock (eds), *The Handbook of Genetics and Society: Mapping the New Genomic Era*. 1st Edition. London: Routledge, pp. 59–75.

Kevles, D.J. (1985) *In the Name of Eugenics: Genetics and the Uses of Human Heredity.* Harvard: Harvard University Press.

Laurent, B. (2017) *Democratic Experiments: Problematizing Nanotechnology and Democracy in Europe and the United States.* Cambridge, Mass, and London: MIT Press.

Laurent, B. (2022) *European Objects: The Troubled Dreams of Harmonization.* Cambridge, Mass: MIT Press.

Lemke, T. (2005) 'From eugenics to the government of genetic risks', in A. Petersen and R. Bunton (eds), *Genetic Governance: Health, Risk and Ethics in a Biotech Era*. 1st Edition. New York: Routledge, pp. 95–105.

Lippman, A. (1993) 'Prenatal genetic testing and geneticization: mother matters for all', *Fetal Diagnosis and Therapy*, 8(Suppl. 1), pp. 175–188. Available at: https://doi.org/10.1159/000263886.

Löwy, I. (2018a) 'Bringing genetics into the clinic: the evolution of genetic testing and counselling', in S. Gibbon, B. Prainsack, S. Hilgartner and J. Lamoreaux (eds), *Routledge Handbook of Genomics, Health and Society.* 2nd Edition. Abingdon, Oxon, and New York: Routledge, pp. 39–46.

Löwy, I. (2018b) *Tangled Diagnoses: Prenatal Testing, Women, and Risk.* Chicago and London: The University of Chicago Press. Available at: https://www.press.uchicago.edu/ucp/books/book/chicago/T/b027949393.html (Accessed: 22 October 2018).

Löwy, I. (2022) 'Non-invasive prenatal testing: a diagnostic innovation shaped by commercial interests and the regulation conundrum', *Social Science & Medicine*, p. 113064. Available at: https://doi.org/10.1016/j.socscimed.2020.113064.

Lupton, D. (2012) '"Precious cargo": foetal subjects, risk and reproductive citizenship', *Critical Public Health*, 22(3), pp. 329–340. Available at: https://doi.org/10.1080/09581596.2012.657612.

Majone, G. (1994) 'The rise of the regulatory state in Europe', *West European Politics*, 17(3), pp. 77–101. Available at: https://doi.org/10.1080/01402389408425031.

Metzler, I. (2020) 'Imaginaries as infrastructures? The emergence of non-invasive prenatal testing in Austria', *BioSocieties*, 15(4), pp. 601–626. Available at: https://doi.org/10.1057/s41292-019-00171-7.

Metzler, I. (2024) 'Bioconstitutional visions in the debate on non-invasive prenatal testing in Germany', *Science as Culture*, 33(2), pp. 205–230. Available at: https://doi.org/10.1080/09505431.2023.2251998.

Nelkin, D. and Tancredi, L.R. (1994) *Dangerous Diagnostics: The Social Power of Biological Information*. Chicago: University of Chicago Press.

Prainsack, B. (2018) 'Power asymmetries, participation, and the idea of personalised medicine', in S. Gibbon, B. Prainsack, S. Hilgartner and J. Lamoreaux (eds), *Routledge Handbook of Genomics, Health and Society.* London and New York: Routledge, pp. 212–220.

Prainsack, B. and Siegal, G. (2006) 'The rise of genetic couplehood? A comparative view of premarital genetic testing', *BioSocieties*, 1(1), pp. 17–36. Available at: https://doi.org/10.1017/S1745855205050106.

Rapp, R. (2000) *Testing Women, Testing the Fetus: The Social Impact of Amniocentesis in America*. 1st Edition. New York: Routledge.

Ravitsky, V. (2017) 'The shifting landscape of prenatal testing: between reproductive autonomy and public health', *Hastings Center Report*, 47(S3), pp. S34–S40. Available at: https://doi.org/10.1002/hast.793.

Ravitsky, V., Roy, M.-C., Haidar, H., Henneman, L., Marshall, J., Newson, A.J., Ngan, O.M.Y. and Nov-Klaiman, T. (2021) 'The emergence and global spread of noninvasive prenatal testing', *Annual Review of Genomics and Human Genetics*, 22(1), pp. 309–338. Available at: https://doi.org/10.1146/annurev-genom-083118-015053.

Raz, A.E., Nov-Klaiman, T., Hashiloni-Dolev, Y., Foth, H., Schües, C. and Rehmann-Sutter, C. (2022) 'Comparing Germany and Israel regarding debates on policy-making at the beginning of life: PGD, NIPT and their paths of routinization', *Ethik in der Medizin*, 34(1), pp. 65–80. Available at: https://doi.org/10.1007/s00481-021-00652-z.

Rose, N. (2001) 'The politics of life itself', *Theory, Culture & Society*, 18(6), pp. 1–30. Available at: https://doi.org/10.1177/02632760122052020.

Rose, N. (2006) *The Politics of Life Itself: Biomedicine, Power, and Subjectivity in the Twenty-First Century*. Princeton: Princeton University Press.

Rothman, B.K. (1993) *The Tentative Pregnancy: How Amniocentesis Changes the Experience of Motherhood*. New York: W.W. Norton & Company.

Rowe, C.A. and Wright, C.F. (2020) 'Expanded universal carrier screening and its implementation within a publicly funded healthcare service', *Journal of Community Genetics*, 11(1), pp. 21–38. Available at: https://doi.org/10.1007/s12687-019-00443-6.

Saltelli, A., Dankel, D.J., Di Fiore, M., Holland, N. and Pigeon, M. (2022) 'Science, the endless frontier of regulatory capture', *Futures*, 135, p. 102860. Available at: https://doi.org/10.1016/j.futures.2021.102860.

Sharon, T. (2016) 'The Googlization of health research: from disruptive innovation to disruptive ethics', *Personalized Medicine*, 13(6), pp. 563–574. Available at: https://doi.org/10.2217/pme-2016-0057.

Sharon, T. (2018) 'When digital health meets digital capitalism, how many common goods are at stake?', *Big Data & Society*, 5(2), p. 2053951718819032. Available at: https://doi.org/10.1177/2053951718819032.

Sharon, T. and Gellert, R. (2023) 'Regulating Big Tech expansionism? Sphere transgressions and the limits of Europe's digital regulatory strategy', *Information, Communication & Society*, 27(15), pp. 2651–2668. Available at: https://doi.org/10.1080/1369118X.2023.2246526.

Van Den Bogaert, K., Lannoo, L., Brison, N., Gatinois, V., Baetens, M., Blaumeiser, B., Boemer, F., Bourlard, L., et al. (2021) 'Outcome of publicly funded nationwide first-tier noninvasive prenatal screening', *Genetics in Medicine*, 23(6), pp. 1137–1142. Available at: https://doi.org/10.1038/s41436-021-01101-4.

van der Meij, K.R.M., Sistermans, E.A., Macville, Stevens, S.J.C., Bax, C.J., Bekker, M.N., Bilardo, C.M., Boon, E.M.J., et al. (2019) 'TRIDENT-2: national implementation of genome-wide non-invasive prenatal testing as a first-tier screening test in the Netherlands', *The American Journal of Human Genetics*, 105(6), pp. 1091–1101. Available at: https://doi.org/10.1016/j.ajhg.2019.10.005.

Wahlberg, A. and Gammeltoft, T.M. (2018) 'Introduction: kinds of children', in A. Wahlberg and T.M. Gammeltoft (eds), *Selective Reproduction in the 21st Century*. Cham: Palgrave

Macmillan, pp. 1–24. Available at: //www.palgrave.com/us/book/9783319582191 (Accessed: 22 October 2018).

Zeng, X., Zannoni, L., Löwy, I. and Camporesi, S. (2016) 'Localizing NIPT: practices and meanings of non-invasive prenatal testing in China, Italy, Brazil and the UK', *Ethics, Medicine and Public Health*, 2(3), pp. 392–401. Available at: https://doi.org/10.1016/j.jemep.2016.06.004.

7 Singularization/mutualization: The emergence of a new form of patient activism around biomedical entities

Madeleine Akrich, Pascale Bourret, Alberto Cambrosio, and Vololona Rabeharisoa

7.1 Introduction, state of the art, and research topic

7.1.1 Patients' Engagement with Biomedical Practices

Steven Epstein, a founding father of contemporary scholarly studies on patient activism, began his 2008 state of the art review of 'Patient Groups and Health Movements' for the Third Edition of the *Handbook of Science and Technology Studies* by noting that when he started working in 1990 on his PhD dissertation on AIDS research and activism, he was only 'able to find little written from an STS or allied perspective on the politics and projects of patient groups, or on health movements more generally' (Epstein, 2008). Clearly, by the late 2000s things had moved on, as evidenced by his detailed 41-page review, and in recent years, the STS literature on patient advocacy has continued to grow and diversify.

STS scholars' interest in patient groups[1] can be traced back to the gradual emergence of groups that were themselves interested in medical knowledge and the development of research. Distinct from the oldest patient associations that focused on mutual support and were often concerned with chronic diseases such as diabetes, hemophilia, and multiple sclerosis, these associations focus on the disease itself. No longer confined to mutual aid, but centering their interventions on the fight against disease, these new organizations brought together patients suffering from pathologies about which no robust knowledge existed, let alone effective treatments, such as HIV/AIDS or rare diseases. These associations by and large joined forces with bio-clinical researchers to advance research into their diseases and, ultimately, find treatments.

Engaging in a fight against disease was not a self-evident activity. STS scholars have documented how patients have transitioned from the passive role of 'clinical material' to the active role of 'engaged patients' (Epstein, 1996; Barbot, 2006), and, beyond that, of research partners (Anglin, 1997; Rabeharisoa, 2003; Heath et al., 2004; Rabeharisoa and Callon, 2004; Keating and Cambrosio, 2012; Timmermans, 2020; Akrich and Rabeharisoa, 2023), while simultaneously deploying peculiar forms of expertise (Epstein, 1995, 2023) and evidence-based activism (Rabeharisoa et al., 2014b). Scholars have also shown how patient groups establish their legitimacy as *bona fide* contributors to therapeutic innovation and drug markets (Novas, 2006; O'Donovan, 2007; Boon and Broekgaarden, 2010; Britten et al., 2015; Rabeharisoa and Doganova, 2021). Echoing the activities of patient advocates, biomedical practitioners from the post-genomic era openly acknowledge and promote their contributions to clinical and translational research (Koay and Sharp, 2013).

7.1.2 Patients' Grouping Around Biomedical Entities

From the turn of the century onwards, we witnessed a subsequent shift in the landscape of patient organizations: the emergence of groups distinctively named after the infra-molecular entities driving their diseases, such as somatic genomic mutations (e.g., oncogenes such as KRAS or EGFR) and chromosomal deletions (e.g., 22q11.2 or 22q13). While also engaging in the war on disease, these novel patient advocacy groups deploy a finer degree of granularity, one that requires the resort to the latest molecular profiling technologies (Campbell et al., 2024). Rare genetic disease[2] associations and oncogene-focused patient advocacy groups are two particularly interesting examples of this novel kind of grouping. Rare genetic disease patient associations gather people with the same mutation in their genome ('constitutional genetics'), whereas oncogene-focused patient advocacy groups gather patients whose tumor has the same mutation ('somatic genetics'). These associations are still little studied, although readers familiar with the anthropology of science will not have failed to notice the potential link with the premonitory notion of biosociality introduced by Paul Rabinow in the early 1990s. Indeed, in a much-cited passage, Rabinow stated that '[i]t is not hard to imagine groups formed around the chromosome 17, locus 16,256, site 654,376 allele variant with a guanine substitution' (Rabinow, 1992, p. 244; for a detailed critical discussion see Hacking, 2006). Yet, focusing on the issue of group identity, Rabinow maintained that while the new categories could 'partially supersede, and eventually redefine' (Rabinow, 1992, p. 245) pre-existing categories such as ethnic or socio-demographic ones, in the end they had no depth or meaning; they amounted to a label without transformative power.

In his book on 'mobilizing mutations,' Navon takes issue precisely with this aspect of Rabinow's argument, noting that 'mutations can acquire meaning when networks of knowledge production and social mobilization are assembled around them.' In addition, Navon shows how, thanks to a looping mechanism, biosociality, as proactively redefined, 'can also transform the way we understand the mutations themselves' (Navon, 2019, pp. 32–33). His detailed monograph significantly extends the analytical reach of the notion of biosociality far beyond its status as a mere label. His analysis, however, also focuses on the problem of identity, the book's central claim being that 'knowledge about genetic mutations can give rise to entirely new categories of human difference and therefore forms of identity.' This argument fits well with Navon's substantive area of investigation, namely rare genetic disease patient organizations, but less so with oncogene-driven patient groups.

The present chapter puts the previous analysis to the test by revisiting our past and recent fieldwork on rare genetic disease associations in France and on oncogene-driven patient advocacy groups in different geographical locations. In the case of rare genetic disease associations, the clinical and social existence of the disease itself (often a syndrome[3]) is constitutively related to the discovery of the biomedical entity, a situation neatly captured by Navon's notion of genomic designation (Navon, 2011), whereas in the case of oncogene-driven patient advocacy groups, the biomedical entity circumscribes finer categories of patients corresponding to specific therapeutic regimens. We can thus ask: from what perspective do these different kinds of associations rally around molecular entities? Is the reference to these entities associated with specific modes of action and relationships patient organizations maintain with basic and clinical research and therapy? As a result, our chapter moves away from an analysis in terms of biosociality as related to the issue of identity to focus on the differential ways in which associations mobilize biomedical entities, and on the forms of collective action triggered by the multiple affordances (Faraj and Azad, 2013) provided by these entities.

7.1.3 Our Analytics: Singularization/Mutualization

Two analytical axes underpin our chapter. A first axis centers on *singularization*. Biomedical entities have meaning for patient associations. The grouping of patients around these entities amounts to a form of singularization of their diseases, a process that parallels the disassembling and reassembling of nosological categories following the investigation of their infra-molecular landscape (Rabeharisoa et al., 2014a; Keating et al., 2016; Cambrosio et al., 2021). Singularization enables patient associations to target their specific problems as evidenced by the phenotypic correlates of genetic deletions (in the case of rare genetic diseases), or to make biomedical entities therapeutically actionable via the development of novel kinds of targeted treatments (in the case of oncogene-driven cancers) (Bourret et al., 2025).

A second axis focuses on *mutualization*. Singularization, by engendering new spaces of comparison, is accompanied by a process of mutualization (Callon, 2012). By comparing the singularities of biomedical entities and their differential effects, patient associations identify shared problems (in the case of rare genetic diseases) or overlaps between treatments targeting different kinds of cancers (in the case of oncogenes). Biomedical entities thus enable patient associations to participate in the networking of patient groups, researchers, clinicians, industrialists, regulators, and healthcare institutions, to pool their efforts around shared problems and overlaps.

This dual process of singularization/mutualization around and across biomedical entities is not exclusive of other grouping modalities, following the differential embedding of those entities in broader biomedical collectives as grounded, for instance, in the very idea of rarity in the case of rare genetic diseases, and, in the case of oncology, with the simultaneous association of innovative roadmaps based on molecular pathology with the traditional, organ-based organization of cancer institutions. To analyze this dynamic, rather than focusing on biosociality we borrow Panofsky's notion of 'sociability' that refers to 'forging close relationships with scientists and orchestrating relationships among them' (Panofsky, 2011, p. 31). In the present case, however, it is more appropriate to speak of sociabilities because of the variable configurations that thrive on different socialization trajectories taken by biomedical entities.

7.2 Grouping and mobilizing around rare genetic mutations

7.2.1 Patient Activism on Rare Chromosomal Syndromes

Before the discovery of their genetic origin, little was known about rare genetic diseases by medical doctors and they were ignored by health policymakers. This prompted patients and families to group and engage in a dialogue with clinical researchers with the aim of understanding the causes of these pathologies, describing their clinical pictures, and ultimately finding cures. The discovery of the genetic or chromosomal origin of a number of these diseases has been a watershed in the development of medical genetics, and later of gene and cell therapies, and has accelerated the creation of patient groups which manifest a vivid interest in biomedical and therapeutic research, notably in Western and Northern countries. Interestingly, some of these groups are named after the genetic mutations or the chromosomal abnormalities involved in their diseases. In France, for instance, 22 groups among the 278 affiliated to Alliance Maladies Rares[4] (the French Rare Diseases Alliance) have done so. What exactly this naming entails may be illustrated with the example of 'Génération 22.[5] Vivre avec la délétion 22q11' ('Generation 22. Living with deletion 22q11'), a French patient group that gathers 'patients with deletion 22q11 and their families.'

Génération 22 was created in 1997 by two families concerned with the syndrome. Its history mimics the 'diagnostic odyssey' experienced by many rare disease patient groups: the long wandering for obtaining a diagnosis, the confrontation with the silo-based functioning of medical specialists, the encounter with an engaged researcher-clinician, and eventually the discovery of the biomedical entity that helps designate the disease. Génération 22 was co-founded by the mother of four girls, the youngest born in 1983 with serious health problems, including angiomas all over her body, cardiac failure, an abnormally low number of platelets, and left varus foot. The young girl was diagnosed with DiGeorge's syndrome, which explained the cardiac failure only. While growing up, she manifested additional somatic problems as well as learning difficulties. The mother knocked on many doors, adamant that her daughter's multiple problems were somehow connected, only to be told by specialists that this was very unlikely. Left with no answers to her questions, she started to read the medical literature and contacted a pediatrician-geneticist in 1996, who thought of deletion 22q11 (located on chromosome 22) discovered five years before. Her daughter, then 13, took the diagnostic test, which turned out positive.

This was a relief for the mother, and the beginning of another adventure: the creation of the patient group. When asked why she named the group after chromosome 22, she explained that 'it was upon the pediatrician-geneticist's suggestion, to signal to the medics that they now have to deal with a new generation of patients who know what the syndrome is they suffer from.' In other words, the naming of the group was meant to denote the genomic designation of a new syndrome and a new kind of people (Hacking, 1986, 2006; Navon, 2019) that have long been ignored by treating physicians. Most importantly, it flagged the syndrome as an entity tabulating hitherto separated diseases and patients, thereby accordingly shaping the group's activism. Génération 22 posted on its website a description of the multiple symptoms of the syndrome and provided links to medical information. For Génération 22 and many other rare disease patient organizations named after genetic mutations or chromosomal deletions, the latter serve to empower patients and families in their search for a diagnosis and to raise awareness among medical doctors on the existence of related syndromes. Hence the continuing effort put forth by patient groups in collecting and formatting patients' and families' experiences and disseminating medical information (Akrich and Rabeharisoa, 2023), to the point that the president of Génération 22 once described the group as a 'library for all' (for patients and specialists) on 22q11 deletion syndrome. Moreover, the biomedical entity is a trigger to further investigate the syndrome, whose clinical picture is very much heterogeneous (there are about 30 genes located at 22q11), with an aim at meeting each patient's needs. Génération 22 considers 22q11 as a 'multiple disability' syndrome which demands personalized multidisciplinary care.

In this perspective, Génération 22 promoted what Panofsky calls 'sociability' (2011), by liaising with different medical communities, setting up a medical advisory board to foster, not without frictions, exchanges between researchers-clinicians, and contributing to research projects and surveys on issues raised by families. Among those issues are psychiatric disorders and intellectual disabilities that may pop up along the way, particularly at adolescence. Within Alliance Maladies Rares, Génération 22 learned that other patient groups with different chromosomal syndromes also encountered similar problems. With those sister organizations, Génération 22 has contributed to set up a network of reference centers for diagnosis and care for 'chromosomal syndromes with psychiatric manifestations,' a brand-new collective gathering different patient groups and specialists.

To put it in a nutshell, Génération 22 and other rare genetic disease patient groups' form of activism showcase the decisive role that genetic mutations or chromosomal deletions play in deciphering both the syndromes at stake and the patient population's needs. Of particular interest is that many of these syndromes, though not always lethal in the short term, come with a vast range of serious disabilities whose understanding is progressively deepened through support for research on and around biomedical entities. Knowing more about biomedical entities and their consequences, and positioning themselves as research partners, is a major route for patient organizations to voice patients' and families' ever-changing and pressing concern with daily care. Biomedical entities offer here one specific affordance, as tools for navigating the complex landscape of multiple disabilities.

7.2.2 Singularization/Mutualization of Syndromes and Patient-Centered Collectives

The naming of Génération 22 after the chromosomal abnormality signals a new syndrome and a new category of patients. Crucial to the group's endeavor towards a personalized multidisciplinary care is to investigate the contours of the patient population. Thanks to its website, families started to identify themselves and join the group. Identification should be understood here as a two-fold operation consisting of comparing patients' situations to the clinical picture displayed on the website, and mutually identifying themselves during group meetings. A telling example is the case of two parents who attended the very first group meeting and who realized that their little boy 'was not like' the other children present. These parents found out later that their child had another deletion on chromosome 22, and joined a group formed in 1993 around deletion 22q13 and named Association française du syndrome Phelan-McDermid (French association on Phelan-McDermid syndrome).

In this respect, as previously mentioned, it is tempting to resort to Rabinow's notion of biosociality (Rabinow, 1992). Indeed, some rare genetic disease patient organizations self-identify as communities built upon biomedical entities. This, for instance, is the case of 'Autour du BPAN. Association de familles et d'aidants liée au gène WDR45. Communauté BPAN' ('Around BPAN. Families and carers' group linked to gene WDR45. BPAN Community.'). However, the term 'community' should not be overstated. For Génération 22 and many other rare genetic disease patient organizations named after biomedical entities, their main concern is to explore the range of manifestations of syndromes that may be similar and yet different, for adjusting care to patients' needs. This singularization process is an ongoing inquiry, associating patients/families/carers and researchers-clinicians. Moreover, this singularization process is one facet of a dual mutualization process, through which patient groups put together their efforts to address shared problems. The network of reference on 'chromosomal syndromes with psychiatric manifestations' mentioned above manifests this mutualization process.

This mutualization process also shows in patient activism around Fragile X syndrome (a mutation on chromosome X) that mainly affects boys. The first French patient group on Fragile X formed in 1990. The syndrome quickly fragmented upon the discovery that a premutation may exist in an earlier generation and transform into a full mutation upon transmission to the next generation. This pattern, called 'mosaic,' prompted the creation of a second group formed around Fragile X mosaics in 1993. This fragmentation, which helped in subdividing Fragile X, also came with the realization that some of its manifestations shared similar characteristics. This resulted in the setting up of a third group named Xtraordinaire in 2006 to address intellectual deficiency linked to Fragile X. This last group gathers patients and families concerned with several biomedical entity-driven syndromes, which liaised with a neuro-pediatrician who coordinates reference centers for intellectual deficiency in rare genetic diseases.

The targeted syndromes are: ARX-Partington; A-TRX-alpha thalassemia linked to chromosome X; Creatine transporter deficiency-SLC6A8; Coffin-Lowry-RSK2; duplication of gene MECP2; Allan Herndon Dudley MCT8; and Re N Penning-PQBP1. Each of those exotic names denotes a singular syndrome, which shares with the others intellectual deficiency that progressively becomes the main concern of families as their children grow up.

In summary, singularization/mutualization is core to the dynamics of patient activism in the field of rare diseases of genetic and/or chromosomal origin (Rabeharisoa et al., 2014a). It comes with the creation of collectives associating patients and specialists within epistemic communities (Haas, 1992; Akrich, 2010) whose contours are not set up once and for all because biomedical entities and their manifestations are highly labile and lend themselves to focusing on diverse issues that patient organizations deem important at certain moments in their trajectories. The formation and transformation of these collectives do not result in fixed identities as the notion of biosociality somehow suggests. There are for sure social bonds developed within these collectives, but social bonds that form and evolve through a dual process of singularization and mutualization: singularization entails differences across biomedical entities (Cambrosio et al., 2021), whereas mutualization points to similarities. 'The same but different' is exactly what patient organizations like Génération 22 strive to explore for patients to get the care they need.

7.2.3 A Dual Sociability Around Biomedical Entities and Around the Rarity of Diseases

Patient activism in the field of rare diseases has become more structured over the years, resulting in patient groups' affiliation to umbrella organizations at national, European, and international levels. In France, many rare disease patient groups are members of Alliance Maladies Rares, set up in 2000 after rare diseases were declared a 'public health priority.' Alliance Maladies Rares is an advocacy organization whose foundational criterion is the rarity of diseases. Rarity was defined as a prevalence threshold, first by the American Orphan Drug Act in 1983, and then by the European Directive on Orphan Medicinal Products in 1999 (Novas, 2009; Rabeharisoa and O'Donovan, 2014; Mikami, 2019), thanks notably to patient advocacy. One mission of Alliance Maladies Rares is the deployment of rare disease reference centers for diagnosis and care at national levels, with the help of its members. It therefore mutualizes efforts in maintaining rare diseases on the political agenda.

Alliance Maladies Rares's gathering of patient groups around the rarity of diseases is shown forcefully in the annual 'March of Rare Diseases' it organizes, where patient groups are asked to wear a sign with the name of a disease other than the pathology they are concerned with. The March is meant to remind public authorities of their pressing common problems beyond the specificities of their conditions, namely poor expertise, dire provision, and lack of treatments. At the first edition of the March, the former president of the Alliance remembers that patient groups were very reluctant to publicize diseases other than theirs. Somehow, they feared that the singularization of their diseases, so critical in their efforts to get finely tuned care and attention, ran the risk of being undermined by such a gesture of mutualization. It took time before they admitted that the political outreach of rarity served the war on their singular disease.

Grouping around the rarity of diseases resorts to a 'politics of numbers' (Rabeharisoa et al., 2014a) compatible with the shaping of public health policy. 'Diseases are rare, but patients are many' is the motto that patient organizations put to the fore to sustain public authorities' attention towards the broad category of rare diseases. That said, this 'politics of numbers' is continuously fueled with the singularization/mutualization around biomedical entities we described in the section above: the more biomedical entities identified, the more diseases discovered (one rare disease is discovered every week according to patient organizations), and the more patients diagnosed. This dual sociability around biomedical entities and around rarity is all the more crucial with the discovery of very rare genetic mutations that raises the issue of ultra-rare diseases:[6] patients and families concerned with ultra-rare diseases cannot afford to detach themselves from umbrella organizations formed around the notion of rarity for their medical, social, and political existence to be recognized. This is why gathering and mobilizing around biomedical entities *and* around the rarity of diseases is today part and parcel of patient activism in the field of rare diseases.

7.3 Oncogene-driven patient groups' activism

7.3.1 'Oncogene-Driven Patient Groups: A New Era for Research Partnerships'

We borrow the title of this section from that of a 2018 paper (Freeman-Daily et al., 2018) co-signed by representatives of four US cancer patient advocacy groups, namely the ROS1ders, the EGFR Resisters, the ALK positive, and the EGFR-HER2 Exon 20 group. As shown by their names (Bourret et al., 2025), a new kind of cancer patient group has emerged during the past decade that characterizes itself primarily by reference to genomic entities rather than its cancer's organ of origin (lung, breast, etc.) as was traditionally the case. ROS1, ALK, or EGFR are oncogenes, i.e., tumor-driving genes harboring various mutations. When identified by genomic testing of tumor cells, these alterations afford novel therapeutic strategies, for instance resorting to 'targeted drugs' that inhibit specific mutations, as contrasted with one-size-fits-all chemotherapies. However, targeted drugs are not available for all oncogene mutations—i.e., not all mutations are *actionable*—and their efficacy is often limited by resistance to targeted therapies appearing after a certain time, requiring the development of new generations of this novel type of drug. Survival through therapeutic innovation is the key *raison d'être* of the new cancer advocacy groups. In addition to patient advocates, the aforementioned 2018 paper was co-signed by two oncologists and two representatives of cancer research foundations, thus associating the agency of biomedical entities with the emergence of advocacy groups and the kind of heterogeneous networks—the 'new era for research partnerships'—that these groups seek to build.

Oncogene-driven groups initially emerged in the US, thanks to social networks like Facebook, which are still their primary mode of existence and which allowed them to quickly mobilize patients from several countries. The first group—the ROS1ders—was born out of a 2015 scientific conference attended by patients with ROS1 positive lung cancer who expressed their concern about the lack of therapies and the poor development of research into this very rare kind of cancer. To remedy this situation, investments in research were deemed to be urgently needed, as well as raising awareness among biomedical practitioners and fellow patients. Naming the group after the oncogene's shorthand was a way to make the mutation visible and actionable, a rallying point for basic and clinical researchers and, beyond the world of research, general practitioners and community oncologists who also had to be made aware of the clinical opportunities offered by the presence of oncogenes. Once sensitized to the need of testing for the presence of oncogenic biomarkers by prescribing molecular profiling, treating physicians would eventually be able to match genomic alterations with specific treatments. In addition to singularizing patient care, this kind of 'precision oncology' could offer further insights into the biopathology of cancer.

The creation of the ROS1ders was closely followed by the emergence of an ALK-positive group, also a rare kind of cancer, and in subsequent years by other US groups for a growing array of oncogenes (i.e., RET, EGFR, MET, BRAF, NTRK, and KRAS, to name a few). This movement spread to Europe (as well as Asian countries and Australia/New Zealand) with a first ALK-positive group in the UK in 2018, followed by numerous ALK groups as well as EGFR, ROS1, and BRAF groups in other countries (see Table 7.1). While remaining connected to the relevant global group as the best provider of information on advances in research, participants in internet networks initially established by US patients created ancillary groups in their own countries, considering that certain issues, notably those having to do with access to new molecules, were specific to national settings.

The relative weight of the groups' various activities—namely information and support for patients, raising public and medical awareness, lobbying regulatory agencies for access to drugs, and participation in patient-centered research—shifted over time and differs from one group to another. However, although different circumstances often presided over the origin and development of oncogene-driven groups, they all share the same key objective: survival through the transformation of their cancers into chronic diseases thanks to the development of innovative therapies, with the perspective of a cure looming on the horizon.

Given the centrality of the biomedical entities—oncogenes and their mutations—in naming patient sub-populations, it is tempting to draw a parallel with rare genetic disease patient groups formed around specific genetic mutations and deletions. In the case of cancer groups, however, oncogenes are present in the tumor, not a patient's genome. They therefore do not lead to the emergence of new kinds of people as is the case with rare genetic diseases, in particular genomically designated ones (Navon, 2019) or, more broadly, to the emergence of 'biosocial' configurations (Rabinow, 1992) whereby biomedical rather than demographic categories define new categories of

Table 7.1 Chronology of emergence of major oncogene groups

Year	Oncogene Group	Country
2015	ROS1ders	US
2015	ALK positive	US
2015	ALK ROS1 Australia/New Zealand	Australia and New Zealand
2016	RET Renegades	US
2017	EGFR Resisters	US
2017	EGFR-HER Exon 20 group	US
2018	ALK Positive UK	UK
2019	MET Crusaders	US
2019	NTRKers	US
2019	EGFR UK	UK
2019	BRAF Bombers	US
2019	ROS1 UK	UK
2019	ALKPOSITIV Deutschland	Germany
2020	KRAS Kickers	US
2020	KRAS mutated colorectal cancer	US
2020	ALK+ Belgium	Belgium
2020	Cáncer ROS1	Spain
2021	ALK+ ROS1 cancer poumon France	France
2021	ALK+ Sverige	Sweden
2021	ALK+ Italia	Italy
2021	ALK+ Finland	Finland
2022	ALK POSITIVE	Denmark
2022	ALK+ International	UK
2023	Breaking BRAF	UK
2023	Oncogene cancer research: patients, caregivers & advocates (all oncogene-driven lung cancers, worldwide)	UK

Source: Authors.

people. Reference by advocacy groups to oncogenes as key actants denotes the kinds of partnerships and networks promoted by these groups to enforce therapeutic actionability as a path to survival. Rather than a marker of identity, oncogenic mutations evolve in a clinical space where they are constitutively connected to the drugs that target them. Moreover, these connections are not necessarily stable as drugs targeting a given oncogene may turn out to also target other oncogenes and thus be relevant for other patient subpopulations and related advocacy groups: crizotinib, initially developed to target the MET oncogene, subsequently proved effective against ALK as well as ROS1, rearranging relations between related groups.

Let us now explore a related issue, namely how oncogene-driven groups negotiate the fact that, despite the recent massive growth of precision oncology and calls to redefine the nosology of cancer on a genomic basis (André et al., 2024), the organization of cancer hospitals and care is still largely grounded in the organ of origin.

7.3.2 Organ of Origin and Oncogenes: A Dual Attachment

While most rare cancer advocacy groups are named after genomic entities, they often display a 'dual attachment' by relating both to the oncogene that characterizes and singularizes their cancer and to the organ of origin of their disease, which, as just mentioned, remains an organizing principle for cancer care. Lung cancer is a case in point. Its incidence has greatly increased in recent decades with survival remaining poor due to a lack of effective therapies. Clinical research, however, has identified several actionable genomic subtypes, followed by the development of effective targeted therapies. Despite the availability of an increasing number of drugs, survival remains poor due to late diagnosis, especially for patients with oncogene-driven lung cancers, who are often non-smokers and therefore excluded from screening programs for high-risk patients. As a result, although oncogenes are found across different types of cancer, several oncogene-driven groups are primarily concerned with lung cancer. Their dual, oncogene/organ attachment is pragmatically related to a range of concrete initiatives, such as funding research for innovative therapies, or awareness campaigns, made possible by strategic alliances with organ-based foundations, such as LUNGevity, the GO2 Foundation for Lung Cancer, or the Roy Castle Lung Cancer Foundation. This dual attachment can follow different modalities, leading to diverse configurations:

1. Most groups focus on a specific oncogene in a specific type of cancer, often lung cancer.
2. Other groups bring together patients with cancers in different organs driven by the same oncogene, and therefore treated with the same targeted therapies and/or sharing similar research challenges. These 'pan-cancers' oncogene-driven groups also feature many lung cancer patients, for the aforementioned reasons.
3. A small number of groups operating at the national level include patients with the same type of cancer, often lung, harboring mutations in different oncogenes that can be targeted by the same difficult-to-access drugs. Patients with these subtypes of lung cancer thus share similar issues of therapeutic actionability.
4. Another, quite peculiar 'pan-oncogene' configuration at a higher level of granularity is provided by the Exon 20 Warriors group, which includes patients whose cancer carries a mutation in Exon 20 of either the EGFR or HER2 oncogenes that renders the long available therapies for EGFR and HER2 mutations ineffective.

This example shows the mutually constitutive connection of oncogenic mutations to the drugs that target them.

The multifaceted configuration of oncogene-driven groups shows that the oncogene as deployed by them is not primarily an identity-building entity. Rather, it amounts to a translational operator aiming at achieving therapeutic actionability at the interfaces between research, care, and regulation. Accordingly, oncogene-driven groups are characterized by an alternation of singularization and mutualization processes, as discussed in the next section.

7.3.3 From Singularization to Mutualization

The French ALK+ ROS1 Lung Cancer group provides an example of a 'mutualization strategy' whereby patients affected by different oncogene-driven cancers join their efforts under a more generic umbrella designation, namely their shared belonging to the category of patients affected by oncogene-driven cancers. The association was created in 2021 by French ALK+ lung cancer patients who met as members of the US-based international ALK Positive group. Inspired by the American model (Barton et al., 2023), the founders of the French group did not want to limit themselves to patient support and mutual help, but to take a more active approach by acting as a mediator between patients, oncologists, and researchers. Accordingly, the document introducing the association listed four main objectives: to raise awareness of their rare form of lung cancer; to support and help patients, namely by referring them to oncologists specializing in ALK lung cancer; to act as privileged partners of treating physicians, thereby promoting access to the best treatments; and to support public and private clinical research for the development of innovative treatments. The aim was to embed the association and its patients within the network of clinicians and researchers working on this type of cancer by partnering with them. To this end, the founders sent out a leaflet and business cards to every hospital in France to notify oncologists of the group's existence 'so that they could mention it to patients who wanted to exchange ideas with other patients.'

The creation of the national group was a response to the twofold imperative of making information accessible in French to promote its circulation *and* of taking into account the specific context of the French access to innovative targeted therapies. Categorized as a priority ('our main activity'), this issue played a role in extending the purview of the association to other oncogene-driven lung cancers. Shortly after its creation, the association included ROS1 patients who are treated with the same targeted therapies as ALK, adding ROS1 to its name. It subsequently included patients with cancers driven by other rare oncogenes (MET, RET, NKTR). As explained by the group's representatives, while these patients did not reach the critical mass to enable them to create their own groups, they were 'fighting the same battles, notably for drug reimbursement.'

Despite being approved by the US Food and Drug Administration and the European Medicines Agency, many innovative treatments are not reimbursed in France. French agencies justify their refusal to reimburse and grant access to those treatments by conflating oncogene-driven cancers with 'the generic lung cancer model' rather than categorizing them as rare diseases. Accordingly, one of the group's priorities is to be involved in the assessment of innovative molecules for early access and reimbursement purposes by aligning the criteria for regulating rare cancers' treatments with those for rare diseases.

Beyond their specific oncogene, ALK+ ROS1 France thus realizes a form of mutualization at a broader level of generality, based on the category of oncogene-driven lung cancers as rare kinds of cancers. This opens up new horizons in terms of action focusing on the administrative and economic dimensions of access to innovative therapies.

The French ALK+ ROS1 Lung Cancer group provides a peculiar mutualization strategy, but other forms of mutualization have also been established at a meta-organizing level, i.e., as coalitions of different groups and associations. Examples include the Oncogene-Driven Lung Cancer Patient Alliance created in 2022, bringing together the EGFR UK, ALK+ UK, and ROS1 UK groups to collaborate on several cross-cutting issues, such as the early diagnosis of lung cancer in non-smokers, or the Biomarker Collaborative, that at the time of this writing included 13 oncogene-driven groups and acts as a portal to direct patients to their relevant oncogene group, as well as advocates for shared issues such as extended biomarker testing and the modernization of clinical trials.

7.3.4 An Unusual Mutualization Modality: The Case of MRCP

In 2014, a French expatriate and breast cancer advocate created a digital network—'Mon Réseau Cancer du Sein' ('My Breast Cancer Network')—to provide reliable information to other patients and overcome their isolation. In 2016, thoracic oncologists suggested she should create a similar network for lung cancer, 'Mon Réseau Cancer du Poumon' ('My Lung Cancer Network') (MRCP). In contrast to the previous lack of effective treatments, the advent of targeted therapies and immunotherapies had extended the life expectancy of patients with metastatic cancer, by the same token making it possible for them to participate in the maintenance of a patient forum and contribute to the continued existence of MRCP. In turn, the availability of targeted therapies was instrumental in the creation of oncogene-focused patient subgroups within MRCP. As mentioned by an interviewee, the EGFR, ALK, and ROS1 subgroups were working very well, and a KRAS subgroup was also emerging because several patients could now be treated with a recently developed drug against this previously undruggable mutation. In contrast, subgroups such as RET and MET, for which treatments were not yet available, had so far failed to recruit.

These oncogene-focused subgroups have remained under the umbrella of the larger lung cancer organization (MRCP), which is part of a network of university hospitals and industrial partners and is called upon by a number of actors to take part in various initiatives, including two projects targeting oncogene-driven cancers.

A dual dynamic is at work in the case of MRCP: on the one hand, the creation of several oncogene-specific groups conforms to a singularization modality internal to the broader organization; on the other hand, an externally driven mutualization process turns the MRCP into the representative of all patients who, beyond their particular oncogene, are concerned by initiatives that range across oncogenes.

At the start of this section, we emphasized the advocacy groups' dual attachment to oncogenes and organs, as manifested in the fact that many groups focus on a single organ and that most groups maintain affiliations with generalist cancer organizations. The shared issue of reliable diagnostic procedures and, in particular, the sought-after integration of biomarkers within these procedures illustrates the importance of this attachment and supports our claim that singularization and mutualization are two intimately linked processes. Although some oncogene groups, with a view to therapeutic innovation, are reluctant to use the notion of rarity so as not to scare off pharmaceutical and biotech companies wary of niche markets, other groups, with a view to regulation, are inclined to move closer to the world of rare diseases, as they feel that such an affiliation would enable them to solve problems of timely access to treatment. In other words, the groups and the networks they mobilize are not locked into a fixed identity: they can adopt variable configurations whereby biomedical entities are, directly or indirectly due to the rarity/specificity with which they are associated, powerful connection operators.

7.4 Discussion

In this chapter, we have investigated the formation and mobilization of patient groups around biomedical entities in the field of rare genetic diseases and of oncogene-driven cancers. These groups, notably those on oncogene-driven cancers, have emerged recently, and there is little research work on their form of activism as of today. Hence our question: what do biomedical entities enable patient groups to do, and what do they make them do?

Our analysis shows that the reference to biomedical entities is associated with a process of singularization: the biomedical entity acts as a flagship both for rallying patients and their families and for creating affordances towards the scientific and medical communities. From this point of view, there are strong similarities between the two types of groups, even if this singularization process occurs as the outcome of different stories.

In the case of rare genetic diseases, singularization has been explored by several scholars, who have shown that this process reflects patients' desire to move on from situations marked by the lack of robust medical knowledge and interest in their conditions. For Génération 22, to stick with a DiGeorge syndrome diagnosis would have meant settling for a truncated description of the disease that excludes both a certain number of symptoms and a certain number of patients who do not present the curtailed symptom profile associated with it. In addition to being part of the most advanced medicine, the reference to the 22q11 deletion has enabled the organization to bring together patients suffering from a syndrome with very heterogeneous manifestations. The biomedical entity made it possible to designate the syndrome, to create the group, to set the syndrome apart from others (22q11 *versus* 22q13), and to work towards managing the multiple disorders that accompany the syndrome.

Oncogene groups have emerged from a slightly different landscape: innovative treatments have given consistency to the biomedical entities behind which some 'otherwise unthinkable patient populations'—to borrow the expression Navon (2019) used for rare genetic disease groups—have rallied, whereas they were previously assimilated with the broader group of patients with organ-defined cancers. The reference to biomedical entities makes mutations visible for the general public and community physicians and enables oncogene groups to join networks of actors working towards therapeutic actionability.

We observe these similarities, despite differences between the two types of pathologies in terms of the nature of the biomedical entities involved: oncogenes represent molecular signatures of tumors, whereas in the case of rare genetic diseases, genetic mutations are embodied in patients' genomes. Consequently, individual and collective identity unfolds differently in the two cases. In the case of rare genetic diseases, biomedical entities are somehow part of the patient's identity. In the case of oncogene-driven lung cancers which affect mostly non-smokers, biomedical entities are significant elements of the patient's self-image and a motivation for taking actions aimed at improving non-smokers' chances of survival by correcting doctors' preconceived ideas that lead them to neglect the cancer hypothesis.

This being said, patient groups are not locked into a unique, fixed, and all-encompassing identity. Indeed, our analysis shows that singularization based on biomedical entities is accompanied by a twin process, mutualization, which has so far received much less attention. Let's think, for example, of the parallel development of a myriad of groups concerned with Fragile X, each of them defined by a very specific biomedical entity, and of an umbrella organization focusing on intellectual disability, a problem they appear to share. In the case of oncogene-driven cancers, mutualization makes it possible to explore the actionability of oncogenes at different levels of granularity: it can operate either between groups concerned with the same oncogene as found in different types of cancers and targeted by the same therapy, or between groups concerned with different oncogenes mostly prevalent in specific kinds of tumors.

In all cases, each form of mutualization is a way of building an agency that presents some sort of affordance to specific networks involving researchers, clinicians, industrialists, regulators, healthcare providers, and payers. These networks are associated with different forms of action: they may be oriented at different degrees towards a combination of research, care, and regulation for accessing treatments. These groupings are not large superstructures that encompass patient groups, but rather lightweight and labile configurations capable of adapting and extending to new groups as the situation and problems evolve. In a way, what is at stake here is the development of different *biosocialities*, in the network-building and mobilization sense Navon (2019) gave to this term.

Moreover, advocacy groups sometimes join collectives formed either around other types of clinical entities or elements other than strictly medical ones, such as rarity, while remaining attached to the biomedical entities driving their diseases. Despite the fact that oncogenes are overturning the organ-based classification of cancers, since a given oncogene can be present in different types of cancers, the attachment to the organ remains present, and is manifested in particular through links with organizations concerned with cancer in a particular organ: the actions they take are varied (research, awareness campaigns, transformation of screening methods to include oncogene testing, etc.) and are part of social, professional, and administrative networks based on organ-definition of cancers.

Rare genetic disease groups are affiliated to umbrella organizations such as the French Alliance Maladies Rares, where rarity—an epidemiological notion—is their common denominator. The message conveyed—if the diseases are rare, the sufferers are numerous—aims to bring all these diseases into the public arena and prevent them from being marginalized; it also aims to highlight the problems shared by these groups, given that each disease affects a relatively small population, and bring forward demands linked to this status. Interestingly, the singularization/mutualization process is not alien to this mode of grouping: the more biomedical entities, the more rare diseases, and the more patients.

To recap, patients' grouping and mobilizing around biomedical entities contributes to the singularization of problems they aim to address and to the mutualization of their efforts on shared concerns, as close as possible to the manifestations of their diseases. This is a dual and dynamic process that intersects with and reshapes other traditional forms of groupings (organ-defined cancers, epidemiological threshold of rarity). Thus, we can fairly say that patient groups formed around biomedical entities do not lock themselves in a biosocial identity. Rather, the singularization/mutualization process leads them to multiply sociabilities (Panofsky, 2011) or, in other words, to engage in different modes of socializing biomedical entities.

7.5 Conclusion

Research on the types of patient groups discussed in this chapter, notably on oncogene-driven patient advocacy groups, is in its infancy. It sheds light on forms of activism that accommodate the latest developments in biomedical and therapeutic research with an aim of coming as close as possible to the specific and often complex manifestations of diseases. To conclude, we would like to offer several lines of future inquiry.

A first line of inquiry is the conjoint dynamics of patient activism and biomedicine. From the late twentieth century onwards, we have witnessed the engagement of an increasing number of patient groups in biomedical research. By focusing on biomedical entities such as the ones we have studied, patient groups bring transformations to the biomedical and patient activism landscape, as well as multiple and changing relationships between them, through multiple sociability practices. The long-term transformative effects of such a collective movement, their local *versus* global outreach, are worth further investigation.

A second line of inquiry is the tight connection between the process of singularization/mutualization we have documented and the targeting of advanced therapeutics and medical products. As we have seen, this is core to the *raison d'être* of oncogene-driven patient advocacy groups, but it is also central to patient activism in other condition areas, including rare genetic diseases. The identification of numerous genetic mutations involved in a rare disease leads to R&D on gene therapies targeting each of these mutations, while putting to the test the clinical and economic feasibility of gene therapy as the main path to cure genetic diseases. In particular, the stratification of the market (Wadmann and Hauge, 2021) that may come with this 'precision medicine' is an emerging issue at the intersection of political science, health economics, and STS. At a more general level, many observers have noticed that the pharmaceutical industry is moving from a 'blockbuster' model to a 'niche-buster' model, but very little is known about how this affects Health Technology Assessment, the design and the regulation of the market, and notably the pricing of these targeted therapeutics (Doganova and Rabeharisoa, 2024), a pressing concern for many patient groups that advocate for accessibility. Whether the singularization/mutualization process we have investigated also constitutes an organizing principle of biomedical entity-driven markets is an open question.

A third line of inquiry is the proliferation of patient groups and epistemic communities that result from the process of singularization/mutualization we have analyzed, and its political consequences. This process sheds light on the multiple modalities of formation of common causes in the domain of health and medicine. One question remains: what does this entail for public health policies, traditionally structured around broad categories of diseases and patient populations? This question invites further studies of the institutional landscape, which is undergoing a complex layering to absorb this multiplicity.

Finally, a methodological challenge is awaiting scholars interested in contemporary patient activism and collective mobilization in the domain of medicine and health: the formation of patient groups through social media, online contacts between them and with a growing number of constituencies, and circulation of medical information on the internet. Digital methods are worth developing further to capture this ever-increasing online activity.

These lines of future inquiry, we believe, will enrich the research agenda on biomedicine and society.

Notes

1. We use 'patient group' as a generic term to designate a group of people concerned with the same disease (patients, parents, families), who engage in collective action for a better knowledge of their disease and for medical and social recognition. To avoid repetitions, we alternatively use other terms such as 'patient association' (the name given to patient group in France), 'patient organization,' and 'patient advocacy group.' We have not investigated philanthropy.
2. As per the 1999 EU Directive on Orphan Medicinal Products, a rare disease is a disease that affects less than 1 person in 2,000 in the general population. Eighty percent of rare diseases are of genetic origin.
3. A syndrome is characterized by a set of symptoms whose occurrence may change over time and whose combination may vary from one patient to another.
4. Rare disease associations are very diverse in size and mode of organizing. Rare genetic disease associations are all interested in research on their diseases.
5. Information about the creation and organization of Génération 22 is drawn upon interviews with the mother who founded the group and the president of the association at the time of our fieldwork. In addition, we have consulted the website of the association https://www.generation22.fr/.
6. As per the EU legislation, an ultra-rare disease is a disease that affects less than 1 person in 50,000.

References

Akrich, M. (2010). From communities of practice to epistemic communities: Health mobilizations on the internet. *Sociological Research Online*, *15*(2).

Akrich, M. & Rabeharisoa, V. (2023). On the multiplicity of lay expertise: An empirical and analytical overview of patient associations' achievements and challenges. In G. Eyal & T. Medvetz (Eds.), *The Oxford Handbook of Expertise and Democratic Politics* (pp. 103–133). Oxford: Oxford University Press.

André, F., Rassy, E., Marabelle, A. et al. (2024). Forget lung, breast or prostate cancer: Why tumour naming needs to change. *Nature*, *626*, 26–29.

Anglin, M. (1997). Working from the inside out: Implications of breast cancer activism for biomedical policies and practices. *Social Science and Medicine*, *44*, 1403–1415.

Barbot, J. (2006). How to build an 'active' patient? The work of AIDS associations in France. *Social Science and Medicine*, *62*, 538–551.

Barton, C., Al Achkar, M., Blender, J.A., et al. (2023). Patient-led advocacy in ALK-positive lung cancer. *Translational Lung Cancer Research*, *12*, 1303–1319.

Boon, W. & Broekgaarden, R. (2010). The role of patient advocacy organisations in neuromuscular disease R&D – The case of the Dutch neuromuscular disease association VSN. *Neuromuscular Disorders*, *20*(2), February 2010, 148–151. https://doi.org/10.1016/j.nmd.2009.10.012. PMID: 20106662.

Bourret, P., Akrich, M., Paterson, F. & Cambrosio, A. (2025). Oncogene-driven advocacy: Collective expertise and therapeutic actionability. *Health* (London), *28*, 13634593251336521. April, 2025 https://doi.org/10.1177/13634593251336521. PMID: 40294041.

Britten, N., Denford, S., Harris-Golesworthy, F., Jibson, S., Pyart, N. & Stein, K. (2015). Patient involvement in drug licensing: A case study. *Social Science & Medicine*, *131*, April 2015, 289–296. https://doi.org/10.1016/j.socscimed.2014.10.024. PMID: 25454636.

Callon, M. (2012). Quel rôle pour les sciences sociales face à l'emprise grandissante du régime de l'innovation intensive? *Cahiers de Recherche Sociologique*, 53, 121–165.

Cambrosio, A., Campbell, J. & Bourret, P. (2021). Beyond nosology? Molecular tumor boards, singularization, and the conflation of diagnosis and therapy. *New Genetics and Society*, *40*(1), 95–111.

Campbell, J., Cambrosio, A. & Basik, M. (2024). Histology agnosticism: Infra-molecularizing disease? *Studies in History and Philosophy of Science*, *104*, 14–22.

Doganova, L. & Rabeharisoa, V. (2024). The temporalities of prices. 'Value-based pricing' in pharmaceutical markets. *Economy and Society*, 53(2), 183–204.

Epstein, S. (1995). The construction of lay expertise: AIDS activism and the forging of credibility in the reform of clinical trials. *Science, Technology and Human Values*, *20*, 408–437.

Epstein, S. (1996). *Impure Science. AIDS, Activism, and the Politics of Knowledge.* Berkeley: University Press of California.

Epstein, S. (2008). Patient groups and health movements. In E.J. Hackett, O. Amsterdamska, M. Lynch & J. Wajcman (Eds.), *The Handbook of Science and Technology Studies* (3rd Ed.), (pp. 499–538). Massachusetts: MIT Press.

Epstein, S. (2023). The meaning and significance of lay expertise. In G. Eyal & T. Metvetz (Eds.), *The Oxford Handbook of Expertise and Democratic Politics* (pp. 76–102). Oxford: Oxford University Press.

Faraj, S. & Azad, B. (2013). The materiality of technology: An affordance perspective. In P. Leonardi, B. Nardi & J. Kallinikos (Eds.), *Materiality and Organizing: Social Interaction in a Technological World* (pp. 237–258). Oxford: Oxford University Press.

Freeman-Daily, J., Elkins, I., Greco, L., et al. (2018). Oncogene-driven patient groups: A new era for research partnerships. *Journal of Thoracic Oncology*, *13*(10S), S343.

Haas, P.M. (1992). Epistemic communities and international policy coordination. *International Organization*, *46*, 1–35.

Hacking, I. (1986). Making up people. In T.C. Heller & C. Brooke-Rose (Eds.), *Reconstructing Individualism. Autonomy, Individuality, and the Self in Western Thought* (pp. 161–171). Stanford: Stanford University Press.

Hacking, I. (2006). Genetics, biosocial groups and the future of identity. *Daedalus*, *135*(4), 81–95.

Heath, D., Rapp, R. & Taussig K.-S. (2004). Genetic citizenship. In D. Nugent & J. Vincent (Eds.), *A Companion to the Anthropology of Politics* (pp. 152–167). Oxford: Blackwells.

Keating, P. & Cambrosio, A. (2012). Cancer research and protocol patients: From clinical material to committee advisors. In C. Timmermann & E. Toon (Eds.), *Cancer Patients, Cancer Pathways: Historical and Sociological Perspectives* (pp. 161–185). London: Palgrave Macmillan.

Keating, P., Cambrosio, A. & Nelson, N.C. (2016). 'Triple negative breast cancer': Translational research and the (re)assembling of diseases in post-genomic medicine. *Studies in History and Philosophy of Science Part C: Studies in History and Philosophy of Biological and Biomedical Sciences*, *59*, 20–34.

Koay, P.P. & Sharp, R.R. (2013). The role of patient advocacy organizations in shaping genomic science. *Annual Review of Genomics and Human Genetics*, *14*, 579–595.

Mikami, K. (2019). Orphans in the market: The history of orphan drug policy. *Social History of Medicine*, *32*(3), 609–630.

Navon, D. (2011). Genomic designation: How genetics can delineate new, phenotypically diffuse medical categories. *Social Studies of Science*, *41*(2), 203–226.

Navon, D. (2019). *Mobilizing Mutations: Human Genetics in the Age of Patient Advocacy.* Chicago: University of Chicago Press.

Novas, C. (2006). The political economy of hope: Patients organizations, science and biovalue. *BioSocieties*, *1*(3), 289–305.

Novas, C. (2009). Orphan drugs, patient activism and contemporary healthcare. *Quaderni. Communication, Technologies, Pouvoir, 68*, 13–23.

O'Donovan, O. (2007). Corporate colonization of health activism? Irish health advocacy organizations modes of engagement with pharmaceutical corporations. *International Journal of Health Services, 37*(4), 711–733.

Panofsky, A. (2011). Generating sociability to drive science: Patient advocacy organizations and genetics research. *Social Studies of Science, 41*(1), 31–57.

Rabeharisoa, V. (2003). The struggle against neuromuscular diseases in France and the emergence of the 'partnership model' of patient organisation. *Social Science and Medicine, 57*(11), 2127–2136.

Rabeharisoa, V. & Callon, M. (2004). Patients and scientists French muscular dystrophy research. In S. Jasanoff (Ed.), *States of Knowledge. The Co-production of Science and Social Order* (pp. 142–160). London: Routledge.

Rabeharisoa, V., Callon, M., Filipe, A.M., Nunes, J.A., Paterson, F. & Vergnaud, F. (2014a). From 'politics of numbers' to 'politics of singularisation': Patients' activism and engagement in research on rare diseases in France and Portugal. *BioSocieties, 9*(2), 194–217.

Rabeharisoa, V., Moreira, T. & Akrich, M. (2014b). Evidence-based activism: Patients', users' and activists' groups in knowledge society. *BioSocieties, 9*(2), 111–128.

Rabeharisoa, V. & O'Donovan, O. (2014). From Europeanization to European construction. The role of European patients' organizations in the shaping of health-care policies. *European Societies, 16*(5), 717–741.

Rabeharisoa, V. & Doganova, L. (2021). War on diseases. Patient organizations' problematization and exploration of market issues. In S. Geiger (Ed.), *Healthcare Activism. Markets, Morals, and the Collective Goods* (pp. 55–85). Oxford: Oxford University Press.

Rabinow, P. (1992). Artificiality and enlightenment: From sociobiology to biosociality. In J. Crary & S. Kwinter (Eds.), *Incorporations* (pp. 234–252). New York: Zone Books.

Timmermans, S. (2020). The engaged patient: The relevance of patient–physician communication for twenty-first-century health. *Journal of Health and Social Behavior, 61*(3), 259–273.

Wadmann, S. & Hauge, A.M. (2021). Strategies of stratification: Regulating market access in the era of personalized medicine. *Social Studies of Science, 51*(4), April 2021, 628–653. https://doi.org/10.1177/03063127211005539. PMID: 33885344.

8 International science collaboration under regulatory capitalism: The corruption of biomedical regulation

Margaret Sleeboom-Faulkner

8.1 Introduction

This chapter draws attention to the roles and dynamics of competition crucial to international science collaboration in biomedicine. Science collaboration tends to be viewed positively in terms of collaboratively striving to attain scientific aims. By showing how international regulatory competition has the potential to harm patients, scientific development and the public in general, this chapter makes clear why research into international science collaborations needs to be part of the research agenda for biomedicine.[1]

There exists little academic work on the practices of international science collaborations. Often, international science collaborations are characterised in terms of 'win-win' outcomes for the collaborative parties involved (Shrum, 2010). Although medical anthropological work examines clinical trials and international development, it usually focus on relations of inequality among collaborative partners (e.g. Petryna, 2009; Sariola and Simpson, 2019), missing the much broader, global dynamics of international scientific collaborations. Most work on international science collaboration, however, is concerned with 'big-data' analysis and focuses on research publications (e.g. Anon, 2023). This chapter, however, by paying attention to the global dynamics of both competition and collaboration in regenerative medicine, shows how science innovation feeds off global inequalities of various kinds, including the availability of science expertise, capital and 'favourable' regulation.

International collaboration is crucial to fortifying the realisation of science ambitions of competitors, including in the field of regenerative medicine. But examples of global science collaborations from Asia and beyond show that global inequalities are crucial to enabling science collaborations, shaping the dynamics of both competition and collaborations in an international context. Therefore, I maintain that competition and collaboration need to be viewed together as part of the global dynamics of regulatory capitalism. Future research in this area, I believe, should explore the following three questions: first, why regulatory and other inequalities are important to science collaboration; second, why there is little transparency about the actual benefits and drawbacks of international collaborative research over time; and, third, why research on the practice of international science collaboration needs to be viewed in an international (rather than a multilateral or national) context of infrastructural resources and science innovation strategies. This chapter introduces concepts, illustrations and analysis that begin to explore these questions.

Though the examples used in this chapter focus on collaboration and competition in the field of regenerative medicine, its conclusions are applicable more broadly to translational research, that is, to biomedical science innovation in general. Like other forms of scientific innovation, regenerative medicine is a fast-moving field characterised by high expectations of and speculation on future profits. Most translational research is driven by huge financial investment and potential economic gain through knowledge assets and industries (Birch, 2016) that are crucial to a political economy of hope (Brown, 2003; Petersen et al., 2017).

In the first section of this chapter, I will situate science collaboration in the global context of regulatory capitalism and clarify what is at stake where science collaboration is incentivised by inequality and becomes a vehicle of gain for non-scientific reasons. In the second section, I will illustrate this with international examples from the field of regenerative medicine. In the third section, I provide examples of how science collaborations are brokered at various levels of organisational contexts. In the concluding section, I will discuss why international science collaboration needs to be placed on the research agenda, especially when based on the convergence of the self-interests of unequal partners.

8.2 Collaboration and regulatory violence in global capitalism

After the Second World War, international economic competition between countries and regions became increasingly based on the power to set the rules and standards for production, also in the field of biomedicine. This form of competition, I refer to as regulatory capitalism (Levi-Faur, 2005; Braithwaite, 2008). As the protection of patients and the quality of therapies depend on these rules and standards, it is foreseeable that altering them in the context of regulatory competition could result in harm to patients. The rise of regenerative medicine, an emergent field of biomedical innovation that aims to restore, maintain or enhance cell, tissue and organ function, is a case in point. It is in the context of regulatory competition in the field of regenerative medicine that I developed the notion of 'regulatory violence' (Sleeboom-Faulkner, 2025).

Research regulation and clinical regulation aim to protect research subjects (often patients) in clinical research trials and other forms of therapy provision. Regulatory violence is about the use and misuse of these regulations for the pursuit of other, illegitimate interests, thereby inflicting not necessarily intended, but foreseeable harm on the people they are meant to protect. Regulatory violence, then, occurs when regulation, meant to protect the quality of treatment and clinical research, is used to satisfy other, often lucrative aims. I use the notion of 'violence' here as understood by philosopher Vittorio Bufacchi (2005), who points out the possible, foreseeable nature of violence and its harm. I speak of violence, here, as one can foresee that harm is likely to be inflicted on patients or clinical trial subjects, who might be receiving unsafe clinical interventions, or, indirectly, when patients/subjects are harmed as a result of suboptimal clinical treatment. This might well be the case where regulations are violated, where they are not implemented as prescribed or envisaged or where they are avoided through collaboration with other jurisdictions.

This relation between regulation and violence may come across as puzzling: people usually think of violence as harmful acts directed against individuals in a direct, physical and intentional way (Bufacchi, 2005). Also, we usually associate regulation with political order and legitimacy. Nevertheless, for over a decade, I have witnessed many instances in which regulatory compromise predictably led to harm to patients. My anthropological research on collaborations among scientists and industry in low- and middle-income countries (LMICs) and high-income countries (HICs) shows how regulation becomes a source of negotiation and manipulation. Here, science collaborations are based on the sharing of a pool of scientific, material and human resources among collaborative partners (Shrum et al., 2007; Shrum, 2010) involving structural inequalities.

Although usually expressing positivity focused on a win-win basis, collaborations also show signs of mutual mistrust, competition and carefully managed dependence. The collaborations I describe here all revolved around *differences in regulations* between countries. As argued above, clinical research regulation is not always used to protect the quality of patient treatment and the quality of scientific research, but can also be manipulated, dodged, reformed and designed to gain an economic competitive edge internationally. What I witnessed was the brokering of collaborations on the basis of regulation: regulation was tinkered with and had *foreseeable* consequences for the quality of patient treatment. For this reason, a naïve belief in the benefits of international science collaboration is not justified: without in-depth understanding of the potential drivers of collaboration, including regulatory and other discrepancies, such as available expertise, financial capital, healthcare provision and equipment, one fails to understand the dynamics of the collaboration, and the conflicting interests that make the collaboration worthwhile. The cumulative evidence for this can be found in the examples given in the next section of this chapter.

Regulatory violence, also when not intended, is a foreseeable symptom of a form of international competition in an international capitalist order. This capitalist order is often presumed to be based on 'competition' and 'global free markets' (Jahan and Mahmud, 2024). Although there is wide awareness of monopolist or oligopolistic relations of power, little attention has been paid to the idea that *collaboration* might be based on the selfish interests generated through a system based on competition. In

'Together in Disharmony', Paul Demouchel (2017) posits that cooperation and conflict are not polar opposites. Rather, they constitute forms of social coordination that partake in social bonds, such as collaborative projects, related in such a way that they grow in parallel. As such, negotiated rules for behaviour are likely to be detrimental to the interests of the weaker of the collaborative partners. Similarly, according to Rene Girard, greater cooperation will lead to more rather than to fewer conflicts (Girard, 1965). To prevent harmful outcomes, both powerful and weaker collaborative partners underplay latent conflict. And, as shown below, because conflict can endanger the success of the collaboration, expressions of good intention, trust and positivity work to stabilise and to structure the collaboration, be it ritually or contractually.

Competition in science is a condition of strife based on the desire to gain possessions and leverage, including money, power, reputation and knowledge, to establish superiority over others. Such 'competitive desire' (Girard, 1965) is a mode of attention (McGilchrist, 2012) cultivated under global capitalism. Scientific innovation when based on competitive desire incentivises collaboration by those that not only share interests, but also have conflicting interests. Competitive desire as a generative principle and subjective force underlying global capitalism is not so much interested in 'cures' as in the possibility of finding therapeutic products that improve economic assets and scientific standing, as well as attracting investment. The competitive drive places patients in a vulnerable position. For, under capitalism, outside the economic contract, there exists no duty of ethical or social duty of care or mutuality (Demouchel, 2017): no reciprocity is required after the exchange, apart from those that have been specified in the contract. Liabilities of clinical trials or other clinical interventions are often covered separately, often with insurance companies, but more usually by national healthcare arrangements, local communities and institutions of social care.

Compromising the regulation that underpins such commercial contracts under global regulatory capitalism (Levi-Faur, 2005; Braithwaite, 2008), the self-interested utilisation and manipulation of regulation translates directly or indirectly into the potential for violence against patients. Thus, by moving clinical research activities deemed illegitimate in one jurisdiction to another through collaborative arrangements for regulatory reasons, it leaves patients vulnerable to exploitation when the target country is not equipped with the appropriate regulation for this kind of clinical research or therapy provision. This, as many journal articles and media reports have evidenced (e.g. Srinivasan, 2006; Kiatpongsan and Sipp, 2008; McMahon and Thorsteinsdóttir, 2010; Brown, 2012; Bianco and Sipp, 2014; Petersen et al., 2017; Montague, 2019; Smith, 2021; Cyranoski et al., 2023), has led to harmful consequences for patients, their families and, often, crowdfunding communities, and, to various extents, to the scientific reputation of the countries that allow the collaborations that are based on such applications. In a world of regulatory capitalism, however, it is not just companies and scientists that are in competition with each other; as will become clear below, nation-states can also change their regulations to accelerate the development of therapies and to attract international collaborations, ultimately so as to satisfy the competitive desire for economic assets, reputation and lower healthcare bills. In the discussion, I will elaborate why this competitive and self-interested mode of attention cultivated under global capitalism deserves to be reconsidered.

8.3 Four examples of international science collaboration, regulatory violence and inequality

The examples below discuss how international science collaborations based on regulatory discrepancies, often accompanied by other discrepancies and inequalities, create the setting for regulatory violence. Examples of science collaboration in Asia and beyond will illustrate collaborative strategies in various regulatory contexts in the field of regenerative medicine. By tracing the collaborative networks and observing the relations of exchange, positions and collaborative advantages of the partners involved, it is possible to identify the conditions under which collaborations emerge. The examples also introduce concepts that could be useful in future research on international science collaboration. Some of these concerns are illustrated through conversations with people engaged in international science collaboration.

8.3.1 Providing Therapy and Developing New Products Through Regulatory Discrepancy and Science Collaboration[2]

This first example shows how regulatory discrepancy is bridged through relatively simple bilateral collaborations for the goals of experimentation, charity and long-term profit.

The Indian-Japanese joint venture, the Z Centre for Regenerative Medicine (ZCRM), is an example of how the perception of restrictive regulation led to collaboration between unequal partners (Sleeboom-Faulkner and Patra, 2011). The founders of ZCRM boasted a large scientific, political and financial network in both Japan and India. In 2005, the Japan-based, Indian-born scientist-entrepreneur Kumar (pseudonyms used throughout for interviewees) and a group of Japanese scientists and companies set up ZCRM as a charitable company in Chennai, India, with Japanese equity. In 2007, the Department of Biotechnology (DBT, India) and the Indian Council of Medical Research (ICMR) implemented jointly developed 'Guidelines for Stem Cell Research and Therapy' (ICMR-DBT, 2007), followed by various reforms and amendments (Sleeboom-Faulkner, 2025: Ch 3). This did not prevent ZCRM from organising clinical stem cell applications for a range of diseases, including spinal cord injury, cardiovascular diseases and cirrhosis of the liver, and immune diseases in India. Settled in Japan and established as a cardiac surgeon at a university there, Kumar commuted between India and Japan to overcome regulatory boundaries. In 2008, Kumar reported how the company's charitable goals had led to long-term profit:

> We now have plans for a lot of years. We have proven that corneal limbal tissues taken from the same patients (are beneficial) on the basis of animal research. Corneal cells have some problems in common with the endothelium. If we do the research here, then we have ten years of research ahead of us, as there are various regulatory complications. The Waseda people gave us the materials and our Indian guys tried the primary culture in the laboratory.

> Then we did the collaboration with an institute in India. There they did the basic study and animal study in the lab, and the tissue engineering before application in the hospital.
>
> *(Interview with Kumar, 5 August 2008)*

Here we find that regulation is brokered by a simple strategic use of regulatory discrepancy and by avoiding regulatory violation where possible, for what was described informally as charitable goals. Although differences in healthcare, wealth and scientific development between the countries played an important role, the regulatory discrepancy between India and Japan was crucial to ZCRM's ability to organise stem cell interventions ('therapy') and to develop their ambitious research ambitions.

8.3.2 Regulatory Discrepancy and Science Collaboration Through Strategic Linking[3]

This second example shows how ZCRM, which in 2008 was formally registered in Japan as a joint venture, created elaborate systems of collaboration. Through a so-called 'hub and spoke model' (O'Kelly, 1998), companies can automatically shift responsibility and risk to collaborating institutions through international 'strategic linking'. I use a later phase in the development of ZCRM as an example here, but other companies, such as the Chinese international giant Beike Biotechnology (Sui and Sleeboom-Faulkner, 2015; Sleeboom-Faulkner, 2016), use the same method. ZCRM provides the coordination of stem cell therapies by providing cell lines, technologies and clients, but they do not actually provide the therapies themselves. This allows them to pass on risk and responsibility to collaborative partners. This system continued to work, even after India in December 2013 introduced relatively stringent guidelines for stem cell research (ICMR-DBT, 2013).

The growth of ZCRM reflected India's regulatory transition, which prompted the company to develop into an entrepreneurial network-based collaborative structure that conditions the abilities of stakeholders to sustain their work successfully and promote experimental therapy. ZCRM carries out research, training, protocol development and clinical applications in regenerative medicine, with an emphasis on stem cells, progenitor cells and autologous adult cells with regenerative capability. ZCRM claims to possess the technology for the processing, expanding and preserving of clinical-grade stem cells, precursor cells and mature cells. ZCRM, as a centre involved in cutting-edge science, has signed academic and research collaborations with universities and research institutes in India to promote basic research or academic training in stem cell science. It has signed a memorandum of understanding with two universities in Andhra Pradesh for stem cell research, and it has also started a web-based training programme in regenerative medicine in collaboration with a training programme in regenerative medicine affiliated with a university in Canada. These kinds of collaborative academic links provide recognition and academic exposure and help maintain global linkages through faculty exchanges and work exposure for young researchers at ZCRM. The collaborating centres in India, in turn, get access to advanced stem cell technology developed in Japan, which enables them to work with world-class scientists.

Central to the functioning of the networks is ZCRM's ability to create strategic connections, which is dependent on its relative centrality as a network hub. Such linking is composed of three elements, which we have described as goal-setting, strategic exposure and the linking of strategic spaces (Patra and Sleeboom-Faulkner, 2017). First, ZCRM had the ability to monopolise the *goal-setting* of the network through its connections with universities and companies in Japan and its access to technologies and other knowledge assets, while in Japan it had a wide network of links with universities, government bureaucracies and hospitals, which in turn had their own links to small-to-medium-sized hospitals and clinics. The interlinked hub could also boast of MOUs with well-known universities abroad and a web-based journal used to publish their research (Patra and Sleeboom-Faulkner, 2017).

The power to *strategically expose* some partners rather than others to clients, training or critique made partners dependent on ZCRM's goodwill. ZCRM could decide to make potential clients aware of the particular expertise of collaborating partners, such as the kinds of techniques they use, their experience or their quality of care, required in a specific entrepreneurial context, such as during negotiations, setting up new scientific ventures and ethical consultation (Patra and Sleeboom-Faulkner, 2017).

Finally, ZCRM has the power to strategically link geographical, scientific and social spaces that it views as conducive to its business. For instance, the official web page of ZCRM explicitly declares that its stem cell treatment and other therapy services are based on advanced technology from Japan:

> One of our core strengths has been the possession of technology for processing, expanding, and preservation of clinically usable stem cells, precursor cells, as well as mature cells. We have a unique advantage of having biomaterial and nanotechnology-based stem cell processing and expansion technology through our collaboration with Japanese institutes.
>
> *(ZCRM, 2024)*[4]

Thus, ZCRM attracts physicians, usually based in small to medium-sized private hospitals, who are keen to have the opportunity to collaborate with partners making use of 'advanced' Japanese technologies (Patra and Sleeboom-Faulkner, 2017).

In short, international collaboration made research and therapy provision possible by making use of regulatory discrepancies. In addition, collaborative networks enabled the passing on of risk to collaborative partners dependent on ZCRM for their business.

8.3.3 Regulatory Brokerage, Unequal Collaboration and Regulatory Capital[5]

This example illustrates how in unequal research collaboration, regulatory capital can serve to broker unequal science collaborations and formalise this bilaterally at state level.

In the 2010s, Japan's life sciences underwent various changes, including the legalisation of clinical research on cells differentiated from pluripotent stem cells and policy strategies such as the 'Highway for the Realisation of Regenerative Medicine', the Japan Revitalisation Strategy and the Plan for the Promotion of Medical Research and Development (Headquarters for Healthcare Policy, 2014). The strategies aimed to increase coordination among the government departments and to enhance Japan's global competitiveness in the pharmaceutical and medical equipment industries, including the areas of medical products and equipment, regenerative medicine and personalised medicine. The final aim was to strengthen competition in the Euro-American market in the field of drugs and devices through technological innovation and to create the infrastructure for regenerative and personalised medicine abroad and at home.

In February 2012, the Minister of Health, Labour and Welfare outlined the five-year strategy intended to serve as the core driver of Japan's economic growth (MoHLW, 2012). It emphasised the bridge-building between industry and academia (*hashi-watashi*) by stimulating venture capital to invest in biomedical science, and it allowed the outsourcing of cell processing and promoted joint research. Another emphasis was on improving the infrastructure for clinical trials and creating an environment that used Japanese-made devices and instruments, making Japan the hub for clinical trials in Asia for the first time. Japan's Department of New Energy and Industrial Technology Development Organisation (NEDO, 2015) was to support industrial applications, both domestically and overseas.

NEDO, in response to 'a recent increase in open and global innovation', had been promoting the establishment of world-standard technology, as well as market development, by drawing on established research networks in collaboration with foreign governments and relevant organisations. One example of a collaborative network supported by NEDO is that between Kawasaki Heavy Industries (KHI) in Japan, with research institutions in Bangkok, where NEDO has an office. In Japan, at the time, only a medical doctor or university involved in a clinical application was allowed to process human cells. KHI, which was developing an automatic cell-processing robot (R-CPX) for upscaling stem cell cultivation, wanted to prove that marketable products could result from clinical trials using the robotic machine. It regarded Japan's regulations, however, as too slow and onerous for its aims.

Thailand's Chulalongkorn University (CU) decided to house KHI's robotic machine for its ability to produce 'clinically graded' cells and to collaborate in clinical research, an opportunity to learn from Japan. As of November 2012, the parties included the Thai Department of Trade Negotiation (DTN), the Ministry of Commerce of Thailand, NEDO, Japan's Ministry of International Trade and Industry (MITI), KHI, DSP Research Co., Ltd., Mukogawa Women's University, the Faculties of Medicine of Chulalongkorn and Srinakharintarawiroj Universities and AESKULAP Clinic (Asia) Co.. The Memorandum of Understanding (MOU) was celebrated with much ritual aplomb in September 2013, in the presence of Crown Princess Sirindhorn and the Japanese ambassador to Thailand (Chulalongkorn University, 2013), and further MOUs were signed between the 'Japanese team' and the 'Thai team'.

A NEDO document illustrates how the collaboration around the R-CPX 'robot' allowed surveillance and control from Japan by means of instructions to and training of Thai scientists, and through electronic CT scan data and X-ray images being sent to Japan (NEDO, 2013). The document presents the project as part of Japan's global expansion strategy, which forecasted an annual market of 3.8 billion Yen in 2050 (£25.8m). While KHI hoped to use the 'donated' R-CPX machine to diversify into medical devices that supported the development of regenerative medicines, Japan's long-term aim was to expand its Asian market and beyond (JSTA, 2015).

When asked why the Japanese wanted to collaborate with a Thai institution, the Thai scientist who had first received the Japanese delegation explained:

> Especially in the beginning we have been wondering why they came to Thailand. They did not go to China, which is understandable. Political relations are not good. But they did not go to Singapore either. This is because they are potential competition. We were skeptical in the beginning. There is no such thing as a free lunch and all that. They now just want to have (Thai) FDA (Food and Drugs Administration) approval or a license.
>
> *(Interview with Wattanapanit, 27 June 2014)*

Here, KHI strategically chose Chulalongkorn University as a collaborative partner, being confident that it would receive permission for conducting a clinical trial using cells cultivated by the robotic machine. Chulalongkorn University, on the other hand, accepted the collaboration because the use of advanced equipment would help it both scientifically and financially.

Although the collaboration was going smoothly according to both the Japanese and Thai partners, there were various potential problems pointed out to me by both researchers from CU and researchers from other universities.

First, relations of dependence made it difficult for the Thai team to insist on their preferential target for clinical applications. Although R-CPX allowed the hospital to have Good Manufacturing Practice (GMP) equipment, various scientists found the planned clinical application for osteoarthritis premature. The MOU specified that the Thai team was in charge of the implementation of the protocol and, according to the Thai orthopaedic surgeon Dr Wilipana, the choice of the condition targeted was made by the Japanese, who 'went straight to the Department of Orthopaedics', which accorded with Dr Sawa's interest in osteoarthritis (Interview with Wilipana, 25 June 2014).

Second, not enough trust had been built to discuss clinical trial permissions frankly. Although the adoption of the R-CPX machine promised an efficient environment for conducting clinical trials, scientific experimentation and the creation of medicinal products, there were wider concerns about the quality of the processed cells.

Nevertheless, the expectation of proving the suitability of using R-CPX in clinical trials made permission for a clinical trial using the cells and a licence to use the cells in a clinical trial a requirement. According to one manager from KHI, 'not allowing it would be *warui* (bad form)' (Interview with Nakasone, 11 November 2013). Although Dr Wilipana thought that KHI hoped that CU would support an application for permissions, he made clear that they would receive it only when there was evidence that the MSc's (mesenchymal stem cells) were safe. He also emphasised that they were not planning to make any exceptions for this particular collaboration. The government, he believed, would want to maintain the high reputation of its laboratories (Interview with Wilipana, 25 June 2014). This, however, had not been made clear to the Japanese partners.

Third, there were worries about being dependent on the Japanese team for the use of the robotic machine, R-CPX. In a situation in which the Japanese team expected permissions for clinical trials and a marketing licence, the Thai team had found it difficult to address issues around the costs that the Thai laboratory was facing. The R-CPX was useless without its software, and because the software updated regularly, the laboratory was presented with hefty bills. In addition, the import costs for assays and other instruments were extremely expensive for Thailand, as it trades under GATT rules (Interview with Sombat, 12 November 2014).

And, finally, doubts were expressed about the wisdom of developing applications using regenerative medicine in the expectation of addressing Thailand's health issues. According to Dr Nantakam (Interview, 26 June 2014), it is because of the high hopes placed on regenerative medicine that the Thai government finds itself in a dilemma: to stimulate high-standard life-science research recognised by the dominant international community, to produce expensive cell products, or to allow less costly research that produces affordable cell products that may not work, or, worse, be harmful. Dr Sombat similarly doubted the imminent large-scale use of regenerative medicine, even in Japan for that matter. Although the Japanese team stressed that the value of affordable medicine is made possible by upscaling through automation, members of the Thai team had doubts about the affordability of the mainstream use of these medical products in Thailand (Interview with Sombat, 27 June 2014); Interview with Nantakam, 26 June 2014). Only in the long run was there hope that conditions such as B Thalassaemia would be cured using regenerative medicine.

As described in this example, KHI with the support of NEDO, a semi-government organisation, in the choice of Thailand as a collaborative jurisdiction, made use of regulatory discrepancies, thereby violating the spirit of the regulation in Japan, as well as harbouring expectations about regulatory permissions for clinical trials. As such, regulation became a form of regulatory capital, similar to the ways in which cheap scientific expertise and a pool of potential patients can become social capital, crucial to collaborative negotiations. The collaboration was based on inequality: although the interests of Japanese and Thai partners converged in the robotic machine, there were differences in aims: key members of the Thai team expressed a preference for different clinical targets, were not happy about Thai regulation being misused, had concerns about dependence on Japanese software and the costs of imported assays and were doubtful about whether the collaboration could address Thai health issues any time soon. In spite of the MOU and the positivity among the teams about the collaboration, the dependent partner had not felt able to address the issues they had to deal with. It seems that both partners underplayed latent conflict and doubts.

8.3.4 Generating International Collaboration Through Regulatory Competition and Regulatory Change[6]

The first three examples involved multiple forms of inequality, including expertise, the level of scientific development and national wealth. In this one, regulatory inequality demonstrates the importance of regulatory competition in the generation of new collaborations. Here the strategic change of regulation is based on a policy of regulatory competition with the aim to stimulate investment and international collaborations. For instance, regulatory 'brokerage' at the level of the Japanese government laid the groundwork for expanded international collaborations in the field of regenerative medicine. A 2012 presentation to a Japanese Cabinet committee on regulation and regulatory reform highlighted how South Korea had approved five times as many cell biologics as Japan had between 2010 and 2012, as an indicator of a purported innovation gap (Toda, 2012). In 2013, Japan's government responded to this competitive challenge by amending the Pharmaceutical Affairs Act to create a new category of medicines ('regenerative medicine products') and a review pathway designed to grant such products accelerated market entry through 'conditional approval'. These regulatory changes aimed to make Japan more attractive for industry interested in developing regenerative medicine and to attract investment from abroad.

In November 2014, Japan promulgated the Pharmaceuticals and Medical Devices (PMD) Act, which established the regulatory framework for pharmaceuticals, medical devices and regenerative and cellular therapy items for the Japanese market. Before this, only two products, J-Tec's JACE and JACC (autologous cultured cartilage cells for cartilage defects and knee joints) had been approved. Shortly after, in 2015, two new cell therapy products obtained approval for marketing: Heartsheet and Temcell; all four products were made eligible for Japan's National Institute of Health (NIH) reimbursement. Another political decision, related to Japan's regulatory reforms, stipulated the creation of Comprehensive Special Zones (CSZs) for industrialisation in 2013, of which Life Innovation in the Keihin Coastal Area CSZ for International Competitiveness is one example. It was set up to stimulate innovation in regenerative medicine and cell therapies (Kanagawa Prefecture, 2016). These CSZs play an important role in the facilitation of international collaboration.

The creation of the CSZs and the eligibility for reimbursement of clinical applications had been designed to attract international collaborators. And, together with the regulatory changes, they led to a flurry of purchases and collaborations. This spurred Japan's pharmaceutical and industrial sectors to further earmark investment for lucrative regenerative medicine ventures. Thus, deregulation made Japan attractive, not only to Japan's pharmaceutical and related industries – some major players include Takeda, Astellas, Sumitomo Dainippon, Fujifilm, Kyowa Kirin, Healios, Terumo and

Eisai – but also to foreign companies. Interest in Japan among foreign companies exploded to such an extent that one scientist referred to it as *kusakariba* (草刈場) or 'cutting from the hay-meadow commons' (Interview with Takeuchi, 5 February 2016), implying a place that anybody can exploit (e.g. RepliCel, 2013; Regeneus, 2014; Cytori, 2015; Athersys, 2016; Cynata Therapeutics, 2016; Densford, 2016; Pluristem, 2016).

The negotiations that took place in the Keihin Coastal Area CSZ in Kanagawa Prefecture illustrate how the particular regulatory features of countries can be combined in international strategies. In this example, Keihin Coastal Area tried to attract industry, with the support of the Forum for Innovative Regenerative Medicine (FIRM). In 2017, ten companies within FIRM formed a taskforce called Regenerative Medicine Industrialisation Task Force (RMIT) to establish a development centre for regenerative medicine in Kawasaki, a city central to the Keihin Coastal Area.

In early 2016, the UK-JAPAN Life Innovation Symposium 'Opportunities for UK-Japan Collaborations in Cell and Gene Therapy' was held in Kawasaki. Representatives of Kanagawa/Keihin and the UK's Cell and Gene Therapy Catapult organisation listed the advantages of their respective science parks in a self-congratulatory display of mutual grooming. Kanagawa/Keihin was presented as close to Haneda airport, allowing one-day round trips to Asian countries and offering 'deregulation', subsidies and tax advantages. Located at a distance from conglomerated areas, it allowed for R&D activities using blood or bacteria. The local government was introduced as being open to industrial applications in regenerative medicine. Kawasaki's closeness to the Tokyo Metropolitan area, with over 40 million people ('one-third of Japan'), it was pointed out, made for attractive access to many patients in a super-ageing society. Conveniently, it was equipped with a Life Innovation Centre (LIC) with a large hospital network counting 15 hospitals and 7,900 beds, and possibilities for integration with other advanced medical technologies. Finally, the Kanagawa Centre for Clinical Research and Strategy boasted PMDA connections that could facilitate early clinical trial permissions. To reassure the audience of its global status, a number of MOUs were mentioned, including with Singapore, various states in the US, France, Germany, Finland, the UK and the World Health Organization.

The British counterparts showcased a similarly long list of attractions, including the Cell and Gene Therapy Catapult, government support for clinical translation in product development and an incubator facility. Representatives of both countries used the occasion to negotiate deals by making use of the regulatory, infrastructural and other 'attractive' features of both countries, including the nature of their patient pools, insurance systems and connections with regulatory institutions.

In the 2000s, many countries, including India, China and Thailand, put great efforts into creating regulation that was at least acceptable to collaborators in 'the West' by developing new regulatory institutions and through regulatory adjustment. But after Japan's 'deregulation', the tables were turned, and companies all over the world started to call for deregulation 'at home' (see Sleeboom-Faulkner, 2025: Ch 8) and tried to find ways to collaborate with Japanese companies. In March 2019, following

Japan and other countries, India published the New Drugs and Clinical Trial Rules, bringing all 'more than minimally manipulated' stem cells as well as stem cell-based products under the Drugs and Cosmetics Act of 1940 (Singh, 2018). The amended regulation both facilitates clinical trials and clinical service providers. On the one hand, it provides for the combination of Phase I and II clinical trials, and it allows conditional approval of cell-based products for unmet needs, if the process or product shows demonstrable safety and efficacy characteristics (Ministry of Health and Family Welfare, 2019, cited in Mathen and Sinnappah-Kang, 2020). On the other hand, it allowed clinical service providers of minimally manipulated stem cell-based therapies to continue their administration in patients, with little oversight. B.N. Manohar, CEO of the company Stempeutics, explained why his company decided to approach the company Novumcella to get approval from the PMDA (Pharmaceutical and Medical Devices Agency) for the commercialisation of its Stempeucel® product for Buerger's Disease:

> Japan is showing a great leadership in innovating regulatory framework for regenerative medicine there by addressing major unmet medical needs faster. The new regenerative medicine law implemented in Japan allows conditional approval of stem cell products thereby enabling more rapid entry into the Japanese market. We would like to leverage this new framework for rapid development of Stempeucel®, a product based on cultured adult allogeneic MSC stromal cells product for the benefits of the patients in Japan in collaboration with Novumcella.
>
> *(Expresspharma, 2020)*

In short, deregulation in Japan turned out to be a major attractor for potential foreign collaborators and, at least, a short-term stimulant for investment by industry into the area of regenerative medicine and its accompanying infrastructural requirements.

8.4 Discussion

Although international science collaboration is crucial to the global dynamics of the development of scientific innovation, its benefits have not usually been queried. Above, I have shown how, under global capitalism, regulatory and other differences encourage collaborations characterised by inequality. I also indicated that collaborations incentivised by regulatory competition foreseeably fail to protect patients and the quality of scientific research.

Examples of international science collaborations with LMICs, which often have small research and health budgets, were driven by relations of dependence. We saw in the first example of ZCRM that, in the name of charity, experimental research was done in India, mainly enabled by regulatory discrepancies and differences in wealth and healthcare provision. In the second example, regulatory discrepancies, differences in the availability of pools of patients and scientific expertise incentivised the same company to create so-called 'hub and spoke' networks of collaborations based on 'strategic linking'. Through strategies of linking, the 'hub' managed to create relations of dependence, while risks and responsibility for the provided stem cell interventions were passed on to the 'partners'. The third example showed how, even though there are convergences in interest in international science collaborations based on inequalities, there are also conflicts of interests whereby the wishes of the dependent partner receive little attention. It became clear that all partners, including those in government positions, were aware of the opportune nature of regulatory discrepancies, turning regulation into regulatory capital. The fourth example showed how governments themselves turn regulatory competition into a policymaking tool to stimulate international collaboration and investment.

But taking advantage of regulatory differences for the sake of financial or economic advantage is a way of avoiding regulation that purportedly protects patients and scientific research quality. Suboptimal regulation and its violation, as many critics have pointed out, carry high risk, played out on the bodies of patients and their financial means, while failing to protect the quality of scientific research. Universities, governments and companies have no business in breaching the trust in the principles that regulation is based on, not even in the name of the 'drug lag' (Wardell, 1973; Sipp and Sleeboom-Faulkner, 2019). But, unfortunately, the primacy of competition is part and parcel of the current world order of regulatory capitalism.

Rather than addressing the most urgent medical and public health needs, governments hope to find medicines that might replenish their economic budgets. As shown above, collaborative partners from LMICs that jump on the bandwagon of translational research through international science collaborations can find themselves in a position of dependence, which can be expensive, decrease their freedom of research and may usurp budgets needed to deal with primary healthcare and more addressable medical conditions. Rather than aiming for high-tech solutions by taking advantage of the rules meant to protect patients and science quality, more attention for preventative measures may be cheaper and more sustainable in the long run; and, rather than trying to 'offer' scientific research in countries that cannot afford the high-tech and regulation available to the rich, an approach more modestly aiming for basic healthcare, disease prevention and local needs could address health in more meaningful ways (Farmer, 2004; Ten Have, 2022).

A 'mode of attention' focused on competition, selfish interest, winning, not lagging behind, promise and bringing salvation through miracle cure seems to lose rationale and human proportion, considering that the huge investments into regenerative medicine, so far, have yielded little in return (Cossu et al., 2018), and are inappropriate considering the problems that can be addressed with little funding through basic healthcare and more sustainable modes of living. In other words, science collaboration needs to be refocused, away from converging self-interests, and towards the interests of the sustainability of the local community.

Considering the risk of harm as a result of regulatory competition, such refocusing of biomedicine needs to be placed on the research agenda. Investigation should focus, first, on the aims and conditions of international science collaborations; second, on the relations of power and dependencies among partners; and, third, on whether the collaborative research actually addresses the health needs of populations rather than the international competitiveness of countries. Such research should look for the strategic use made of 'regulatory discrepancies', the 'strategic linking' with unequal collaborators, and the use made of regulation as 'capital' in its negotiation. Where we suspect that regulatory change serves 'regulatory competition', we need to be vigilant about the signs of 'regulatory violence', i.e. foreseeable harm to patients and scientific research, which can occur on the levels of individual researchers, universities, hospitals, industry and state and international levels.

Although various case studies of international science collaboration have been explored in detail (Sleeboom-Faulkner, 2025), given the importance of regulatory capitalism (Levi-Faur, 2005; Braithwaite, 2008), research into collaborations in other fields of biomedicine, such as genome editing, immuno-cancer therapy and immunotherapy, is likely to yield more insight into the global dynamics of regulatory experimentation with health. Such an approach to international science collaboration would presume that, under global capitalism, the coordination of interests in international science collaboration thrives on and produces conflict and inequality. Furthermore, under regulatory capitalism, collaboration can bind actors in different jurisdictions, *especially* when regulations diverge. The kinds of collaborations regulatory differences afford usually violate the spirit or actual intentions of regulation in one or more of the jurisdictions involved and tend to entail further inequalities.

To gain further insight into the research area, a multi-sited approach to connections and inequalities of collaborative networks can identify and reveal the functions that these links have to and for research collaborations. This would involve internet research and ethnographic research, but also conversations with the collaborating partners themselves and their competitors. Realising that inequality encourages collaborative exchanges could facilitate the exploration of what the shared and diverging interests and needs of partners are. Inequalities here do not just refer to regulatory discrepancies, but also to differences in infrastructures and production resources, including scientific and medical expertise, financial capital, healthcare provision and insurance systems. Keeping in mind that science collaboration is not simply a question of pooling assets and bundling efforts to achieve a shared scientific goal is crucial. Future research needs to involve a scrutinisation of how socio-economic, political and regulatory conditions enable available resources to be used to satisfy a range of goals, many of which may not be shared. Regulation from this angle is a form of capital negotiated, not just between institutions, but also between regulatory jurisdictions and polities.

Notes

1. This chapter draws heavily on my research monograph (Sleeboom-Faulkner, 2025).
2. This example draws on Sleeboom-Faulkner and Patra (2011) and Sleeboom-Faulkner (2025: Ch 3).

3. This example draws on Sleeboom-Faulkner and Patra (2011) and Patra and Sleeboom-Faulkner (2017).
4. The citation and reference have been slightly altered.
5. This example draws on Sleeboom-Faulkner (2025: Ch 5).
6. This example draws on Sleeboom-Faulkner (2019), Sipp and Sleeboom-Faulkner (2019) and Sleeboom-Faulkner (2025: Ch 8).

References

Anon (2023) End the glaring inequity in international science collaborations. *Nature*, 20 December 2023. https://www.nature.com/articles/d41586-023-04022-1

Athersys (2016) Healios and Athersys enter into regenerative medicine partnership for treatment of stroke using MultiStem(R) Therapy. Press Release, 8 January 2016. https://www.athersys.com/investors/press-releases/press-release-details/2016/Healios-and-Athersys-Enter-Into-Regenerative-Medicine-Partnership-for-Treatment-of-Stroke-Using-MultiStemR-Therapy/default.aspx

Bianco, P. and Sipp, D. (2014) Sell help not hope. *Nature*, 510, 336–337.

Birch, K. (2016) Rethinking value in the bio-economy: Finance, assetization and the management of value. *Social Studies of Science*, *42*(3). https://doi.org/10.1177/0162243916661633

Braithwaite, J. (2008) *Regulatory Capitalism: How it Works, Ideas for Making it Work Better.* Cheltenham and Northampton: Edward Elgar Publishing.

Brown, C. (2012) Stem cell tourism poses risk. *CMAJ*, *184*(2), E121–E122.

Brown, N. (2003) Hope against hype – Accountability in biopasts, presents and futures. *Science and Technology Studies*, *16*(2), 3–21.

Bufacchi, V. (2005) Two concepts of violence. *Political Studies Review*, *3*(2), 193–204.

Chulalongkorn University (2013) HRH Princess Maha Chakri Sirindhorn presided over grand opening for robotic stem cell processing laboratory at Faculty of Medicine, 8 October 2013. http://www.chula.ac.th/en/archive/681 (No longer available. Last visited 20/06/2015.)

Cossu, G., Birchall, M., Brown, T., De Coppi, P., Culme-Seymour, E., Gibbon, S., Hitchcock, J., Mason, C. et al. (2018) Lancet Commission: Stem cells and regenerative medicine. *The Lancet*, *391*, 883–910.

Cynata Therapeutics (2016) Proactive: Cynata Therapeutics and Japan's Regience K.K. in stem cell alliance. https://www.proactiveinvestors.co.uk/companies/news/135034/cynata-therapeutics-and-japans-regience-kk-in-stem-cell-alliance-67327.html

Cyranoski, D., Sipp, D., Malik, S. and Rasko, J. (2023) Too little too soon: Japan's experiment in regenerative medicine regulation. *Cell Stem Cell*, *30*(7), 913–916.

Cytori (2015) Japanese approval trial for stress urinary incontinence using Cytori Therapeutics, Inc. cell therapy announced. https://www.biospace.com/article/releases/japanese-approval-trial-for-stress-urinary-incontinence-using-cytori-therapeutics-inc-cell-therapy-announced-/

Demouchel, P. (2017) Acting together in dis-harmony. Cooperating to conflict and cooperation in conflict. *Studi Di Sociologia*, *4*, 303–318.

Densford, F. (2016) MassDevice. http://www.massdevice.com/avita-medical-eyes-japan-south-korea-for-recell/

Expresspharma (2020) Stempeutics India and Novumcella Japan to work on development co-operation of Stempeucel product for Japanese market. *Expresspharma*, 1 June 2020. https://www.expresspharma.in/stempeutics-india-and-novumcella-japan-to-work-on-development-co-operation-of-stempeucel-product-for-japanese-market/

Farmer, P. (2004) *Pathologies of Power.* Berkeley: University of California Press.

Girard, R. (1965) *Deceit, Desire and the Novel: Self and Other in Literary Structure* (Y. Ferrero, trs.). Baltimore: Johns Hopkins University Press.
Headquarters for Health Policy (2014) The plan for promotion of medical research policy. http://www.kantei.go.jp/jp/singi/kenkouiryou/en/pdf/plan.pdf
ICMR-DBT (Indian Council of Medical Research, Department of Biotechnology) (2007) *Guidelines for Stem Cell Research and Therapy*. New Delhi: ICMR-DBT.
ICMR-DBT (Indian Council of Medical Research, Department of Biotechnology) (2013) *National Guidelines for Stem Cell Research*. New Delhi: ICMR-DBT.
Jahan, S. and Mahmud, A.S. (2024) What is capitalism. IMF. https://www.imf.org/en/Publications/fandd/issues/Series/Back-to-Basics/Capitalism
JSTA (2015) Research Center Network for Realization of Regenerative Medicine. http://www.jst.go.jp/saisei-nw/en/
Kanagawa Prefecture (2016) Life innovation in Keihin coastal areas. https://bit.ly/3S3iTDn (No longer available. Last visited: 03/01/2024.)
Kiatpongsan, S. and Sipp, D. (2008) Offshore stem cell treatments. *Nature Reports Stem Cells*. https://www.nature.com/articles/stemcells.2008.151
Levi-Faur, D. (2005) The global diffusion of regulatory capitalism. *The Annals of the American Academy of Political and Social Science*, 598, 12–32.
Mathen, C. and Sinnappah-Kang, N.D. (2020) Stem cell research and therapy in India: General awareness for the public and stem cell therapy providers. *CHRISMED*, *7*(2), 90–94. https://journals.lww.com/chri/Fulltext/2020/07020/Stem_Cell_Research_and_Therapy_in_India__General.2.aspx
McGilchrist, I. (2012) *The Master and His Emissary: The Divided Brain and the Making of the Western World*. New Haven and London: Yale University Press.
McMahon, D. and Thorsteinsdóttir, H. (2010) Regulations are needed for stem cell tourism: Insights from China. *The American Journal of Bioethics*, *10*(5), 34–36.
MoHLW (2012) *Kakuseiteki Yiryōhin-yiryōkikai sōsakushutsu no tame no 5 ka nen senryō wo harikaete* (Outline of a Five-Year Strategy for the Innovation of Drugs and Medical Devices (materials 2)).
Montague, J. (2019) The 'unwarranted hype' of stem cell therapies. BBC *Future*, 21 August 2019. https://www.bbc.com/future/article/20190819-the-unwarranted-hype-of-stem-cell-therapies-for-autism-ms
NEDO (2013) *Saisei saibō iryō gijutsu oyobi seizō infura saiteki-ka no kenkyū kaihatsu* (Research and development of regenerative therapy, technology and the optimization of the manufacturing infrastructure). https://www.nedo.go.jp/content/100873753.pdf)
NEDO (2015) NEDO project activities. https://www.nedo.go.jp/english/introducing_pja.html
O'Kelly, M.E. (1998) A geographer's analysis of hub-and-spoke networks. *Journal of Transport Geography*, *6*(3), 171–186.
Patra, P.K. and Sleeboom-Faulkner, M. (2017) Bionetworking and strategic linking between India and Japan: How clinical stem cell intervention continues despite new regulatory guidelines. *East Asia Journal for Science and Technology Studies*, *11*(3), 353–372.
Petersen, A., Munsie, M., Tanner, C., MacGregor, C. and Brophy, J. (2017) *Stem Cell Tourism and the Political Economy of Hope*. Basingstoke: Palgrave MacMillan.
Petryna, A. (2009) *When Experiments Travel*. Princeton: Princeton University Press.
Pluristem (2016) Pluristem Therapeutics Inc. http://www.pluristem.com/wp-content/uploads/2016/05/Japan_Approves_Cells_isa.pdf (No longer available. Last visited: 08/02/2019)
Regeneus (2014) Press Release. https://regeneus.com.au/wp-content/uploads/141126-rgs-new-japanese-laws-take-effect.pdf (No longer available. Last visited: 14/07/2024.)
RepliCel (2013) Press release, 28 May 2013. https://bit.ly/4azZVeS
Sariola, S. and Simpson, B. (2019) *Research as Development. Biomedical Research, Ethics, and Collaboration in Sri Lanka*. Ithaca and London: Cornell University Press.

Shrum, W., Joel, G. and Ivan, C. (2007) *Structures of Scientific Collaboration*. Baskerville: MIT.

Shrum, W. (2010) Collaborationism. In J. Parker, N. Vermeulen and B. Penders (Eds.), *Collaboration in the New Life Sciences*. Farnham & Burlington: Ashgate, 247–258.

Singh, M. (2018) India proposes to regulate stem cells as drugs; to require clinical trials, licenses. https://www.indiaspend.com/india-proposes-to-regulate-stem-cells-as-drugs-to-require-clinical-trials-licenses-80799/

Sipp, D. and Sleeboom-Faulkner, M. (2019) Downgrading the regulation of regenerative medicine. *Science*, *365*, 644–646.

Sleeboom-Faulkner, M. and Patra, P.K. (2011) Experimental stem cell therapy: Biohierarchies and bionetworking in Japan and India. *Social Studies of Science*, *41*(5), 696–707.

Sleeboom-Faulkner, M. (2016) The large grey area between 'bona fide' and 'rogue' stem cell interventions—Ethical acceptability and the need to include local variability. *Technological Forecasting and Social Change*, *109*, 76–86.

Sleeboom-Faulkner, M. (2019) Regulatory brokerage: Competitive advantage and regulation in the field of regenerative medicine. *Social Studies of Science*, *49*, 355–380.

Sleeboom-Faulkner, M. (2025) *Regulatory Violence. The Global Dynamics of Regulatory Experimentation in Biomedicine and Health*. Cambridge: Cambridge University Press.

Smith, R. (2021) Time to assume that health research is fraudulent until proven otherwise? *BMJ*. https://blogs.bmj.com/bmj/2021/07/05/time-to-assume-that-health-research-is-fraudulent-until-proved-otherwise/

Srinivasan, S. (2006) Rogue research in the guise of stem cell therapy. *Infochange Public Health*. http://infochangeindia.org/public-health/features/rogue-research-in-the-guise-of-stem-cell-therapy.html (No longer available. Last visited: 03/02/2017.)

Sui, S. and Sleeboom-Faulkner, M. (2015) Governance of stem cell research and its clinical translation in China. *EASTS*, 9, 1–16.

Ten Have, J. (2022) *Bizarre Bioethics*. Baltimore: Johns Hopkins University Press.

Toda, Y. (2012) *Saisei iryou sangyōka sokushin e no kadai* (Issues in accelerating the commercialization of regenerative medicine). Presentation by the Forum for Innovative Regenerative Medicine to the Cabinet Committee on Regulation and Reform, 29 November 2012. https://www.cao.go.jp/sasshin/kisei-seido/meeting/2012/togi/life/121129/item2.pdf

Wardell, W.M. (1973) British usage and American awareness of some new therapeutic drugs. *Clinical Pharmacology and Therapeutics*, *14*, 773–790. https://doi.org/10.1002/cpt19731461022

ZCRM (2024) https://www.zcrm.org/ (No longer available. Last visited: 12/07/2024.)

9 An agenda for research on the biopolitics of testing in healthcare

Alan Petersen and Kiran Pienaar

9.1 Introduction

Testing in healthcare, involving the analysis of blood samples or scans, colonoscopies, biopsies or other procedures, is generally viewed as the first step to medical intervention and/or recommended lifestyle changes. It tends to be undertaken for purposes of diagnosis, risk assessment or monitoring the progression of a disease. However, the concept of testing is rapidly expanding to encompass an increasingly diverse array of practices performed within or outside the clinic such as in population-wide screening (especially for cancer and infectious disease) and for behavioural or cognitive assessment (for example, Attention Deficit Hyperactivity Disorder (ADHD), dementia) and self-care. In recent decades, the varieties of 'testing' have rapidly expanded in the wake of the advance of new technologies of genome sequencing, genetic testing and artificial intelligence (AI), with more and more spheres of life becoming subject to biomedicalisation (Clarke et al., 2010) and the medical gaze (Foucault, 1975).

The practices of testing, we contend, are bound up with the exercise of 'biopower', involving 'the administration of bodies' and 'management of life' (Foucault, 1980: 140). These practices shape decisions about when life begins and ends and who is accorded or denied access to healthcare and other resources. Testing, no matter what form it takes, also carries responsibilities to oneself and to others who may be affected by what it reveals, whether this be an underlying pathology or risk of infection or susceptibility to disease. If testing is undertaken for diagnosis and credentialed experts judge the results to be unequivocal, it may provide the affected individual with the certainty that they need (and often seek) to guide decisions on medical intervention and/or lifestyle changes. However, the results of testing are often ambiguous and individuals are left in a state of uncertainty and heightened anxiety, especially when further investigation is called for. While, at the population level, testing in the form of population screening (typically for cancer) may save many lives and much suffering, it may also contribute to over-diagnosis and over-treatment which produce their own harms and increase financial costs. In short, the biopolitics of testing has complex effects which, we suggest, tend to be overlooked by both researchers and policymakers in societies that have come to rely heavily on health technologies.

In this chapter, we consider the dimensions and significance of the biopolitics of testing in an era increasingly utilising AI-enabled technologies that combine personal genetic, lifestyle and other information to identify and evaluate 'risk' and 'disease'. As we observe, trends in testing are concerning in many respects, especially regarding growing intrusions into bodies and lives, but as the history of technologies indicates, paths of innovation are neither linear nor inevitable. While we recognise that the reliance on testing technologies entails a form of path dependence and technological lock-in (Barnes et al., 2004) where previous technological practices and processes set in motion chains of events with a predictable sequence (Mahoney, 2006), there is always potential to forge alternative, less technologically mediated futures. We conclude by discussing some potential scenarios for testing in the future and identifying possible avenues for research on the biopolitics of testing.

To set the scene, we begin with some brief comments on sociological and other social science research on testing in healthcare and the observations that stimulated our own interest in this field, before laying out our proposed agenda for research on the biopolitics of testing in healthcare. We suggest that future studies should aim to widen the lens of research—which has been dominated by certain concerns and disciplinary perspectives—and pay greater cognisance to history and changes in the biopolitical order laid bare by the COVID-19 pandemic. Features of this order include the increased blurring of the line between 'risk' and 'disease', growing reliance on technological interventions (especially AI-based or -assisted) to manage health and illness and the generation of unintended consequences of interventions undertaken in the name of public health. We illustrate our argument with reference to some specific examples of testing for obesity, ADHD and dementia.

9.1.1 Social Research on Testing in Healthcare

The topic of testing in healthcare is not new in sociology and other social sciences, and we acknowledge the many important contributions made by colleagues to date, including investigations of population-based screening and routine diagnostic practices in the clinic, specifically prenatal genetic testing, and direct-to-consumer genetic testing (e.g. *Sociology of Health and Illness* special issues edited by Armstrong and Eborall, 2012 and Bell et al., 2024; Boardman and Thomas, 2023; Hallowell, 1999; Jutel, 2009, 2019, 2024; Mol, 2000, 2002; Tutton and Prainsack, 2011). Indeed, sociological and other social science (including historical) interest in medical testing and diagnosis stretches back many decades (e.g. Brown, 1987, 1995; Conrad, 1975; Rosenberg, 2002; Scheff, 1963). This work has focused on discrete diseases/conditions or specific populations, screening and/or diagnostic practices and the experiences of those who receive or deliver diagnoses. However, other important issues are rarely or never explored in the literature and we aim to highlight these in this chapter.

We cannot do justice in this relatively short contribution to the wide-ranging issues that require greater research, which include the actors and actor-networks involved in the design, funding, production and marketing of technologies of testing, how different professional groups ascribe meaning to and assess the utility of the tests they deploy in their day-to-day work and how lay citizens deploy tests to monitor their health and/or manage their conditions. Rather, we identify some broad trends in the biopolitics of testing and encourage research on some important questions that we believe have been largely neglected to date.

9.2 The observed rise in testing

Our own research arises from an Australian study that we undertook from 2017 to 2024 to help explain observed increases in testing in a number of contemporary societies. We sought to understand the sociocultural processes that underpin optimism for the use of testing technologies in healthcare, and specifically in Australia's national cancer screening programmes (focusing on breast cancer and bowel cancer) and in clinical practice. (For details of the research and the findings see, e.g. Petersen and Pienaar, 2021, 2024; Pienaar et al., 2021; Pienaar and Petersen, 2022.) In its formal definition, a medical test is 'a medical procedure performed to detect, diagnose, or monitor diseases, disease processes, susceptibility, or to determine a course of treatment' (Wikipedia, 2024). However, while this definition may seem uncontentious, it provides no guide to the meanings and expectations that attach to the use of tests by different actors, including health professionals and ordinary citizens in different settings through time. Since we commenced our study in 2017, testing has rapidly evolved, gaining impetus with the development of genomic sequencing and the rapid adoption of rapid antigen (RAT) devices during the COVID-19 pandemic which, some researchers predict, could potentially serve as the basis for new tools for detecting various respiratory viruses, thereby enhancing global surveillance efforts (Moso et al., 2024).

Many researchers and health professionals also expect that recent advances in AI, notably generative AI following the launch of OpenAI's ChatGPT in 2022, will 'revolutionise' healthcare by integrating it into medical practice (Alowais et al., 2023). AI is rapidly finding application in healthcare, with researchers investigating its potential in areas such as screening for breast cancer (Ahn et al., 2023) and prostate cancer (Satturwar and Parwani, 2024). High hopes and hyped claims are as common in the field of testing as they are in other technological domains, but what is often unacknowledged is that their applications have unforeseen consequences, such as the creation of increased rates of testing and related over-diagnosis (including self-diagnosis) and over-treatment (and self-treatment), often resulting in rising healthcare costs and personal harms. While the hopes ascribed to novel technologies of testing may not be fulfilled in the future, they are performative in the sense of profoundly shaping actions in the present; for example, regarding investment in certain technologies and/or systems and individual healthcare decisions.

In recent years, some sections of the medical profession have expressed concerns about the implications of over-testing and over-diagnosis, which led to the American Board of Internal Medicine launching the Choosing Wisely initiative in the US in 2012 (Cassel and Guest, 2012). In our own research we have sought to bring a wider lens to the field of testing by exploring the factors that may account for the optimistic expectations for tests among at least some medical specialists such as oncologists for certain types of cancer (Soletti et al., 2018) and testing in general in healthcare. As sociologists with an interest in the biopolitics of health and disease and the ways in which medical practices serve to govern populations, our research has been driven by the question: what does the optimism for testing in healthcare reveal about contemporary processes of governance?

9.3 Widening the lens

Funding, influence and scholarly work on testing thus far have been dominated by the perspectives of biomedicine, bioethics and psychology, which is not surprising given the institutional status of medicine and the forms of commentary (and critique) on its practices that it is willing to acknowledge. However, we believe this bioscientific focus has served to narrow understanding of the biopolitical implications of testing, i.e. how medical testing is involved in the governing of bodies and the management of life itself via, among other processes, its role in shaping diagnosis and determining access to limited healthcare resources. Social science scholarship has offered valuable sociohistorical perspectives on the development of testing technologies and the social and political impact of particular regimes of testing (notable examples include Rapp's (1999, 2014) influential research on the reproductive technology of amniocentesis and its consequences for pregnant women and their foetuses, Nicolson and Fleming's (2013) social history of obstetric ultrasound imaging and Rothman's (1997) prescient analysis of the role of medical technology in producing the inequities in American healthcare policy that mean the poorest citizens have no access to health insurance). While this research provides important insights into the sociohistorical development and consequences of specific technologies of testing, we suggest that future work could usefully build on this literature to explore a wider range of technologies and advances in medical testing, focusing on their implications for social and biopolitical life (Marres and Stark, 2020) and the governance of populations. Some of the issues that need greater attention in this regard are discussed in the following paragraphs. They include the historical processes whereby diseases or conditions become classified or are reclassified as a consequence of growing corporate influence in healthcare (so-called 'biomedicalisation' (Clarke et al., 2010)); broad and/or imprecise diagnostic criteria that increase the scope to pathologise certain conditions and lifestyles; the increased blurring of the distinction between 'diagnosis' and 'screening' that is accelerating with genome sequencing; the intensification of consumer-oriented healthcare as reflected in the growing array of self-tests available for purchase online; and the contestations that accompany these processes. These processes are often interconnected and their intertwining calls for investigation of the conditions, actors and networks that shape regimes of testing, the kinds of tests that are developed and how they are used in the spheres of health and medicine and, more broadly, to govern populations and shape social relations (Marres and Stark, 2020).

Historical investigation is needed to reveal the 'stakeholders' involved in the definition of diseases or conditions and the issues at stake in decisions surrounding the adoption of certain tests to diagnose or screen for them (notable exceptions that have taken up these questions are discussed below). The contestants are diverse and dependent on the condition at stake, but may include the producers of tests, pharmaceutical companies, researchers, health professionals, and patients and their communities who demand action on 'their' disease/condition. Such interests are evident in the case of prostate-specific antigen (PSA) testing. As medical historian Robert Aronowitz (2021) has shown, once approved by regulators in 1985, PSA testing quickly reinforced the prevalence of prostate cancer and preventive and treatment efforts—what he calls the 'looping effect'—along with fear, among those detected with cancer. Historical investigation reveals how certain paths of technological development become settled (Barnes et al., 2004) and may shape subsequent innovations and investments via a process termed 'path dependency' (Barnes et al., 2004; Mahoney, 2006). Once technologies are approved and enter clinical practice, they very often find newer applications, and early reservations may be cast aside in the light of the newly discovered or assumed benefits of their use. Professional groups may undertake 'boundary work' to defend their preferred technologies drawing on certain kinds of evidence to provide credibility for their claims (Gieryn, 1999).

The historical development of pharmaceuticals, especially 'blockbusters', highlights that commercial influence may shape the practices of testing, particularly via the classification (especially widening) of disease categories and the redefining of what counts as credible evidence. This can be seen in the case of Viagra, for which the 'little blue pill' for 'erectile dysfunction' was eventually repackaged and marketed as the 'little pink pill' for 'female sexual dysfunction', which considerably widened the market (and the profit margins) of its manufacturer (Loe, 2004; Moynihan, 2003, 2005; Moynihan and Cassels, 2005). In this case, considerable effort went into developing a new classificatory system for 'female sexual dysfunction' through, for example, changes to the International Classification of Diseases and a series of (unsuccessful) drug trials, all of which were part of an endeavour to medicalise female sexual response and promote pharmacological treatments (Bancroft, 2002; Loe, 2004: 138–143). Professionals often also play an important role in installing practices of testing through, for example, making diagnoses that fit the treatment they believe is most appropriate. As Casper and Clarke (1998) have shown, in their analysis of the history of the Pap Smear for cervical cancer screening in the US, making a test the 'right tool for the job' may involve multiple actors, actor-networks and strategies, who work together, sometimes over a long period of time, to ensure that the test is successfully adopted with a clearly stated purpose.

ADHD clearly illustrates the workings of biomedicalisation and, specifically, pharmaceuticalisation whereby a purported condition becomes an opportunity for pharmaceutical intervention (Gabe and Martin, 2023). Diagnosis for ADHD has skyrocketed over the last two decades, which can be linked to a combination of campaigns by Big Pharma to market ADHD medications, demand from parents seeking a medical explanation for their child's behavioural issues (Singh, 2006) and the use of imprecise diagnostic criteria drawn from the DSM-5 (the American Psychiatric Association's Diagnostic and Statistical Manual), which is the authoritative medical source for classifying mental disorders (see, e.g. Centers for Disease Control and Prevention, 2024). In Australia, the prescription rate for ADHD across all age groups and genders grew significantly between 2013 and 2023, accelerating from 2019. Whereas the average annual growth rate of prescriptions since 2013 was just under 18 per cent, it increased to more than 25 per cent between 2019–20 and 2022–23 (Department of Health and Aged Care, 2023a).

The number of ADHD scripts and diagnoses more than doubled from 1.4 million scripts given to 186,000 people in 2018 to 3.2 million prescriptions issued to 414,000 people in 2022 (Department of Health and Aged Care, 2023b). The Australian Government Department of Health and Aged Care attributes this growth to:

> an increased use of all ADHD medications with the highest increases found in the prescribing of guanfacine (which was Pharmaceutical Benefits Scheme (PBS) listed on 1 September 2018), and lisdexamfetamine (which had a restriction change allowing use in the >18-year-old population without prior diagnosis on 1 February 2021).
>
> *(Department of Health and Aged Care, 2023a)*

The COVID-19 pandemic-induced lockdowns, along with increased popularity of TikTok (36 billion views of #ADHD as of March 2024) and celebrity diagnoses appear to have contributed to the post-2019 global surge in prescriptions, including for large numbers of adults (for a condition traditionally seen as linked to childhood) and females across all ages (it was previously diagnosed mostly in males) (Hooton, 2024).

As the above examples highlight, diagnostic testing can only be properly understood with reference to factors such as commercial and professional interests and regulatory changes that shape investment decisions, clinical practices and individual conduct. In many instances, decisions are underpinned by the promise that testing will produce a definitive diagnosis pointing the path to treatment or ongoing surveillance; for example, 'watchful waiting' (or active surveillance) in the case of a persistently high PSA test results in men. Through its history, PSA testing has been shrouded in controversy and the benefits of population-wide screening have been hotly debated with concerns raised about the potential for over-diagnosis and over-treatment, which is reflected in the absence of clear guidelines among various organisations around the world (see, e.g. Faulkner et al., 2000; Tidd-Johnson et al., 2022).

Yet for some diseases/conditions there is no available 'treatment', or the therapeutic options are limited. Dementia screening is one such example: it is contentious because there is no generally accepted efficacious 'treatment' or 'cure' for the condition, and the path to testing relies greatly on subjective assessments from the patient and/or their family members or caregivers for whom cognitive decline may be seen as something to be feared and hence relatively minor changes magnified because of fears of developing the condition (Hugo and Ganguli, 2014). Despite this, dementia organisations encourage people to get tested if they or those whom they care for show behavioural or emotional changes. Dementia Australia, for example, encourages people to get tested for changes in 'memory, thinking, behaviour and mood', noting that 'There isn't one single test that tells you have or don't have dementia' and that 'doctors will do several different kinds of tests', which will 'help them rule out some conditions, and get closer to working out what's causing your changes'. It adds, 'The process can take time. Even after testing, your doctor may tell you it's "possible" or "probable" that you have one or more conditions' (Dementia Australia, 2024). Similarly, the UK's National Health Service (NHS) stresses the importance of an early diagnosis, which 'may help you get the right treatment and support in place in good time' (NHS, 2019).

However, current 'treatments' for dementia are limited to at best easing some of the symptoms, rather than 'curing' the condition or reversing memory loss. The testing itself is complicated and lengthy, often involving assessments of behavioural, functional and psychosocial changes, along with radiological and laboratory tests, undertaken over three to six months (Dementia Australia, 2024). Given the optimism surrounding AI, it is hardly surprising that the technology is being trialled for Alzheimer's diagnosis, using data from MRI images and PET scans from healthy patients (Seo, 2022)—the assumption being that, given enough data, the disease can be accurately identified. Perspectives on age-related cognitive impairment have shifted over the twentieth century, from being seen as an inevitable part of ageing—according to some due to the isolation of the elderly and their deprivation of meaningful interactions with friends and relatives—to being defined as a clinical category, mostly attributable to Alzheimer's disease in the 1990s (Fotuhi et al., 2009). Critical to this shift was the coining of the concept of 'mild cognitive impairment', described as a 'transitional stage between normal cognitive aging and dementia', which was devised as an attempt to develop secondary preventive therapies based on a biomedical understanding of Alzheimer's disease (Moreira, 2010: 32–33).

Viewed from a historical perspective, one may ask how did this biomedicalisation of dementia come about? Who are the key stakeholders in the research on and diagnosis of dementia—and how have they shaped responses to and experiences of dementia? Could an alternative history of dementia have been written—if so, what would this have meant for how dementia is understood and addressed? (For examples of recent research that engages with these questions, see Grenier et al., 2017; Shakespeare et al., 2019.)

9.3.1 Non-Diagnostic Forms of Testing

Many applications of testing are unrelated to diagnosis. They may include evaluating susceptibility to disease (preventive screening) or the severity of a condition (prognostic test), or gauging changes in health status (monitoring tests). Formal definitions of medical testing, such as that cited earlier, make references to procedures and their purposes; viz., to detect, diagnose or monitor diseases, disease processes and so on. However, testing may also be classified according to whether it is undertaken by a credentialled expert, such as a medical physician or nurse, or self-administered (self-tests) (e.g. rapid antigen (or 'at-home') tests, monitoring of glucose levels, blood oxygen saturation (pulse oximeter), pregnancy self-tests, or faecal occult tests) and/or according to the instantaneity of the results (for example, whether they need to be analysed in a laboratory (which may take hours or days) or can produce quick results (as with rapid antigen or point-of-care testing (POCT) (laboratory testing undertaken at the site of patient care or treatment) which may take only a few minutes to enable timely intervention)).

Such classifications are undergoing change with technological advances such as 'lab-on-a-chip' technologies, widespread use of smartphones and health apps, and AI-driven, chatbot-based symptom checkers (Arshavsky-Graham and Segal, 2022; You et al., 2023). Increasingly, individuals are ascribed responsibility for self-testing with the advance of consumer-oriented healthcare, with many companies, including Big Tech and pharmaceutical industries, keen to exploit the potential of AI innovations that promise huge profits to those able to 'corner the market'. The COVID-19 pandemic has served to accelerate the shift from reliance on centralised, laboratory-based diagnostics to decentralised self-diagnosis via the widespread use of rapid antigen tests, with potentially profound implications for individuals' conceptions of health, self and contemporary forms of biological citizenship (Petersen and Pienaar, 2024).

The recent rapid advance of POCT would appear to represent a critical juncture in the history of surveillance medicine (Armstrong, 1995) in that it can be performed by healthcare professionals and, in certain circumstances, by individuals themselves (Larkins and Thombare, 2023). This form of testing potentially reinforces what we call 'liminal bio-citizenship', whereby citizens are made responsible for self-managing their condition or risk without the diagnostic certitude this demands (Petersen and Pienaar, 2024). As mentioned earlier, once technologies of surveillance are introduced, they may become subject to 'path dependency', with earlier decisions affecting later ones, and 'lock-in' whereby it becomes difficult to change the general direction of technological development given the investments and stakeholder interests involved. Many examples of path dependency and technological lock-in can be found in the domain of testing practice, including ultrasound and magnetic resonance imaging (MRI), both of which had limited applications to begin with but have found wider deployment supported by many vested interests over time (Blume, 1992). The adoption of tests may have, and very often has had, less to do with proven clinical effectiveness or patient safety than with sociocultural, political, economic and historical factors; for example, cultural ideas about technologies and visualisation ('seeing is believing'), commercial imperatives, healthcare policies, health insurance premiums and pressure exerted by interest groups. Commercial interests have played a significant role in the adoption of many tests, which is evident in the case of PSA tests and MRI (Joyce, 2008).

9.3.2 The Blurred Distinction Between 'Diagnosis' and 'Screening'

As we noted earlier, and as historical investigation of testing practices makes clear, the boundary between 'diagnosis' and 'screening' is becoming increasingly blurred. While professionals may draw a firm line between screening—which targets populations that are otherwise well (the asymptomatic) but may have an underlying disease, risk or 'susceptibility' of which they are not aware—and diagnosis—which generally occurs in clinical contexts where individuals report with signs and symptoms—this line is becoming less and less distinct for various reasons. In particular, whole genome sequencing, which looks set to find more regular application in healthcare—especially following its critical role in understanding the biology of SARS-CoV-2 and its origin and evolution (Saravanan et al., 2022)—promises to provide comprehensive, potentially universal risk profiles covering the entire population for a host of conditions. This predicted intervention into our biophysical lives would seem to reflect a much longer and wider trend in biomedicine, presciently observed by Armstrong (1995), involving the blurring between 'risk' and 'disease'. This phenomenon can be seen as early as the twentieth century in the labelling of hypertension as a specific condition in the 1940s. Identified as a risk factor for heart failure, stroke and renal failure, the modern management of hypertension is now seen as a success of preventive medicine (Moser, 2006).

This convergence of 'risk' and 'disease' has various consequences. At the level of populations, it creates new categories of the 'pre-symptomatically ill': those who are presumed to potentially harbour disease and seen in need of ongoing surveillance and likely early biomedical intervention. Thus, even those who feel well are drawn into biomedical surveillance and intervention and called upon to play their role as presumed responsible citizens in the surveillance of health (Armstrong, 1995; Foucault, 1975) through engagement in practices of regular screening and self-vigilance. With economies becoming increasingly reliant on technologies of prediction—founded upon big data analytics using citizens' personal genetic and other health information—and on automated systems of risk analysis, a growing number of citizens are likely to become subjects of surveillance (Zuboff, 2019).

9.3.3 Taking Healthism to a New Level

This blurring of 'risk' and 'disease' has the potential to radically transform citizens' conceptions of self and their relationship to 'health' and 'risk'. Writing some decades ago, in the US context and before social media and the widespread use of self-tracking devices, Robert Crawford (1994) observed the rise of an obsessive attention to healthy lifestyles, which he termed 'healthism'. Healthism, he noted, promised salvation of the self: a resurrection or transcendence through intensive work on the self by attention to diet, exercise, lifestyle and so on. Crawford (1994) characterised healthism as a political ideology enabling the middle class, who at the time were experiencing an identity crisis linked to falling real incomes and standards of living, to create a distinct identity, 'the healthy self'. This ideology prescribes pursuit of an idealised conception of health that is both unattainable and may lead to an unhealthy obsession with diet and weight (Petersen, 2015: 7–8). If new predictive tests, assisted by AI and genomic sequencing, find general adoption in healthcare, as anticipated by many commentators, citizens' anxieties about 'health' and 'risk' will likely be raised to unprecedented levels, and help underpin a new, consumer-driven economy of testing. As testing becomes increasingly reliant on big data-driven algorithms—that have been found to be biased in terms of gender, ethnicity and other characteristics (e.g. Noble, 2018; O'Neill, 2016)—the potential for insidious surveillance, discrimination and exclusion will increase. One does not need to look too far into the future to envisage some of the likely implications. A recent 'breakthrough' in the form of a genetic test for obesity provides some pointers in this regard.

9.3.4 The Case of Genetic Testing for Obesity

The search for the 'obesity gene' has a long history but has been given considerable impetus by developments in genomics, IT and data science over the last two decades. Research on the genetics of obesity has been used to argue that genetic factors may be involved in 40–70 per cent of the development of obesity (e.g. Herrera and Lindgren, 2010). Developing a test for predicting obesity risk—which may allow health professionals to identify high-risk individuals to be offered timely interventions to prevent or at least contain weight gain through, say, changes to diet or physical activity or the use of medications—has evident great appeal to many policymakers who seek economic efficiencies, using technological solutions to complex problems and shifting more responsibility onto citizens for health and other matters. The idea of a genetic test also holds great appeal among the many commercial interests who aim to capitalise on major health problems such as the purported 'epidemic of obesity'. Not surprising then that the news of a new genetic test that uses several million genes to 'predict' obesity, published in the journal *Cell* in 2019, attracted great interest (Khera et al., 2019). The test is described as a 'prognostic test' whose value depends on its ability to achieve prevention of the condition by providing a warning of the need for changes in lifestyle or the use of specific drugs (Torkamani and Topol, 2019: 519). The researchers drew on data from a previous genome study, that examined the genomes of 300,000 people for 2.1 million genetic variants affecting body mass index (BMI), to develop a single number, the 'polygenic risk score'. The 'breakthrough' promised to enable scientists to understand why those exposed to the same or similar diets may end up with very different weights. It also suggested that individual 'will power' may not be enough and that some may find it more difficult than others to control their weight (Guglielmi, 2019).

According to the researchers, the polygenic risk score has particular application with children when preventive opportunities are optimal and will enable those at high risk to be targeted (Khera, 2019). However, the editors of the issue in which this article appeared offered some important qualifications: there is 'no proven medication or intervention for obesity', the score relies on BMI as a proxy for obesity when there are known to be better metrics to quantitatively define obesity, and the study is limited to only those of European ancestry (Torkamani and Topol, 2019: 520). One issue not mentioned in the original article, the editorial and the associated media commentary is that obesity is heavily stigmatised. Developing a test for obesity has the potential to reinforce the stigmatisation and marginalisation of those so classified, especially children for whom, according to the test's inventors, the test will have most applicability. One reporter commenting on the findings points out, 'Detecting health problems before they start is a major selling point for consumer genetics'; however, people may not recognise that the test is likely to be inaccurate and a poor indicator of future health (Flam, 2019: para 3).

Setting aside questions of accuracy, if the obesity test were to become routinely used by health professionals in clinical practice as part of 'precision medicine'—for example, using genetic risk scores based on the number of risk alleles across all genetic variants to assess one's genetic susceptibility to becoming obese (Loos and Janssens, 2017: 537)—it will likely serve as a tool for genetically discriminating against those classified as 'obese' (depending on the national regulatory regime), denying them insurance coverage and future healthcare for perceived related diseases or leading to exclusion from certain types of employment. Asymptomatic 'obese' individuals might become targets of active surveillance, creating a new class of citizens denied what are currently considered to be basic rights to privacy and self-determination. The idea that a genetic test for 'obesity' could be useful for preventive health is underpinned by a series of highly questionable assumptions regarding this purported problem. It also obscures the role of social inequities in health outcomes and effectively shifts blame on to and stigmatises individuals for their failure to meet a culturally normative ascribed ideal of body size and weight (Houtz, 2024).

9.3.5 The Uncertain Future of Testing and Avenues for Future Research on the Biopolitics of Testing

One of the key lessons to be drawn from Science and Technology Studies (STS) is that technologies, as social products, rarely develop as envisaged. Innovations may and often do diverge from expected paths and are inclined to have unforeseen, unintended consequences. The potential implications of the recent trends we have described will only be realised if individual citizens continue to contribute their personal information to the big data projects that underpin genomics research and consumer genetics, and this ultimately relies on generating and sustaining public trust in the new technologies. Future 'digital healthcare' is ultimately dependent on citizens' *active* engagements with new technologies, including social media platforms, apps and mobile devices that rely on the harvesting of personal data. It presupposes certain practices of the self, whereby individuals use technologies in certain prescribed ways. The Cambridge Analytica scandal in 2018 highlighted considerable public concerns about the collection and sharing of personal data, and a growing mistrust of the Big Tech companies that exist only by virtue of monetising citizens' personal data, including medical data (Petersen, 2019).

While, in the past, ordinary citizens have played an active, 'bottom-up' role in the development of some new tests and treatments—as seen most clearly in the case of breast cancer and HIV/AIDS communities—it is by no means certain that they will play such a role in the future. Growing calls for 'algorithmic accountability', pockets of data activism (with citizens developing their own databases to offer alternative sources of data to those offered by technology companies) and calls for greater regulatory control of Meta/Facebook, Amazon and other Big Tech companies, point to limits on some of the developments flagged above. Given as STS scholars observe, technologies and users are 'co-produced' (Oudshoorn, 2005), citizens may use innovations in totally unexpected ways. If we examine just one sector that is projected to increase in the future, the personal wearable market, while this appears huge (according to the marketing hype of the producers of Fitbit and other wearables), the compliance rate is poor, with reports of a large number of people abandoning them over time because they do not find them useful or get bored with them (Petersen, 2019: 85). If the future testing economy is to be a personal data-driven one, then new ways may need to be found to encourage citizens to contribute their data. The question is, will citizens comply? However the future testing economy materialises, there is a need for critical, sociologically informed scholarship that builds on the insights of the literature reviewed here to explore the biopolitics of specific testing technologies and broader regimes of testing. Such work might be animated by the following kinds of questions:

- How does testing shape social life by calling into being particular subjects and populations?
- What role does testing play in creating new social categories (e.g. the pre-symptomatically ill) and what are the implications of these categories for governing certain groups (e.g. targeting them for surveillance)?
- How are regimes of testing implicated in decisions about healthcare access? And with what consequences?
- How do certain tests function as biopolitical technologies to regulate individual bodies and manage life?

Acknowledgements

The research that informed this chapter was funded by an Australian Research Council Discovery Grant (DP170100504), awarded to Alan Petersen and Diana Bowman for a project entitled, 'Expectations of healthcare testing: A sociological study'. Kiran Pienaar was the researcher for the duration of the project. Parts of this chapter were previously published in a special issue of *Science, Technology and Society*, guest edited by Alan Petersen and Kiran Pienaar. For the original article, please see Petersen, A. and Pienaar, K. (2021) Testing for life? Regimes of governance in diagnosis and screening. *Science, Technology and Society*, *26*(1): 7–23. We are grateful to the editors and the journal for granting permission to republish sections of the article in this chapter.

References

Ahn, J. S., Shin, S., Yang, S.-A., Park, E. K., Kim, K. H., Cho, S. I., Ock, C.-Y. and Kim, S. (2023) 'Artificial intelligence in breast cancer diagnosis and personalised medicine', *Journal of Breast Cancer*, *26*(5): 405–435.

Alowais, S. A., Alghamdi, S. S., Alsuhebany, N., Algahtani, T., Alshaya, A. I., Almohareb, S. N., Aldairem, A., Alrashed, M., et al. (2023) 'Revolutionising healthcare: The role of artificial intelligence in clinical practice', *BMC Medical Education*, 23, 689.

Armstrong, D. (1995) 'The rise of surveillance medicine', *Sociology of Health and Illness*, *17*(3): 393–404.

Armstrong, N. and Eborall, H. (2012) 'The sociology of medical screening: Critical perspectives, new directions', [Special issue] *Sociology of Health and Illness*, *34*(2): 1–150.

Aronowitz, R. (2021). 'Prostate cancer: People transforming a diagnosis, a diagnosis transforming people', *Science, Technology and Society*, *26*(1): 41–63.

Arshavsky-Graham, S. and Segal, E. (2022) 'Lab-on-a-chip devices for point-of-care medical diagnostics', *Advances in Biochemical Engineering Biotechnology*, *179*: 247–265. https://doi.org/10.1007/10_2020_127

Bancroft, J. (2002) 'The medicalization of female sexual dysfunction: The need for caution', *Archives of Sexual Behaviour*, *35*(4): 451–455.

Barnes, W., Gartland, M. and Stack, M. (2004) 'Old habits die hard: Path dependency and behavioral lock-in', *Journal of Economic Issues*, *38*(2): 371–377.

Bell, A. V., Jutel, A., Weinberg, D. and Young, J. (2024) 'The sociology of diagnosis: Critical distance', [Special issue] *Sociology of Health and Illness*, *46*(S1): 1–7.

Blume, S. S. (1992) *Insight and Industry: On the Dynamics of Technological Change in Medicine*. MIT Press: Cambridge, MA.

Boardman, F. and Thomas, G. (2023) 'Expressive objections to prenatal screening and testing: Perceptions of people living with disability', *Sociology of Health and Illness*, *45*(6): 1223–1241.

Brown, P. (1987) 'Diagnostic conflict and contradiction in psychiatry', *Journal of Health and Social Behaviour*, *28*(1): 37–50.

Brown, P. (1995) 'Naming and framing: The social construction of diagnosis and illness', *Journal of Health and Social Behaviour*; *34*(52): 34–52. PMID: 7560848.

Casper, M. J. and Clarke, A. E. (1998) 'Making the Pap smear into the 'right tool' for the job: Cervical cancer screening in the USA, circa 1940–95', *Social Studies of Science*, *28*(2): 255–290.

Cassel, C. K. and Guest, J. A. (2012) 'Choosing wisely: Helping physicians and patients make smart decisions about their care', *JAMA*, *307*: 1801–1802.

Centres for Disease Control and Prevention (2025) 'Diagnosing ADHD'. https://www.cdc.gov/adhd/diagnosis/index.html (Accessed: 10 November 2025).

Clarke, A. E., Shi, J. K., Fosket, J., Fishman, J. and Mamo, L. (2010) *Biomedicalization: Technoscience and the Transformation of Health and Illness in the U.S.* Duke University Press: Durham, NC.

Conrad, P. (1975) 'The discovery of hyperkinesis: Notes on the medicalization of deviant behaviour', *Social Problems*, *23*(1): 12–21.

Crawford, R. (1994) 'The boundaries of the self and the unhealthy other: Reflections on health, culture and AIDS', *Social Science and Medicine*, *38*(10): 1347–1365.

Dementia Australia (2024) 'Testing and diagnosis'. https://www.dementia.org.au/about-dementia/testing-and-diagnosis (Accessed 10 November 2025).

Department of Health and Aged Care (2023a) *Attention Deficit Hyperactivity Disorder: Utilisation Analysis*. https://www.pbs.gov.au/industry/listing/participants/public-release-docs/2023-09/Lisdexamfetamine-review-DUSC-PRD-2023-09.pdf

Department of Health and Aged Care (2023b) *Senate Community Affairs References Committee: Inquiry into Barriers to Consistent, Timely and Best Practice Assessment of ADHD and Support Services for People with ADHD*. https://www.health.gov.au/sites/default/files/2023-09/foi-4507-documents-released.pdf (Accessed 10 November 2025).

Faulkner, A., Brookes, S. T., Donovan, J., Selley, S., Gillatt, D. and Hamdy, F. (2000) 'The use of prostate-specific antigen testing in the detection of localized prostate cancer: Current opinion and urological practice in the United Kingdom', *European Journal of Public Health*, *10*(4): 289–295.

Flam, F. (2019) 'Don't get sucked in by the fat gene', *The Australian Financial Review*, 5R, 24 May.

Fotuhi, M., Hachinski, V. and Whitehouse, P. J. (2009) 'Changing perspectives regarding late-life dementia', *Nature Reviews*, *5*. https://neurogrow.com/wp-content/uploads/2020/07/2009_-_fotuhi_-_nature_reviews_neurology.pdf (Accessed: 19 February 2025)

Foucault, M. (1975; orig. 1963) *The Birth of the Clinic: An Archaeology of Medical Perception*. Vintage Books: New York.

Foucault, M. (1980) *The History of Sexuality. Volume One: An Introduction*. Vintage Books: New York.

Gabe, J. and Martin, P. (2023) 'Pharmaceuticalisation: Origins, drivers and new developments', in Petersen, A. (Ed.), *Handbook of the Sociology of Health and Medicine*. Edward Elgar Publishing: Cheltenham, UK and Northampton, MA, pp. 170–186.

Gieryn, T. F. (1999) *Cultural Boundaries of Science: Credibility On the Line*. Chicago University Press: Chicago, IL.

Grenier, A., Lloyd, L. and Phillipson, C. (2017). 'Precarity in late life: Rethinking dementia as a 'frailed' old age', *Sociology of Health and Illness*, *39*(2): 318–330.

Guglielmi, G. (2019) 'New genetic 'risk score' could predict obesity odds', *Science*, 18 April. https://www.sciencemag.org/news/2019/04/new-genetic-risk-score-could-predict-obesity-odds (Accessed 10 November 2025).

Hallowell, N. (1999). 'Doing the right thing: Genetic risk and responsibility', *Sociology of Health and Illness*, *21*(5): 597–621.

Herrera, M. and Lindgren, C. M. (2010) 'The genetics of obesity', *Current Diabetes Reports*, *10*(6): 498–505.

Hooton, A. (2024) 'Why has everyone suddenly got ADHD?', *The Age*, 9 March. https://www.theage.com.au/national/why-has-everyone-suddenly-got-adhd-20240214-p5f4rr.html (Accessed 10 November 2025).

Houtz, C. (2024) 'Weighty matters: Considering the ethics of genetic risk scores for obesity', *Genetics in Medicine*, *26*(9): 101196.

Hugo, J. and Ganguli, M. (2014) 'Dementia and cognitive impairment: Epidemiology, diagnosis, and treatment', *Clinics in Geriatric Medicine*, *30*(3): 421–442.

Joyce, K. (2008) *Magnetic Appeal: MRI and the Myth of Transparency*. Cornell University Press: Ithaca, NY, and London.

Jutel, A. G. (2009) 'Sociology of diagnosis: A preliminary review', *Sociology of Health and Illness*, *31*(2): 278–299.

Jutel, A. G. (2019) *Diagnosis: Truths and Tales*. University of Toronto Press: Toronto, Canada.

Jutel, A. G. (2024). *Putting a Name to It: Diagnosis in Contemporary Society* (2nd Ed.). Johns Hopkins University Press: Baltimore, MD.

Khera, A. V., Chaffin, M., Wade, K. H. Zahid, S., Brancale, J., Xia, R., Distefano, M., Senol-Cosar, O., et al. (2019) 'Polygenic prediction of weight and obesity trajectories from birth to adulthood', *Cell*, *177*(3): 587–596.

Larkins, M. C. and Thombare, A. (2023) 'Point-of-care testing', in StatPearls (Internet). StatPearls Publishing: Treasure Island, FL. https://www.ncbi.nlm.nih.gov/books/NBK592387/ (Accessed 10 November 2025).

Loe, M. (2004) *The Rise of Viagra: How the Little Blue Pill Changed Sex in America*. New York University Press: New York and London.

Loos, R. J. F. and Janssens, A. C. J. W. (2017) 'Predicting obesity using genetic information', *Cell Metabolism*, *25*: 535–543.

Mahoney, J. (2006) 'Analyzing path dependence: Lessons from the social sciences', in Wimmer, A. and Kössler, R. (Eds.), *Understanding Change*. Palgrave Macmillan: London, pp. 129–139.

Marres, N. and Stark, D. (2020) 'Put to the test: For a new sociology of testing', *British Journal of Sociology*, *71*: 423–443. https://doi.org/10.1111/1468-4446.12746

Mol, A. (2000) 'What diagnostic devices do: The case of blood sugar measurement', *Theoretical Medicine and Bioethics*, *21*(1): 9–22.

Mol, A. (2002) *The Body Multiple: Ontology in Medical Practice*. Duke University Press: Durham, NC.

Moreira, T. (2010) 'Prologue: Preventing Alzheimer's disease: Health, ageing and justice', in Mathar, T. and Jansen, Y. J. F. M. (Eds.), *Health Promotion and Prevention Programmes in*

Practice: How Patients' Health Practices are Rationalised, Reconceptualised and Reorganised. Transcript Verlag: Bielefeld, pp. 29–52.

Moser, M. (2006) 'Historical perspectives on the management of hypertension', *The Journal of Clinical Hypertension*, *8*: 15–20. https://doi.org/10.1111/j.1524-6175.2006.05836.x

Moso, M. A., Talaroa, G., Steinig, E., Zhanduisenov, M., Butel-Simoes, G., Savic, I., Taouk, M. L., Chea, S., et al. (2024) 'Non-SARS-CoV-2 respiratory viral detection and whole genome sequencing from COVID-19 rapid antigen test devices: A laboratory evaluation study', *The Lancet Microbe*, *5*(4): E317–E325.

Moynihan, R. (2003) 'The making of a disease: Female sexual dysfunction', *British Medical Journal*, *326*: 45–47.

Moynihan, R. (2005) 'The marketing of a disease: Female sexual dysfunction', *British Medical Journal*, *330*: 192.

Moynihan, R. and Cassels, A. (2005) *Selling Sickness: How Drug Companies Are Turning Us Into Patients.* Allen & Unwin: Crows Nest, AU.

NHS (2019) 'Dementia guide'. https://www.nhs.uk/conditions/dementia/

Nicolson, M. and Fleming, J. E. E. (2013) *Imaging and Imagining the Fetus: The Development of Obstetric Ultrasound.* Johns Hopkins University Press: Baltimore, MD.

Noble, S. U. (2018) *Algorithms of Oppression: How Search Engines Reinforce Racism.* New York University Press: New York.

O'Neill, C. (2016) *Weapons of Math Destruction: How Big Data Increases Inequality and Threatens Democracy.* Allen Lane: London.

Oudshoorn, N. and Pinch, T. (Eds.) (2005) *How Users Matter: The Co-production of Users and Technology.* MIT Press: Cambridge, MA.

Petersen, A. (2015) *Hope in Health: The Socio-Politics of Optimism.* Palgrave Macmillan: London.

Petersen, A. (2019) *Digital Health and Technological Promise.* Routledge: London and New York.

Petersen, A. and Pienaar, K. (2021) 'Testing for life? Regimes of governance in diagnosis and screening', *Science, Technology and Society*, *26*(1): 7–23. https://doi.org/10.1177/0971721820964889

Petersen, A. and Pienaar, K. (2024) 'Competing realities, uncertain diagnoses of infectious disease: Mass self-testing for COVID-19 and liminal bio-citizenship', *Sociology of Health and Illness*, *46*(1): 242–260.

Pienaar, K. and Petersen, A. (2022) 'Searching for diagnostic certainty, governing risk: Patients' ambivalent experiences of medical testing', *Sociology of Health and Illness*, *44*(1): 25–40.

Pienaar, K., Petersen, A. and Bowman, D. M. (2021) 'Managing risks or generating uncertainties? Ambiguous ontologies of testing in Australian healthcare', *Health*, *25*(6): 669–687.

Rapp, R. (1999) *Testing Women, Testing the Fetus: The Social Impact of Amniocentesis in America.* Routledge: London and New York.

Rapp, R. (2014). 'Constructing amniocentesis: Maternal and medical discourses', in Lamphere, L., Ragone, H. and Zavella, P. (Eds.) *Situated Lives.* Routledge: London and New York, pp. 128–141.

Rosenberg, C. E. (2002) 'The tyranny of diagnosis: Specific entities and individual experience', *The Milbank Quarterly*, *80*(2): 237–260.

Rothman, D. J. (1997) *Beginnings Count: The Technological Imperative in American Health Care.* Oxford University Press: Oxford.

Saravanan, K. A., Panigrahi, M., Kumar, H., Rajawat, D., Nayak, S. S., Bhushan, B. and Dutt, T. (2022) 'Role of genomics in combatting COVID-19 pandemic', *Gene*, *823*: 146387.

Satturwar, S. and Parwani, A. V. (2024) 'Artificial intelligence-enabled prostate cancer diagnosis and prognosis: Current state and future implications', *Advanced Anatomic Pathology*, *31*(2): 136–144.

Scheff, T. J. (1963) 'Decision rules and types of error, and their consequences in medical diagnosis', *Behavioral Science*, *8*(2): 97–107.

Seo, Y., Yang, H. and Lee, H. (2022) 'Potential applications of artificial intelligence in clinical trials for Alizheimer's Disease', *Life* (Basel), *12*(2): 275. https://doi.org/10.3390/life12020275

Shakespeare, T., Zeilig, H. and Mittler, P. (2019) 'Rights in mind: Thinking differently about dementia and disability', *Dementia*, *18*(3): 1075–1088. https://doi.org/10.1177/1471301217701506

Singh, I. (2006) 'A framework for understanding trends in ADHD diagnoses and stimulant drug treatment: Schools and schooling as a case study', *BioSocieties*, *1*(4): 439–452. https://doi.org/10.1017/S1745855206004054

Soletti, P., Sanna, P., Gabutti, L. and Ghielmini, M. (2018) 'Choosing wisely in oncology: Necessity and obstacles', *ESMO Open*, *3*(5): e000382.

Tidd-Johnson, A., Sebastian, S. A., Co, E. L., Afaq, M., Kochhar, H., Sheikh, M., Mago, A., Poudel, S., Fernandez, J. A., Rodriguez, I. D. and Razdan, S. (2022) 'Prostate cancer screening: Continued controversies and novel biomarker advancements', *Current Urology*, *16*(4): 197–206.

Torkamani, A. and Topol, E. (2019) 'Polygenic risk scores expand to obesity', *Cell*, *177*(3): 518–520. https://doi.org/10.1016/j.cell.2019.03.051

Tutton, R. and Prainsack, B. (2011) 'Enterprising or altruistic selves? Making up research subjects in genetic research', *Sociology of Health and Illness*, *33*(7): 1081–1095.

Wikipedia (2024) 'Medical test'. https://en.wikipedia.org/wiki/Medical_test (Accessed 10 November 2025).

You, Y., Chun-Hua, T., Li, Y., Ma, F., Heron, C. and Guio, X. (2023) 'Beyond self-diagnosis: How a chatbot-based symptom checker should respond', *ACM Transactions on Computer-Human Interaction*, *30*(4): 1–44. https://digitalcommons.unomaha.edu/isqafacpub/161 (Accessed 10 November 2025).

Zuboff, S. (2019) *The Age of Surveillance Capitalism: The Fight for a Human Future at the New Frontier of Power*. Profile Books: London.

10 Assembling CAR-T cancer therapies for the clinic: Craftwork, socio-technical practices, and the challenges of a 'process' technology

James Mittra

10.1 Introduction

Significant advances in our understanding and treatment of cancer have been made in the past two decades, with innovative immunotherapies having contributed to this progress. Immunotherapy encompasses a range of biological technologies that modify the patient's immune system to fight disease. There is understandable hope and expectation that these treatments will improve outcomes for patients with cancer. However, immunotherapies are complex and costly in terms of how they are manufactured and delivered to patients, so they face significant barriers to clinical adoption. This makes them an important and interesting focus for a research agenda in biomedicine and society, as they can improve our empirical and conceptual understanding of how novel and transformative therapies navigate the complex and uncertain pathway from laboratory to clinic.

In this chapter I explore how a specific type of immunotherapy – the chimeric antigen receptor T-cell (CAR-T) – foregrounds a number of salient manufacturing, regulation, pricing, and access challenges. I focus mainly on autologous CAR-T, which uses the patient's own genetically modified T-cells to target their cancer, and reveal how innovation and regulation pathways for the first marketed products may have limited scope for increasing availability and broadening access to treatment. Nevertheless, as an emerging and promissory technology, where sustainable R&D pathways and routes to clinic have not yet become institutionally embedded and ossified, CAR-T provides an opportunity to reflect on the ways that novel therapeutic products and different patients' lives are valued within health systems. The current challenges and limitations of CAR-T also enable us to consider the merits of alternative innovation and governance options that might shape the future of the technology.

I also make an important contribution to theory by articulating a conceptual framework that explains CAR-T as part of a continuous biological, clinical, and social process, rather than a discrete and stable object like a conventional drug. Here, I build on Dupré's (2020, 2021) account of a 'process ontology' for biology to illustrate the implications of CAR-T therapy existing only as part of a broader socio-technical system. I suggest that each component of the CAR-T therapy is best understood as part of a complex process within a system of overlapping practices, which includes the often invisible 'miscellaneous care' provided by non-clinical actors (Briz Hernández, 2025). I also draw on conceptual and empirical work around 'craftwork' (Meskus, 2018) and 'modes of bioavailability' (Argudo-Portal, 2025) to illustrate and explain the processual nature of CAR-T and its material consequences.

My main argument is that what most distinguishes CAR-T from conventional therapies is the fact that it can only be understood as an assemblage of multiple and sometimes ephemeral biological, social, and institutional practices and processes; a crucial point when considering its value and limitations. The fact that the patient is an integral part of the CAR-T manufacturing and clinical system – as both the source and recipient of the T-cells – means their variable biological status determines whether the assembly and stabilisation of a viable therapy is successful. This conceptual understanding of CAR-T has broader implications for a research agenda in biomedicine, because this question of ontology and its material affordances is relevant to most biological therapies. I tease out these broader lessons throughout the chapter.

In the following section I explain the nature of CAR-T therapy, provide a brief history of product development, and highlight the current and most salient challenges and limitations. In the next section, I explore the implications of recognising and treating CAR-T as a process, drawing on the concepts of process ontology, craftwork, and socio-technical practices. I also reflect on pertinent empirical work to substantiate the conceptual argument. Finally, I discuss the different modes of delivery for CAR-T and address the implications for access and value. Here, I consider the more practical implications of the processual nature of CAR-T, particularly the need to stabilise the therapy so it can be made ready for the clinic. I also consider the future for CAR-T, and novel therapies more broadly, in the context of how choices about different innovation and regulatory options and the ways they are enacted can promote or undermine equity in access to treatment.

10.2 Background to CAR-T therapy: Product development opportunities, challenges, and limitations

The first CAR-T therapies received regulatory approval from the US Food and Drug Administration (FDA) and the European Medicines Agency (EMA) in 2017, and as of 2025 there are six approved products available to patients (see Table 10.1 for details). All target relatively simple blood cancers (lymphoma, myeloma, and leukaemia) and there are currently no CAR-T therapies effective against more complex solid tumours, which account for more than 90% of cancer deaths worldwide (Rafiq, Hackett, and Brentjens, 2020).

Table 10.1 FDA-approved CAR-T therapies

Therapy	Manufacturer	Indication	Mode of Delivery	Approval Date	List Price (USD)
Kymriah/ Tisagenlecleucel	Novartis	Lymphoblastic leukaemia (B-ALL)	Leukapheresis followed by genetic modification at external manufacturing centre	2017	475,000 (one-time infusion)
Yescarta/Axicabtagene ciloleucel	Kite Pharma	Diffuse large B-cell lymphoma (DLBCL); primary mediastinal large B-cell lymphoma (PMBCL); and follicular lymphoma (FL)	Leukapheresis followed by genetic modification at external manufacturing centre	2017 (orphan drug status)	373,000
Breyanzi/Lisocabtagene maraleucel	Juno Therapeutics (a Bristol-Myers Squibb Company)	Large B-cell lymphoma (LBCL), including diffuse large B-cell lymphoma (DLBCL)	Leukapheresis followed by genetic modification at external manufacturing centre	2021 (orphan drug status, priority review, and breakthrough therapy designation)	410,000
Abecma/Idecabtagene vicleucel	Bristol-Myers Squibb and Bluebird Bio	Multiple Myeloma (targets B-cell maturation antigen) Idecabtagene is a second generation CAR product	Leukapheresis followed by genetic modification at external manufacturing centre	2021	545,000 (per infusion)

Therapy	Manufacturer	Indication	Mode of Delivery	Approval Date	List Price (USD)
Tecartus/ Brexucabtagene autoleucel	Kite Pharma	Adults with mantle cell lymphoma or acute lymphoblastic leukaemia	Similar to Yescart, but includes additional manufacturing step to purify T-cells from circulating tumour cells	2020	373,000
Carvykti/Ciltacabtegene autoleucel; cilta-cel	Janssen-Cilag International (a Johnson & Johnson company)	Adults with relapsed and refractory multiple myeloma	Leukapheresis followed by genetic modification at external manufacturing centre	2022 (orphan designated)	465,000 (one-time infusion)

Source: Author-generated from publicly available information from company websites, FDA regulatory documents, and news sources.

Although CAR-T therapies might appear novel, they build on more than a century of basic research in cell biology and immunology. The nineteenth-century New York surgeon William B. Coley was an early pioneer of cancer immunotherapy through his work using the bacterial toxins *streptococcus erysipelas* and *bacillus prodigiosus* to treat patients with rare sarcomas, and he achieved some moderate but inconsistent success (Russkamp and Zenz, 2019; Singh and McGuirk, 2020). Limited knowledge of the mechanism of action and recurrent risk of infection meant Coley's treatment served more as a proof of basic concept than a viable therapy (Zhang and Zhang, 2020, p. 808).

The following decades witnessed incremental progress in the development and understanding of immunotherapies for cancer, but it was the discovery of T-cells and the role of the thymus in immune function in the 1960s that galvanised interest in targeting the cellular components of the immune system (Singh and McGuirk, 2020). Haemopoietic stem-cell transplantation (bone marrow transplant) provided the evidence that T-cells could induce an anticancer immune response, and this became an established therapy by the 1970s for the treatment of leukaemia and lymphoma.

By the 1980s, advances were made in the biological understanding of lymphocytes and new techniques for transferring immune cells were developed, but a crucial limitation was the inability of scientists to generate enough immune cells sensitive to specific cancers. The discovery that interleukin 2 (a protein that regulates white blood cells) could be activated in peripheral blood cells did enable the production of human lymphokine-activated killer cells in the 1980s with some success. However, the biggest breakthrough came with T-cell engineering, which enabled scientists to create cells with high specificity. These were developed throughout the 1990s with the use of viral vectors, eventually leading to the manufacture of synthetic receptors and the CAR-T therapy. In addition to the six FDA-approved CAR-T therapies, there are hundreds of active clinical trials testing new CAR-T products, mainly in the United States, Europe, and China. Nevertheless, alongside the promissory benefits of this technology there are numerous barriers and limitations.

10.2.1 Scientific, Clinical, and Institutional Challenges

CAR-T is currently proving quite effective in treating cancer using a patient's own (autologous) genetically modified white blood cells (lymphocytes). Combining gene therapy and cell therapy, it is generating hope among patients, oncologists, and the biopharmaceutical industries. However, the promissory value of cancer immunotherapies like CAR-T, as Morrison (2012) and others (Gardner et al., 2017) have usefully articulated in the context of regenerative medicine, is tempered by ongoing challenges of complexity and cost of manufacture and supply. Another limitation is the invasive clinical procedure for extracting lymphocytes from the peripheral blood of patients (leukapheresis), many of whom are very sick from undergoing lymphodepleting chemotherapy and taking bridging therapies to avoid rejection when their modified cells are reinfused. The processes of cell extraction, modification, activation, expansion, and reinfusion present both temporal and geographical challenges, so optimisation and coordination of these processes will be crucial if CAR-T is to become a routine therapy (Qayed et al., 2022).

Although there is interest and potential long-term value in 'off-the-shelf' allogeneic CAR-T therapies, which avoid some of the limitations of autologous treatments by using donors for the source material, they bring their own development challenges in terms of poor immunological safety and efficacy (Depil et al., 2020). There is perhaps less hype around them because they are not currently seen as a viable near-term therapy. The current focus, hype, and expectation continue to coalesce around the delivery of autologous CAR-T therapies. However, there are still outstanding questions facing these treatments, which include: (1) the relative benefits and costs of centralised manufacturing (cells transported to a facility for modification) versus decentralised manufacturing (closed systems for cell manipulation in local clinical settings); (2) pricing and value compared to more conventional therapies; and (3) appropriate regulation and governance for what are 'disruptive' therapies (Banda, Tait, and Mittra, 2019). What this means is they disrupt, or at least challenge, conventional processes and practices for the manufacture and delivery of medicines. This can include clinical workflows, payment and reimbursement systems, and the very hospital infrastructure where treatment is provided.

The concept of 'institutional readiness' nicely captures some of these challenges, which most novel biological therapies must overcome (Webster and Gardner, 2019; Webster and Terzic, 2021). Specifically, 'readiness' draws our attention to the user-side as opposed to the supply-side of technology adoption. Rather than ask whether a product is 'ready' for the market, which has traditionally been addressed through crude Technology Readiness Levels (TRLs) and prioritises the role of the producer, instead we should ask 'how far are those seeking to engage with, develop and embrace an innovative product themselves "ready" to meet the new challenges it may pose for them?' (Webster and Terzic, 2021, p. 189). Here we look at adopters or users of the technology. In the case of CAR-T therapies, these will be institutions such as hospitals and their associated service providers, clinical, and auxiliary staff, as well as the individual patients receiving treatment. Specific clinical specialities relating to CAR-T will include oncologists, haematologists, and immunologists, alongside specialist nurses for T-cell extraction, so there is an institutional cost and challenge in terms of labour and staffing.

Within the scientific and clinical literature, it is the manufacturing, cost of goods, safety, and efficacy challenges of CAR-T that have been the main focus of discussion. On the issue of efficacy, Zheng et al. (2018) report that a significant number of patients taking Kymriah relapsed a few months after treatment, and 30% of patients taking Yescarta achieved only a partial response to the treatment. Furthermore, with many CAR-T therapies the long-term efficacy of single treatments is uncertain, because cancer cells develop resistance to the cytotoxic T lymphocytes. There is also a growing safety concern that CAR-T therapies may themselves induce malignant secondary cancers, which was reported to the FDA in late 2023 and is being monitored (FDA, 2023). As with most novel biological therapies, regulatory authorities may struggle to keep pace with innovation and ensure regulations are appropriate to the known and potential risks (Banda, Tait, and Mittra, 2019). Regulations designed for conventional small-molecule drugs are not always appropriate for these advanced therapies, a point I will pick up on again later.

It is, however, the complexity and cost of manufacturing CAR-T therapies that are often cited as the most significant challenges and limiting factors for the treatment becoming more widely available. Rafiq et al. (2020) suggest the current personalised autologous approach to CAR-T limits the number of patients who can benefit, mainly due to the manufacturing complexities. They argue that the process for harvesting cells from patients sets a natural limit to the number of viable cells that can then be modified for the treatment. Furthermore, the time constraints for manufacturing a personalised treatment mean patients with advanced cancers can deteriorate or die before their cells can be modified and reinfused. Since these patients are already quite ill with advanced cancer, the T-cells that are extracted by apheresis may also be dysfunctional or suboptimal and therefore result in an inferior CAR-T product (Rafiq, Hackett, and Brentjens, 2020, p. 161). This point illustrates how the patient is an essential part of the process for the assembly and manufacture of CAR-T. Both the quality and efficacy of the therapy are partially dependent on their unique and highly variable biology.

Ran et al. (2020) focus on the centralised nature of manufacturing, and related costs, as an important limiting factor for CAR-T therapy. Based on estimated costs for a potential not-for-profit organisation delivering CAR-T therapy in a German context, they show how developing a closed, decentralised system for manufacturing CAR-T within a local clinical setting could significantly reduce manufacturing time and associated clinical costs (Ran et al., 2020, p. 3442). Specifically, a closed system (a machine within the clinic is used to modify the cells for immediate infusion) avoids the need for cryopreservation and shipping, both of which add costs and delays to a centralised process.

Papathanasiou et al. (2020) explain this in terms of a complex supply 'chain of custody', which requires multiple processing and quality control steps. Scaling this process to service an increasing demand for the therapy could potentially introduce new risks for this operational model, so a dynamic and adaptable supply chain must be established. Furthermore, the recurrent process of freezing and thawing cells reduces their quality, so a decentralised system that does not depend on cryopreservation can bring additional benefits in terms of product quality. The key point is that decisions around centralised or decentralised manufacturing, and their associated benefits and limitations, will determine the success or failure of CAR-T business models (Medcalf, 2016).

These time, cost, and quality benefits of a decentralised system should in theory make CAR-T therapy available to more patients, if local clinical settings can manage the additional demand and a cost-effective technology for local cell modification can be scaled out. This approach may be important for achieving greater equity and access, which I discuss in more detail in the final section. However, Ran et al. (2020) acknowledge that for-profit commercial production, which rests on a system of centralised manufacturing, does bring efficiencies and economies of scale that are difficult to achieve in a not-for-profit decentralised setting. Nevertheless, the commercial drivers of the centralised approach will always demand a high price for the treatment and may limit access as healthcare payers struggle with affordability.

Given the substantial challenges facing CAR-T, which I address further throughout this chapter, I now want to unpack the assembly of CAR-T through the conceptual lens of process ontology and craftwork, where the stabilisation of a viable therapy through the coordination of multiple socio-technical practices becomes salient.

10.3 Assembling the CAR-T therapy: Process ontology, craftwork, and socio-technical practices

In explaining his own approach to 'process ontology' – a theory of change generally attributed to the ancient Greek philosopher Heraclitus – Dupré suggests that the properties of certain things change over time and so what we intuitively think of as 'constant things' are in reality more like 'temporary stabilities in this constant flux of change, eddies in the flux of process' (Dupré, 2020, p. 97). The idea of process, which is inherent to all living things, is something that is not constant or static but continually undergoing change. Dupré suggests that a process ontology is fundamental to our understanding of the nature of all living things, and he gives primacy to this element of change. Dupré espouses an anti-reductionist approach to biology, arguing that reductionism only makes sense within what he calls 'closed systems'. Biological systems are necessarily open in that they are always interacting with an external and relatively boundless environment (Dupré, 2021, p. 12). Stabilisation of what Dupré characterises as temporally ordered structures 'requires a range of activities both in the systems ("mechanisms") that make up the thing, and in the larger systems in which they are embedded' (Dupré, 2021, p. 12).

The key distinction for Dupré is that conventional 'things', like most non-biological objects we are familiar with (e.g. a table or a chair), have clear boundaries and are both independent and durable. In contrast, a biological phenomenon is a process which 'is either simply a sequence of changes, or it is an arrangement of matter that cannot persist without undergoing changes' (Dupré, 2021, p. 15). Dupré illustrates his point by asking us to consider an animal organism:

> For it to continue being the animal it is a vast number of activities must be occurring: the heart beats; haemoglobin molecules pick up oxygen; genes are transcribed and translated; metabolic reactions are catalysed; and so on. An animal in which nothing is happening must be dead and probably deep frozen.
>
> *(Dupré, 2021, p. 15)*

Dupré rightly resists the tendency to reduce the complexity of biological systems or processes to the supposedly stable, mechanistic unit of the cell or one of its constituent components. He uses the example of the ribosome (a macromolecular assembly that synthesises proteins) to argue that it is simplistic and misleading to describe it as a machine, or a fixed structure, because its very existence and function depend on a confluence of other processes and entities within which it is embedded (Dupré, 2021, p. 50). The key point is that macro biological entities are not reducible to individual structures or things (a ribosome, a protein, an enzyme, or a cell, for instance) interacting with each other in a machine-like fashion, but a 'dynamic system in which the inventory of objects is itself a target variable that the system is constantly working to stabilise or adapt to varying conditions' (Dupré, 2021, p. 53).

Dupré's argument for a process ontology is mainly focused at the level of a species or whole organism, but I suggest it can usefully be used alongside the well-established Science and Technology Studies (STS) concepts of craftwork and socio-technical practices/assemblages to help us better understand the nature of CAR-T therapies as well as their challenges and limitations. In doing so, I want to extend the idea of process beyond the biological material itself to include the institutional and clinical practices and processes that intervene in the construction and maintenance of the CAR-T therapy as a stable and viable treatment for patients with cancer.

10.3.1 Craftwork and Socio-Technical Practices in Cell Biology

In the introduction to their influential edited book *The Right Tools for the Right Job*, Clarke and Fujimura (1992) emphasise the importance of 'practice' and 'craft' in the sciences, which I suggest is crucial for exploring the processual nature of biological products like the CAR-T therapy and its *material* impact on the clinic. For Clarke and Fujimura, the 'situatedness' of scientific work, that is its geographical, institutional, and temporal context, helps us better understand science and its material practices. They write: 'anyone who has worked in science, observed in a laboratory or other research site, or read scientists' accounts … understand[s] that scientific practice is multifaceted, changing, and highly contingent' (Clarke and Fujimura, 1992, p. 6). The authors reflect on the social and organisational practices scientists use to construct scientific tools that are 'right' for the problem or question being addressed. This involves crafting, tinkering, making ad hoc arrangements, and standardising or stabilising the laboratory. Importantly, Clarke and Fujimura suggest that scientists bring to the laboratory everyday skills, knowledge, and abilities they have acquired in their lives outside of it (1992).

There is also an important element of 'tacit knowledge' related to the craft of science, which Harry Collins explained in his now classic paper 'Tacit Knowledge, Trust and the Q of Sapphire' (Collins, 2001). He revealed how different research teams using 'resonance' to determine the quality of sapphire crystals for precision instruments achieved very different results, and that this was contingent on tacit knowledge and the local milieu of the different laboratories. Clarke and Fujimura note that these craft aspects of science were often ignored because they were considered obvious and therefore banal, but they are now rightly seen as central to the conduct of science and our understanding of it (1992).

These concepts of craftwork and tacit knowledge are particularly important in cell biology, which Meskus (2018) nicely illustrates in her work on stem cell science. Based on her extensive ethnographic study of the production of pluripotent stem cells, which have important synergies with CAR-T therapies, Meskus reveals how cell biology involves craft labour (hands as well as brains) and human interaction with tools and other material objects that are often variable and unstable. Our modern notions of advanced techno-science often obscure this underlying subjectivity and nuance to work with biological materials. Furthermore, Meskus argues that the craft element of scientific practice has been marginalised as scholars have prioritised instead the construction and validation of 'scientific knowledge'.

Craftwork focuses on the 'thing in itself' or the object of craft, which Meskus suggests requires discipline and commitment. The stem cell scientist interacts with live and unstable living material where 'viability' is the goal. An important craft skill in cell biology, according to Meskus, is the ability to judge the 'quality' of cells and cell lines. Because pluripotency (the ability of a cell to differentiate into multiple cell types) is a transient and dynamic state (a process in Dupré's terms), a significant part of daily life in the stem cell lab involves the laborious work of culturing and maintaining stable and consistent cell colonies for experimental work.

In talking about their cells, Meskus's scientists described them to her as 'delicate, easily offended, slow, and picky' among other characterisations (Meskus, 2018, p. 131). One postdoctoral researcher told the author, 'like people are different from each other, so it seems also with every cell line' (Meskus, 2018, p. 131). This humanising of the cells is quite common in accounts of cell biologists and, according to Meskus, reflects an important duality. The vitality of these cells intrigues the scientists, but it also presents a problem when they try to compare research findings or reproduce scientific work, because results are so dependent on the specific research group and their tacit understanding of culturing and growing the cell lines. Here, the local milieu is important, as it was for the scientists in Collins's case study. Meskus claims that studying stem cells involves not only the laboratory set-up and its techno-material extensions, but also the 'attentive orientation and embodied presence of the researchers and other lab personnel' (Meskus, 2018, p. 133).

10.3.2 CAR-T Therapy As a Process Technology: Empirical Case Examples

So, what does this mean for the process ontology that characterises CAR-T therapies for cancer? We can see the practical implications illustrated in the recent empirical work of both Briz Hernández (2025) and Argudo-Portal (2025). In her ethnographic study of Chinese hospitals conducting clinical trials and providing CAR-T therapy to international patients, Briz Hernández offers a rich account of the craftwork and embodied practices that are carefully mediated and coordinated in the production of a therapy. She draws our attention to the invisible translational labour of trial coordinators, translators, and other support staff who provide 'miscellaneous care', which she describes as 'intersubjective practices learned in-between the experience of accompanying trial patients and the interactions with lab technicians' (Hernández, 2025, p. 253).

Miscellaneous care has particular salience in the context of apheresis. Translators and coordinators bridge the clinician-patient relationship by performing both social/administrative and clinical functions. In this dual role, Briz Hernández found they acquired important tacit knowledge from being present in both clinical meetings and supporting patients at the bedside. For example, Briz Hernández recounts that they developed good knowledge of how blood volumes collected from patients affected the viability of the T-cells and used this knowledge to facilitate patient care. By encouraging and supporting patients through the procedure, and using their acquired tacit knowledge, they effectively helped the clinical staff (doctors and specialist nurses, etc.) optimise the treatment protocols. This also helped the researchers minimise negative results that could compromise the trial's success. As Briz Hernández argues, 'the biological material in oncology clinical trials for immunotherapy is scarce and its collection requires the effort not only of patients, nurses, and doctors but also workers considered as support staff' (Hernández, 2025, p. 252). These important practices of support and auxiliary staff are ephemeral, I suggest, because they are often fleeting, informal conversations or exchanges that function as a conduit between the patient experience and the demands of the clinic. Because they are not formally recorded, this translational labour is often invisible, unrecognised, and unrewarded.

This example also nicely illustrates how the CAR-T is a socio-technical assemblage. The treatment and its success are intimately connected to interweaving technologies and social and clinical practices that must be carefully orchestrated, both temporally and geographically, to generate the 'product'. The product itself – modified T-cells of sufficient number and viability – depends on both the variable biological status of the patient and the efforts of both them and the clinical staff to successfully 'achieve' apheresis, which is not a given. The variability and uncertainty of this process further supports my contention that CAR-T treatments are ontologically different from conventional drugs, or 'things' in Dupre's sense of the term. Patients must undergo assessment prior to apheresis because their suitability for the CAR-T treatment is affected by their age, cancer history, immunological suppression status, infection status, prior treatment with CAR-T, and any co-morbidities they may have (Qayed et al., 2022, p. 870).

Briz Hernández's work draws attention to the relational aspects of these advanced therapies, which Gardner et al. (2017) have also explored in the context of regenerative medicine. They argue:

> the meaning of an entity (whether it be a molecule, a technology, or social organisation) is not the result of its inner 'essence'; rather, it is a consequence of its immersion within

> networks of other technologies and systems of meaning making ... the intelligibility of an entity such as a healthcare technology depends on the context within which it is immersed.
> *(Gardner et al., 2017, p. 71)*

From this perspective, we might say the CAR-T, as a processually constructed therapy, has meaning and materiality only in the context of the broader network of biological and non-biological processes, activities, and ephemeral practices that constitute it.

Shifting perspective now from the patient and the clinic to the manufacturing of cell therapies, Argudo-Portal's (2025) research on immunotherapy in Spain uses the concepts of 'readiness' and 'modes of bioavailability' to reflect on the diverse practices and strategies through which these complex biologicals are made available to patients. For Argudo-Portal, 'bioavailability' is a companion concept to 'readiness'. Offering an alternative to the more commercially-oriented approach to assessments of readiness, she reveals how biological therapies are made available for different uses and actors (Argudo-Portal, 2025, p. 277). Her empirical focus is on the biobanking of donor T-cells, so these are allogeneic rather than autologous and not technically CAR-T. Nevertheless, this work is useful for our understanding of process ontology and the more generic challenges of T-cell manufacturing, which depend on ephemeral practices and craftwork.

Argudo-Portal's study, based on two years of fieldwork with an immunotherapy project trying to set up and characterise a donor registry based on leukocyte antigens to different viruses, reveals how the project team sometimes recalibrated its work to create and capitalise on different 'modes of bioavailability'. According to Argudo-Portal (2025, p. 277), there were two modes of bioavailability that the research team were attempting to craft: 'In bioavailability mode I, T cells are banked in donors and extracted for fresh infusion when needed (donors as walking biobanks). In bioavailability mode II, T cells are expanded and cryobanked in a cell bank for thawed infusion'.

This idea of different modes of bioavailability – one for fresh infusion from live donors and the other for expansion, cryopreservation, and thawed infusion – illustrates how manufacturing decisions shape different availability options as well as the 'institutional readiness' described by Webster and Gardner (2019). Furthermore, it exemplifies the processual nature of T-cell therapy by emphasising how these different options depend on a constantly changing and unstable source material (the white blood cells) and the coordination of multiple and relational socio-technical practices to deliver a viable treatment.

The assembly of a T-cell therapy in Argudo-Portal's study involves what she calls 'translational labour'. The researchers performed work to understate the notion of novelty in their allogeneic approach to bring it closer to reality and appear less promissory. The research team switched between the two types of bioavailability to realise both short and long-term commercial, clinical, and technological goals. For instance, the benefit of mode 1 fresh infusion was low infrastructural and manufacturing costs and better human leukocyte antigen (HLA) matching, which meant the product had greater specificity. This was the preferred option when the team had limited funding.

The challenge for mode 1 was to create a full and usable donor registry so patients could be quickly matched to a suitable donor, and the donor (as a walking cell bank) could be made available to the patient. This was a difficult logistical problem to solve, but brought the benefit that transfusion could be performed with little delay. Mode 2, which requires cryopreservation and thawing, had the limitation that it provided poorer HLA matching than mode 1. It also required significant infrastructure to deliver. Nevertheless, it was the preferred option when the team had secured more funding, because this more 'industrial method' through a national virus-specific T-cell bank could be more easily scaled up to deliver greater 'availability' for patients (Argudo-Portal, 2025, p. 289). Nevertheless, Argudo-Portal suggests the mode 1 option, which was not entirely abandoned by the team, demonstrates that 'virus specific T cells do not necessarily require techniques of accumulation and cryopreserved manufacture to be available for patients—these are just additional possible modes of bioavailability' (Argudo-Portal, 2025, p. 291).

These different empirical case examples illustrate how the process ontology of cell therapies, including CAR-T, shapes different options or modes of development and delivery, which brings both benefits and limitations. I will now interrogate further these different options for delivery and address the broader implications for pricing, access, and value. How does the processual nature of CAR-T shape its potential readiness for the clinic, and with what implications for equity and health justice?

10.4 Modes of delivery, access, and value: How CAR-T as process shapes 'institutional readiness'

Scepticism about the promissory claims of CAR-T therapy is perhaps justified by the continuing challenge of cost and affordability, which limits patient access and undermines the principle of health equity and justice. The processual complexities of different manufacturing options and modes of bioavailability exacerbate this challenge. Constructing and coordinating complex socio-technical assemblages and practices to extract, modify, and deliver these therapies at scale remains too difficult and costly. The craft element of CAR-T, coupled with the personalised aspect of autologous treatment, means these products require very different business models and innovation pathways than the conventional drugs to which our health systems have become accustomed.

In their review of the cost-effectiveness of two CAR-T therapies – tisagenlecleucel and axicabtagene – Fiorenza et al. (2020) note that efficacy does not always determine value as measured through standard cost-effectiveness criteria such as quality-adjusted life year (QALY), which has become a standard economic tool for assessing whether a treatment should be offered by healthcare providers. The authors argue that therapies with high upfront costs like CAR-T can significantly impact healthcare budgets if they do not reduce downstream costs of managing and treating disease (Fiorenza et al., 2020, p. 1708). Innovative and more efficient processes like decentralised local systems for cell modification could potentially decrease the costs of manufacture and clinical delivery of CAR-T. However, these advanced therapies also impact hospital practices and workflows, which can undermine 'institutional readiness' and continue to hinder clinical adoption. As Ellis et al. note, the costs associated with CAR-T go far beyond the headline price set by the developer, but also incur the costs of specialised training for hospital staff to deliver the therapy (Ellis et al., 2021, p. 91). We must also acknowledge the costs of bridging therapies, hospital stays, and the time and administrative costs of delivering a treatment for very sick patients with cancer, which requires they undergo invasive procedures punctuated by at least a two-week interval while their cells are modified.

Hospitals approaching or exceeding capacity to deliver existing services may find the delivery of therapies like CAR-T highly disruptive, placing already limited resources under additional pressure. These issues also apply to regenerative medicine therapies as they struggle to meet conventional cost-effectiveness criteria and become adopted by hospitals (Banda, Tait, and Mittra, 2019). This problem of adoption also affects developers of relatively simple and inexpensive antimicrobial drugs. Market barriers to new antimicrobials are partly due to the cost and impact of diagnostic testing on hospital practices and reimbursement systems that are not sufficiently covered by the price of the antimicrobial drug (Mittra et al., 2021). Such barriers create disincentives for commercial innovation, despite the recognised urgency to deal with antimicrobial resistance as a global challenge (Do and Whittaker, 2026). What both the examples of antimicrobial drugs and advanced cellular therapies show is that regardless of their promissory value or benefit, any treatment that disrupts existing hospital workflows and practices, or brings idiosyncratic reimbursement or pricing issues, can find clinical adoption difficult if not impossible.

Recent work in valuation studies, which recognises the need to adopt broader definitions of value beyond the purely economic (Mittra, 2016), challenges standard cost-benefit calculations for advanced therapies and offers alternative adoption pathways for disruptive technologies. This work highlights how value has a strong social and political dimension, exemplified by the recognition within the Health Technology Assessment (HTA) community that the 'multidimensional worth of treatments is significantly broader and indeed at odds with narrower yet high-profile perspectives of value defined by medical outcomes' (Faulkner and Mahalatchimy, 2018, p. 229). Faulkner and Mahalatchimy suggest that an institutional politics perspective encourages us to consider the nature of payment systems as well as the various methods for assessing the value of innovative medicines and medical devices. Their analysis reveals that debates about valuation bring into play different principles and regimes of value (socio-economic, clinical, and ethical), and that these are shaped by the nature of the therapies and their broader clinical and social impacts. CAR-T therapies, I argue, are particularly useful for reflecting on the conflicting views and approaches to valuation, pricing, and equity in terms of access to lifesaving or life-extending treatments.

Jacobson et al. (2019) rightly argue that CAR-T therapy does not raise profoundly new issues in terms of healthcare access and equity, but it does illuminate existing health inequalities. While difficult choices have always been made around availability and access to costly treatments, if we wish to ensure CAR-T is made available to all those who need it or could benefit from it, this perhaps ought to be stated as an explicit policy goal. Furthermore, Jacobson et al. (2019) note that concerns about reimbursement in the United States have left many hospitals and insurers unwilling to cover the costs for CAR-T therapy. Medicare coverage has been highly prescriptive in terms of the criteria it uses to assess eligibility for the therapy to keep down costs.

This challenge of affordability and access in a wealthy nation like the United States has deeper socio-economic and racial elements, which are important to recognise. Ahmed et al. (2022) argue that geographical limits to CAR-T availability – fewer than 300 academic medical centres have accreditation to offer the therapy and most are clustered in particular urban regions – create additional costs for patients who may need to travel to access treatment and spend many weeks near the hospital for routine monitoring. Ahmed et al.'s study, which used a database capturing 95% of in-patient and out-patient billing data for CAR-T infusions between 2018–2020, also explored the impact of race, ethnicity, and socio-economic status on access to the treatment. They discovered that the overwhelming majority of patients accessing the treatment were white (68.7%) while only 5.9% were African-American (Ahmed et al., 2022, p. 359). Furthermore, of 81 clinical centres included in the study, only 29% of CAR-T transfusions were provided to patients living more than 2 hours' travel time from the hospital.

This study, which included both patients enrolled on clinical trials and those paying privately for the therapy, revealed enduring disparities in access to treatment for specific minority groups, even when controlling for income and insurance level. This suggests there is a structural barrier to access for some minority groups. If we want more patients to derive benefit from CAR-T and avoid further entrenching existing socio-economic and racial disparities in healthcare, greater effort will need to be made to better manage the process of assembling and distributing the therapy. Furthermore, alternative pricing and reimbursement options may need to be considered.

Of course, the very decision to regulate and price CAR-T therapy as we do for conventional drugs, rather than say a surgical procedure, inevitably embeds it within a commercially driven system for delivery and access; one based on expensive centralised manufacturing (Chalasani, Hershey, and Gellad, 2020). I raise again my earlier point that a local point of care option of manufacturing might help reduce costs and increase access. However, this does require a different regulatory approach, as the time and costs of going through full FDA or EMA approval make it almost impossible for small public hospitals or academic centres to both manufacture and deliver the therapy.

Alternative options, like 'hospital exemption', where health providers can offer experimental treatments to named patients on a non-routine basis without a licensing authorisation, are available throughout the EU and could be considered as a mechanism to deliver CAR-T. However, these kinds of regulatory exceptions also bring different challenges in terms of monitoring safety and meeting efficacy standards. Furthermore, these approaches do not allow for routine use of the therapy, as we have seen in the field of regenerative medicine (Mittra et al., 2015), so unless they are adapted for the specific needs of CAR-T they may fail to increase access and availability. In the UK, the Medicines and Healthcare products Regulatory Agency (MHRA) has started a consultation on new regulations for point of care manufacturing (MHRA, 2023). This could help clinical adoption of CAR-T and other advanced therapies without having to rely on exemptions, which are limited in scope and have proved controversial. Bicudo and Brass have reflected on hospital exemptions and these regulatory proposals in the context of 'point of care manufacturing readiness', where they suggest the MHRA proposal may indeed provide the proportionate and adaptive approach needed to support the use of these therapies in the clinic (Bicudo and Brass, 2022, 2023).

Beyond specific regulatory changes to help optimise the manufacturing process and reduce the cost for CAR-T, what is needed are pricing and reimbursement options that better capture the broader value(s) that these kinds of therapies engender. A more 'value-based assessment' approach might consider criteria such as the impact of the therapy on the ability to work, or its capacity to reduce other costs for the treatment and care of patients with advanced cancer. There is increasing interest among health policymakers and payers to consider alternatives to crude QALY approaches as means of addressing access issues to advanced cell therapies, such as the National Institute for Health and Care Excellence's (NICE) use of Incremental Cost-Effectiveness Ratio (ICER). However, more radical policies for value assessment and pricing have struggled to gain traction due to the complexity and additional costs that arise when additional data are required to make the case for value beyond conventional and simple standardised metrics.

These issues around value, pricing, and access also return us to the concept of institutional readiness and the challenge of process technologies. To get complex and advanced therapies like CAR-T into patients requires readiness not only on the part of the hospitals that deliver the treatment, but our entire health policy and regulatory systems as they provide the social and economic infrastructure and frameworks that shape the journey of novel treatments from the laboratory to the bedside.

10.5 Conclusion

In this chapter I have reflected on the assembly of CAR-T therapy through the conceptual lens of process ontology, craftwork, and socio-technical practices. I have demonstrated how exploring these kinds of cell therapies as complex processes of change, rather than relatively predictable and stable things (like many conventional drugs), affects broader issues of accessibility, cost, and access. Once we recognise that the CAR-T product is a socio-technical process – requiring coordination and manipulation of biological entities as well as social, clinical, and other institutional practices – we are much better placed to critically assess its benefits and limitations. I have reviewed various options for delivery of CAR-T, and the recognised translational barriers, to illustrate some of the key issues that must be addressed if these therapies are to be scaled up and made 'ready' for the clinic.

However, this requires significant changes to conventional clinical practices and patient-care pathways, reimbursement mechanisms, as well as manufacturing processes. On the latter point, it may demand a move to decentralised manufacturing and a more non-commercial route to clinic. Additionally, the future viability of different CAR-T options will require us to adopt a broader approach to value(s), valuation, and governance, given these types of advanced therapies challenge conventional, and often crude, cost-effectiveness criteria as well as broader regulatory and governance systems.

The conceptual approach I have outlined in this chapter, and the empirical case examples relating specifically to the CAR-T therapy I have discussed, have much broader lessons for an emerging research agenda in biomedicine and society. The switch from relatively simple small-molecule drugs to new biological-based therapies has been disruptive not only to the pharmaceutical industries that had to adapt to this new paradigm of drug development, but also to our regulatory and healthcare delivery systems. The processual nature of these advanced therapies, which are not limited to CAR-T, requires both novel conceptual frameworks and methods. I have outlined the usefulness of the 'process ontology' theoretical framework to help us better understand the unique and inherent features of these new technologies, which most distinguish them from conventional small-molecule drugs. Coupled with established STS concepts of craftwork, socio-technical practices/assemblages, and readiness/availability, we can develop new empirical studies that better reveal and help us understand the different elements of the process through which these new therapies are made to work, or not, in a range of different contexts. Importantly, this approach encourages us to look across the board at scientific, clinical, social, regulatory, and institutional processes, and their interdependencies, as only in this way can we capture the full story of how these technologies travel from the bench to the bedside.

In conclusion, a few key themes are worth highlighting. First, the idea of miscellaneous care, and the ephemeral practices through which it is provided, is crucial to the delivery of many advanced cellular therapies. However, it is often marginalised or made invisible as an important translational activity. Perhaps the ephemeral nature of these practices makes it easier for them to be taken for granted. Yet, to stabilise a complex and variable process, where the patient and their unique biological status will determine the success of treatment, the role of non-clinical staff becomes crucial to linking the patient experience with the prevailing norms and practices of the clinicians and researchers. Second, and following from this, the particular way in which these therapies are currently being manufactured and delivered raises issues specific to the notion of autologous patienthood, given the patient is both the source and recipient of the therapeutic T-cells. This is perhaps quite different to the concept of 'donorship', which would apply to allogeneic CAR-T, and may need further unpacking and explanation in future studies. Finally, through the case example of CAR-T I have revealed important tensions between the disruptiveness of this technology and the readiness of hospitals to adopt it for patient benefit. The focus on autologous approaches brings this tension to the fore, and I have addressed the impacts this has for resource allocation, valuation, and equity. The different options and pathways for future development of CAR-T will need to address these important issues of health justice, if indeed cancer immunotherapy is to be made more widely available.

References

Ahmed, N. et al. (2022) 'Socioeconomic and racial disparity in chimeric antigen receptor t cell therapy access', *Transplantation and Cellular Therapy*, *28*(7), pp. 358–364. https://doi.org/10.1016/j.jtct.2022.04.008.

Argudo-Portal, V. (2025) 'Fresh or thawed T cells?: How modes of bioavailability matter in the study of translational medicine', *Science, Technology, & Human Values*, pp. 274-298. https://doi.org/10.1177/01622439231171972.

Banda, G., Tait, J. and Mittra, J. (2019) 'Regenerative medicine as a disruptive technology: Implications for manufacturing & clinical adoption', *Cell and Gene Therapy Insights*, *5*(10), pp. 1287–1303.

Bicudo, E. and Brass, I. (2022) 'Institutional and infrastructure challenges for hospitals producing advanced therapies in the UK: The concept of "Point-Of-Care Manufacturing Readiness"', *Regenerative Medicine*, *17*(10), pp. 719–737. https://doi.org/10.2217/rme-2022-0064.

Bicudo, E. and Brass, I. (2023) 'Advanced therapies, hospital exemptions & marketing authorizations: The UK's emerging regulatory framework for point-of-care manufacture', *Cell and Gene Therapy Insights*, *9*(1), pp. 101–120.

Briz Hernández, I. (2025) 'Miscellaneous care: Bridging the in-between of translational medicine', *Science, Technology, & Human Values*, pp.251-273. https://doi.org/10.1177/01622439231223787.

Chalasani, R., Hershey, T.B. and Gellad, W.F. (2020) 'Cost and access implications of defining CAR-T therapy as a drug', *JAMA Health Forum*, *1*(7), p. e200868. https://doi.org/10.1001/jamahealthforum.2020.0868.

Clarke, A.E. and Fujimura, J.H. (Eds.) (1992) *The Right Tools for the Job: At Work in Twentieth-Century Life Sciences*. Princeton University Press.

Collins, H.M. (2001) 'Tacit knowledge, trust and the Q of sapphire', *Social Studies of Science*, *31*(1), pp. 71–85. https://doi.org/10.1177/030631201031001004.

Depil, S. et al. (2020) '"Off-the-shelf" allogeneic CAR T cells: Development and challenges', *Nature Reviews Drug Discovery*, *19*(3), pp. 185–199. https://doi.org/10.1038/s41573-019-0051-2.

Do, T. and Whittaker, A. (2026) 'Medical travel for AMR treatment', in *A Research Agenda for Biomedicine and Society*. Faulkner, A (Ed.), Edward Elgar Publishing.

Dupré, J. (2020) 'Life as process', *Epistemology and Philosophy of Science*, *57*(2), pp. 96–113.

Dupré, J. (2021) *The Metaphysics of Biology* (1st Ed.). Cambridge University Press. https://doi.org/10.1017/9781009024297.

Ellis, K. et al. (2021) 'Understanding the feasibility of implementing car T-cell therapies from a Canadian perspective', *Healthcare Policy | Politiques de Santé*, *16*(3), pp. 89–105. https://doi.org/10.12927/hcpol.2021.26430.

Faulkner, A. and Mahalatchimy, A. (2018) 'The politics of valuation and payment for regenerative medicine products in the UK', *New Genetics and Society*, 37(3), pp. 227–247. https://doi.org/10.1080/14636778.2018.1487282.

FDA (2023) 'FDA investigating serious risk of T-cell malignancy following BCMA-directed or CD19-directed autologous Chimeric Antigen Receptor (CAR) T cell immunotherapies', FDA [Preprint]. https://www.fda.gov/vaccines-blood-biologics/safety-availability-biologics/fda-investigating-serious-risk-t-cell-malignancy-following-bcma-directed-or-cd19-directed-autologous

Fiorenza, S. et al. (2020) 'Value and affordability of CAR T-cell therapy in the United States', *Bone Marrow Transplantation*, 55(9), pp. 1706–1715.https://doi.org/10.1038/s41409-020-0956-8.

Gardner, J. et al. (2017) 'Promissory identities: Sociotechnical representations & innovation in regenerative medicine', *Social Science & Medicine*, 174, pp. 70–78. https://doi.org/10.1016/j.socscimed.2016.12.018.

Hernández, I.B. (2024) 'Miscellaneous care: Bridging the in-between of translational medicine', *Science, Technology, & Human Values*, p. 01622439231223787. https://doi.org/10.1177/01622439231223787.

Jacobson, C., Emmert, A. and Rosenthal, M.B. (2019) 'CAR T-cell therapy: A microcosm for the challenges ahead in medicare', *JAMA*, 322(10), p. 923. https://doi.org/10.1001/jama.2019.10194.

Medcalf, N. (2016) 'Centralized or decentralized manufacturing? Key business model considerations for cell therapies', *Cell and Gene Therapy Insights*, 2(1), pp. 95–109. https://doi.org/10.18609/cgti.2016.012.

Meskus, M. (2018) *Craft in Biomedical Research*. Palgrave Macmillan. https://doi.org/10.1057/978-1-137-46910-6.

MHRA (2023) *Consultation on Point of Care Manufacturing*. UK Government.

Mittra, J. et al. (2015) 'Identifying viable regulatory and innovation pathways for regenerative medicine: A case study of cultured red blood cells', *New Biotechnology*, 32(1), pp. 180–190. https://doi.org/10.1016/j.nbt.2014.07.008.

Mittra, J. (2016) *The New Health Bioeconomy*. Palgrave Macmillan. https://doi.org/10.1057/9781137430526.

Mittra, J. et al. (2021) 'Regulatory and market influences on innovation pathways for the development of new antimicrobial drugs', *Technology Analysis & Strategic Management*, 33(3), pp. 283–295. https://doi.org/10.1080/09537325.2019.1634253.

Morrison, M. (2012) 'Promissory futures and possible pasts: The dynamics of contemporary expectations in regenerative medicine', *BioSocieties*, 7(1), pp. 3–22. https://doi.org/10.1057/biosoc.2011.24.

Papathanasiou, M.M. et al. (2020) 'Autologous CAR T-cell therapies supply chain: Challenges and opportunities?', *Cancer Gene Therapy*, 27(10–11), pp. 799–809. https://doi.org/10.1038/s41417-019-0157-z.

Qayed, M. et al. (2022) 'Leukapheresis guidance and best practices for optimal chimeric antigen receptor T-cell manufacturing', *Cytotherapy*, 24(9), pp. 869–878. https://doi.org/10.1016/j.jcyt.2022.05.003.

Rafiq, S., Hackett, C.S. and Brentjens, R.J. (2020) 'Engineering strategies to overcome the current roadblocks in CAR T cell therapy', *Nature Reviews Clinical Oncology*, 17(3), pp. 147–167. https://doi.org/10.1038/s41571-019-0297-y.

Ran, T. et al. (2020) 'Cost of decentralized CAR T-cell production in an academic nonprofit setting', *International Journal of Cancer*, 147(12), pp. 3438–3445.https://doi.org/10.1002/ijc.33156.

Russkamp, N. and Zenz, T. (2019) 'The CAR T cell story', *Oncology Hematology*, 1, pp. 22–27.

Singh, A.K. and McGuirk, J.P. (2020) 'CAR T cells: Continuation in a revolution of immunotherapy', *The Lancet Oncology*, *21*(3), pp. e168–e178. https://doi.org/10.1016/S1470-2045(19)30823-X.

Webster, A. and Gardner, J. (2019) 'Aligning technology and institutional readiness: The adoption of innovation', *Technology Analysis & Strategic Management*, *31*(10), pp. 1229–1241. https://doi.org/10.1080/09537325.2019.1601694.

Webster, A. and Terzic, A. (2021) 'Regenerative readiness: Innovation meets sociology', *Regenerative Medicine*, *16*(3), pp. 189–195. https://doi.org/10.2217/rme-2021-0034.

Zhang, Y. and Zhang, Z. (2020) 'The history and advances in cancer immunotherapy: Understanding the characteristics of tumor-infiltrating immune cells and their therapeutic implications', *Cellular & Molecular Immunology*, *17*(8), pp. 807–821. https://doi.org/10.1038/s41423-020-0488-6.

Zheng, P.-P., Kros, J.M. and Li, J. (2018) 'Approved CAR T cell therapies: Ice bucket challenges on glaring safety risks and long-term impacts', *Drug Discovery Today*, *23*(6), pp. 1175–1182. https://doi.org/10.1016/j.drudis.2018.02.012.

11 Understandings of commercial and open-source 3D bioprinting: The politics of metaphors and metonymies

Edison Bicudo

11.1 3D bioprinting and normalised understandings

What are the relations between technology governance and the ways in which technologies are implicitly (and often unconsciously) understood? To what extent is the pathway followed by technologies shaped by the linguistic strategies used by various social players to speak of these technologies? These questions can be faced by combining sociological interpretation and insights from cognitive linguistics – a conversation that can open up new avenues in future research agendas.

This chapter proposes this theoretical conversation, drawing on foundational insights from Johnson and Lakoff (Johnson, 1987; Lakoff, 1987; Lakoff & Johnson, 1980, 1999) who are considered among the fathers of cognitive linguistics. For so doing, the logics of metaphors and metonymies will be analysed from the viewpoint of 3D bioprinting. In line with points made in a previous publication (Bicudo, 2023, 2025), it will be claimed that technology and scientific development involve not only technical factors but also cognitive processes that carry the seeds of social and political life.

3D bioprinting derives from the application of additive manufacturing techniques to the domain of tissue engineering. Bioprinting researchers construct functional organoids or tissues via deposition of successive layers of cells, embedded in an enabling medium, forming 3D structures (Ahadian & Khademhosseini, 2018; Gao et al., 2018; Garcia-Garcia & Rodriguez-Salvador, 2018; Mandrycky et al., 2016; Mironov et al., 2008). They rely on a range of resources, including: so-called bioinks (gels laden with cells), bioprinters (devices that deposit bioinks automatically), software packages, and various reagents and laboratory equipment.

Biopronting can potentially be used in various scientific and clinical tasks, including the production of biomimetic microsystems (sometimes called organ-on-a-chip) useful for understanding particular aspects of tissues or how candidate drugs act on specific tissues (Knowlton & Tasoglu, 2016; Sun et al., 2020), as well as the construction of micromodels for the comprehension of diseases (Ma et al., 2018). Even though scientists believe that at some point, it will be possible to bioprint whole organs for transplants (Mironov et al., 2008), the technology is at present far from reaching this level of maturation (Gao et al., 2018). However, some researchers have indeed conducted successful studies enabling partial organ transplantation (Noor et al., 2019). Furthermore, the drug-testing potential of bioprinting can eventually reduce the number of animals sacrificed in drug development (Ioannidis et al., 2020; Yun et al., 2019).

As we showed elsewhere (Bicudo et al., 2021), the bioprinting market is still in its infancy, being constituted, for the most part, by small and medium-sized companies manufacturing bioprinters for academic researchers. There has been a consistent proliferation of companies developing bioprinters operating with various printing approaches (Choudhury et al., 2018). A few companies have gained international reputation and success (Bicudo et al., 2021), such as EnvisionTEC (Germany), Revotek (China), Cellink (Sweden), and Organovo (United States), the latter being generally regarded 'as the leading company in 3D bioprinting' (Rodríguez-Salvador et al., 2017, p. 12).

In parallel to these market trends, there is a recent, international, academic-led, open-source bioprinting movement with twofold motivation. On the one hand, those researchers are conscious of the technical limitations of the bioprinters currently sold on the market, and are therefore willing to produce innovative customised bioprinters (Darwish et al., 2021; Engberg et al., 2021; Garciamendez-Mijares et al., 2021; Koch et al., 2021). On the other hand, this bioprinting community is concerned with the high prices of commercial bioprinters (Cortez et al., 2022; Garciamendez-Mijares et al., 2021; Honiball et al., 2021; Lanaro et al., 2021), which hinders technology access. Hence the search for technical solutions aimed at 'reducing the inherent costs for more affordable bioprinting systems' (Cortez et al., 2022, p. 151).

Bioprinting, in these commercial and open-source branches, holds two sets of understandings. In this chapter, we claim that two political stances are thus being formed. It will be claimed that the commercial side of bioprinting draws on the ADDITIVE BIOMANUFACTURE IS PRINTING metaphor, mobilised to set up the scientific discipline theoretically and methodologically. This metaphoric reasoning has to a large degree informed the relations and schemes of commercialised science. Additionally, it will be claimed that the emerging open-source bioprinting movement rests on the BIOPRINTER FOR THE BIOPRINTING metonymy, highlighting a socially or ideologically problematic aspect of the bioprinting discipline. This problematising metonymic approach aims to denounce and oppose the commercialisation of science.

Previous analyses, carried out from a cognitive linguistics point of view, have claimed that political disagreements are motivated by discordant metaphors. For example, Goatly (2007, p. 28) claimed that 'conventional metaphors,' along with the 'ready-made linguistic and cultural categories and the ontologies and ideologies which they manifest,' are challenged by new, 'original metaphors.'

Alternatively, it will be claimed here that today's most fundamental political oppositions lie, not in the differences between discordant metaphors, but in the cognitive *division* between metaphorical and metonymic understanding. Furthermore, it is argued that political dissidence is generally brought about, not by newly created metaphors, but by metonymies that come to be socially disseminated. This interpretation – which points to a fundamental division between metaphoric and metonymic understandings – resonates with linguistic insights coming from Jakobson (1956) and reverberating in the domains of philosophy of language (Bartsch, 2003) and cognitive linguistics (Dirven & Pörings, 2003).

To conduct this analysis, the remainder of this chapter is organised as follows. Initially, our research methods are outlined. Subsequently, the proposed theoretical framework, combining sociology and cognitive linguistics, is explained. The potentialities of metaphors are then reviewed in an analysis of the discourses deriving from the bioprinting market. Next, the potentialities of metonymies are reviewed in an analysis of the open-source bioprinting movement. The following section illuminates points of convergence between the metaphoric and the metonymic approaches. The final section brings some closing considerations, briefly expanding the conclusions to other biomedical domains, and suggesting that the approach proposed here can expand the research agenda for the years to come.

11.2 Research methods

This paper is based on a research project called *Biomodifying technologies: governing converging research in the life sciences*, carried out in the School of Global Sciences, University of Sussex, from 2019 to 2021, in collaboration with researchers based in the Universities of Oxford and York (Bicudo et al., 2022). This study aimed to understand the regulatory, governance, and social dimensions of three biomedical technologies: 3D bioprinting, induced pluripotent stem cells, and gene editing.

In addition to a literature review, this study drew on qualitative interviews with academics, entrepreneurs, regulators, and regulatory experts. With approval from the Central University Research Ethics Committee, University of Oxford, fieldwork was carried out in the UK, Brazil, and Italy, involving professionals based in these countries but in other countries as well. Eventually, 31 bioprinting-related interviews were conducted, as summarised in Table 11.1.

These interviews dealt with different aspects of bioprinting research, development, and regulation, including institutional aspects (such as research partnerships), market aspects (such as marketing strategies and companies' client base), and technical aspects (such as challenges entailed by product design).

For identifying metaphors and metonymies in interview transcripts, the method proposed by the Pragglejaz Group (2010) was used, with three steps: 1. Recognise relevant units of a sentence; 2. Understand such units' meaning in that context; and 3. Ask

Table 11.1 Summary of qualitative interviews

Position	Number
Entrepreneurs	8
Academic researchers	17
Regulators	6
TOTAL	31

Source: Author.

whether some unit (such as the verb 'print' in the sentence 'We are printing cells') has a more basic meaning in a different context, in which case a metaphor or metonymy is likely to occur.

Following the requirements of the Ethics Committee, interviewees and their organisations are not identified in this chapter. Interviewees are identified with codes whose structure depends on the country where the interviewee is based. This is why, although 31 interviews were conducted, some interviewees have numbers greater than 31.

11.3 The politics of metaphors and metonymies

Cognitive linguistics, whose theoretical pillars were initially established in the late 1970s and early 1980s (Fillmore, 1985; Lakoff & Johnson, 1980; Rosch, 1978), argues that language and understanding are products of human cognition, which encompasses the skills with which people make sense of their interactions in social groups and the physical environment. Its main ideas can be summarised as follows: 1. The human mind has no specialised linguistic functions, for the cognitive processes required for linguistic operations are not different from those used in everyday tasks; 2. Linguistic capacities are not purely intellectual, because every linguistic activity (like the classification of objects) draws on lessons learned through bodily experiences; 3. Linguistic operations (like metaphors and metonymies) are not limited to the linguistic realm but are manifested in various human activities; we are not simply dealing with figures of speech and stylistic choices, as these operations reflect deeply ingrained ways to make sense of the world by means of analogies and analytical views; 4. Frequently, these cognitive approaches are normalised to the point of becoming unconscious; eventually, people are fully aware of the cognitive and linguistic operations they mobilise to make sense of their lives; and 5. There is no objective reality independent of people, because entities called 'reality' make no sense without the understandings which people create.

By considering the capacities highlighted by cognitive linguistics (such as categorisation, perception, and identification of structure), sociologists can better interpret high-level elements of human cognition such as ideologies, political motivations, and discourses, which are endowed with structure. 'The key word here is "structure," for there can be no meaning without some form of structure or pattern that establishes relationships' (Johnson, 1987, p. 75). It will be seen below, for example, that key concepts are organised in particular ways when different people speak of a certain scientific discipline, creating a conceptual structure that ushers in a discursive structure.

It is proposed here that social players involved in 3D bioprinting frequently endow this discipline with a metaphoric or a metonymic structuration, as analysed below.

11.4 Conceptualising the field: The politics of metaphors

In Lakoff and Johnson's (1980, p. 5) definition: '*The essence of metaphor is understanding and experiencing one kind of thing in terms of another.*' This is manifested, for example, when one claims that 'The virus is an enemy.' Metaphors link up a target domain, that is, the entity explained or delimited – in this case, *virus* – and a source domain, that is, the entity explaining or delimiting the target – in this case, *enemy*. What connects target and source, or entities A and B, is a set of similarities that the speaker focuses on. In other words, 'metaphorical thinking of a target in terms of a source involves establishing some similarity or analogy linking A and B' (Goatly, 2007, p. 11).

Metaphors are particularly useful for dealing with abstract concepts – such as virus, fairness, and love – as they relate these concepts to more concrete ones – such as enemy, balance, and journey (Lakoff & Johnson, 1980; Sweetser, 1990). Kövecses contended that metaphors are useful not only for abstract concepts but also for concepts referring to 'complex systems,' including entities such as: 'The mind, economic systems, careers, social organizations, relationships, society, and a company' (Kövecses, 2010, p. 155), that is, things, institutions, and relations with several constituent parts and interrelationships. Not surprisingly, then, metaphors have been extensively used in scientific practice, especially for defining and conceptualising novel disciplines.

Additive biomanufacturing (frequently called 3D bioprinting), as a discipline, does involve several devices, professionals, and institutional relations which are combined to constitute the domain of additive biomanufacture. To conceptualise this complex domain, a metaphor has been created: ADDITIVE BIOMANUFACTURE IS PRINTING. Interestingly, the metaphorical blend is reflected in the discipline's name itself: if *biomanufacture* = *printing*, then one can speak of *bioprinting*. The neologism consolidates the metaphor while hiding it, because it covers the blend with a unified word.

According to the main definition given by the Cambridge dictionary,[1] *printing* is 'the activity or business of producing writing or images on paper or other material with a machine.' This definition does not fit the world of additive biomanufacture and tissue engineering where there is no activity aimed at 'producing writing or images'; nor can the use of any 'paper' be identified. Nevertheless, the metaphor is effective because it smoothly maps the *printing domain* onto the *additive biomanufacture domain* via some analogies, as illustrated in Figure 11.1.

A complex scientific discipline (bioprinting) is thus cognitively related to a concrete process (printing) which many people have at least basic knowledge of and physical experience with.

Let us consider three manifestations of the ADDITIVE BIOMANUFACTURE IS PRINTING metaphor. First, the concept of (ORDINARY) PRINTER is mapped onto the concept of BIOPRINTER. The latter, including its component parts, is then referred to with printing vocabulary. For example, the word *cartridge* is used to refer to the containers storing bioinks.

At the same time, some components of bioprinters find no counterpart in ordinary printers, and therefore keep their clinical or biomedical names.

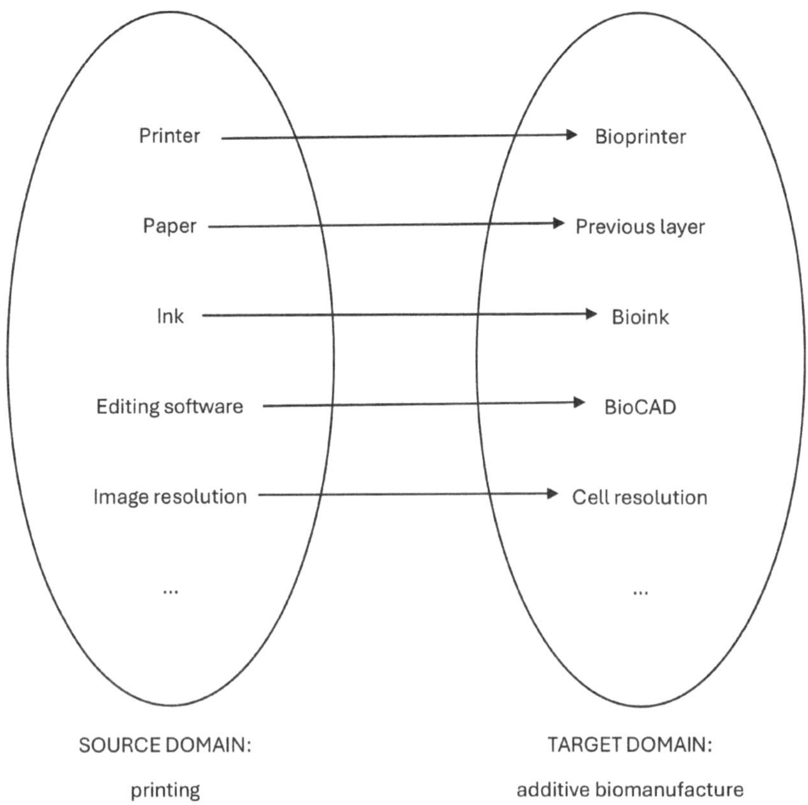

Source: Author.

Figure 11.1 Metaphoric mappings of 3D bioprinting

> A bioprinter is a syringe … It's a hand with a syringe that deposits material where I want it, the way I want it, and in the proportion I want it … If I handle a syringe, I can print with it. With a syringe that you buy in a pharmacy.
>
> *Interviewee 23, research institute, Brazil*

Therefore, normal syringes (which keep their original name) may be used in the bioprinting process for the deposition of bioinks. Thus the metaphorical blend (biomedical domain + technical domain) is corporified in both the bioprinter as an object and the terminology used to describe it.

Second, the metaphor manifests itself in the names used to talk about bioprinting techniques.

> If I want to print with an extrusion printer or inkjet printer, or laser-induced printer, then the material, the bioink material you need, is going to be different, because they are different applications and they require different physical requirements in the ink.
>
> *Interviewee 01, bioink company, UK*

As seen above, bioprinting approaches inherit the terminology employed in ordinary printing – inkjet, extrusion, laser printing – even though such technologies need to be modified for the deposition of fragile living cells. For example, some extrusion bioprinters may have cooling systems to maintain low temperatures, keeping cells alive – while no such system is found in ordinary printers.

Finally, it is known that ordinary printers generate images with different resolutions, the best images being obtained with high-resolution printers, able to deposit tiny drops of ink very close to each other. This concept has also been taken to bioprinting: tissues that mimic natural tissues the most closely are those produced with high-resolution bioprinters, able to deposit cells very close to each other. To a great extent, the evolution of bioprinting depends on the development of bioprinters with higher and higher resolutions.

> A serious problem is the resolution of devices. We, nowadays, still don't have devices which allow us to work at the same resolution, or at the same scale, which is found in [natural] tissues.
>
> *Interviewee 10, academic laboratory, UK*

How can a process aimed to produce three-dimensional biological constructs be understood as printing, a two-dimensional operation?

This is possible because of the way in which tissues are computationally modelled in additive manufacture. On the computer screen, the 3D model is segmented in such a way that the object is 'cut' into slices or layers that are sufficiently thin (for human eyes) to be considered as a flat or two-dimensional object. For this reason, the software used in this operation is sometimes called 'slicer.' '[T]his software … prepares a 3D model by splitting it into layers, also termed slices; hence, the name of the type of program' (Garciamendez-Mijares et al., 2021, p. 21). In this way, the computer instructs the machine to deposit the first layer onto the flat printing surface, as if onto a sheet of paper. This first layer becomes the new printing surface on which the second layer is added. Gradually, via the addition of successive thin – practically two-dimensional – layers, a 3D construct comes to be. This allows specialists to talk about printed 'cell layers,' as Interviewee 24 (bioprinting company, Brazil) put it.

Text-related metaphors have also been extensively used in biomedical domains like genomics and cell and gene therapies. It has been noted, for example, that the concept of editing is central in genomics, creating expressions such as 'gene editing' (Maben, 2016; O'Keefe et al., 2015). If DNA molecules are formed by letters (A, T, C, and G), and if cells can be altered through 'editing' operations, then it is coherent to assume that cells and tissues can be 'printed.'

Metaphors have implications or 'entailments' to use the concept proposed by Lakoff and Johnson (1980). A crucial entailment of the ADDITIVE BIOMANUFACTURE IS PRINTING metaphor is that this scientific practice is framed as a highly accurate and reproducible technique. For example, this is how regenHU, a Swiss company developing bioprinters and bioprinting software, describes its products:[2]

> The high-level of accuracy in material placement when printing using our industrial robotic systems, even when using multiple print technologies in one print run, enables the reproducibility of the process.

In this example, references to printing procedures ('printing technologies' and 'print run') are coupled with concepts suggesting the process' mechanical robustness ('industrial robotic systems'), its precision ('accuracy in material placement'), and consistency ('the reproducibility of the process'). As Interviewee 01 (bioink company, UK) claimed:

> The other thing is reproducibility. It's not just a question of working well once, but in a year's time, when I buy this [bioprinted] product, is it going to be the same product? Because, again, if you're doing research, you don't want material change, batch to batch. Batch to batch variability kills research in this area.

Another crucial entailment of the metaphor analysed here is that in order for bioprinting products and tools to be accurate, they must be developed and produced by highly skilled professionals who tend to be gathered by resourceful institutions, especially large corporations. For example, Interviewee 21 (academic laboratory, UK) was asked why his academic team decided to buy a commercial bioprinter instead of building up their own device, when in-house expertise was in place for such endeavour:

> Of course, it would be much cheaper if we produced our own device, but the quality wouldn't be the same as that of the company, very probably. We wouldn't have technical support ... So we would be acting like amateurs.

The recognition of this academic limitation is frequently matched with a suspicion towards non-commercial products, including the open-source software frequently used in bioprinting.

> [A]t some point, you will need to transmit that patient-specific data from … the doctor to the printer, so therefore you will need some proof that actually you can't ... that cannot be open-access to anybody … Does open-access printing increase that risk?
>
> *Interviewee 03, government agency, UK*

This uncertainty regarding data safety in open-source software, as voiced by interviewee 03, is frequently justified with reference to the collective and distributed ways in which open-source software is developed.

> What we've observed, in terms of open-source software, is that, because development can receive … many actions, many interventions from several users who can modify the code freely, what ends up happening is that the code becomes too complicated and too unstable. When the code is simple, instabilities are less frequent and you can correct them … A package like a CAD [Computer-Assisted Design], which is a much more complex tool, with much more complex functions, would require a much bigger group to do it, which is precisely what you have in companies, but, because of that, they close the package.
>
> *Interviewee 25, research institute, Brazil*

Therefore, the entailments of the ADDITIVE BIOMANUFACTURE IS PRINTING metaphor stress the technical competence required for equipping the field with the precision it depends on. As this competence is said to be concentrated in companies, this approach can be used to justify the preference for proprietary software and the strategies of companies which 'close the package.'

Historically, this view was strengthened by software developer Eric Raymond, who identified two models of software development. The 'bazaar model' is said to be practiced by open-source communities and characterised by spontaneous relations between programmers moved by altruistic and creative impulses. In the 'cathedral model,' generally adopted in companies, software development would follow a hierarchical structure with clear rules and rational organisation (Raymond, 2001). Interestingly, Raymond's view is reflected in his implicit use of metaphors: PROPRIETARY SOFTWARE DEVELOPMENT IS CATHEDRAL, and OPEN-SOURCE SOFTWARE DEVELOPMENT IS BAZAAR.

Nevertheless, when open-source and proprietary software are compared under systematic criteria, open-source is sometimes described as more innovative (Lamastra, 2009), a conclusion that may surprise some readers. Equally, some of the claims and explanations presented above may sound self-evident. These possible impressions point to the social force of metaphors such as ADDITIVE BIOMANUFACTURE IS PRINTING. 'The acceptance of the metaphor, which forces us to focus *only* on those aspects of our experience that it highlights, leads us to view the entailments of the metaphor as being *true*' (Lakoff & Johnson, 1980, p. 157).

Metaphorically created 'truths' are always limited in scope. Therefore, the aim of this section is not to denounce or regret the metaphor's reductionist effect. This has been realised by some authors who, for example, pointed out that editing metaphors simplify the genomics field, giving the impression of simple and easy biological interventions (Maben, 2016; O'Keefe et al., 2015). Instead of adopting this stance, this section contends, in line with Kövecses' explanation, that metaphors always have their 'meaning focus.' 'When a source domain is applied to a target, only some (but not all) aspects of the target are brought into focus' (Kövecses, 2010, p. 91). In the case of the ADDITIVE BIOMANUFACTURE IS PRINTING metaphor, a technical view – that is, an understanding organised around ideas such as precision and reproducibility – comes to constitute the bioprinting domain, emphasising technical rigour and commercial capabilities.

To challenge this metaphorical stance, some emerging open-source bioprinting communities have proposed an alternative, metonymic understanding.

11.5 Criticising the field: The politics of metonymies

Metonymy is the linguistic operation that involves a reference to part-whole relations. An example is: 'The company is in need of new hands.' Here the part (hands) is chosen to represent the whole (employees). The PART FOR THE WHOLE is the most basic form taken by metonymies. According to Lakoff (1987, p. 77): 'It is extremely common for people to take one well-understood or easy-to-perceive aspect of something and use it to stand either for the thing as whole or for some other aspect or part of it.' There are various kinds of metonymic reference (Kövecses, 2010), including THE PLACE FOR THE INSTITUTION metonymy where one would, for example, use 'Westminster' (the place) to make reference to 'the UK's government' (the institution). Another example would be THE SYMBOL FOR THE INSTITUTION metonymy, like in the sentence 'The case has shaken the legitimacy of the Crown,' where the symbol ('the Crown') refers to the institution it symbolises (the Monarchy).

A certain concept can be alluded to by means of different metonymic references. Let us consider, for example, the following sentences: 1. 'The country needs to get more vaccines into arms.' 2. 'The virus is constantly looking for new lungs to infect.' In both sentences, the meaning is the same, but in sentence 1 we have THE ARM FOR THE BODY metonymy whereas in sentence 2 we have THE LUNGS FOR THE BODY. Thus the same whole – in this case, *body* – can be referenced by different parts – *arm* or *lung*.

For the concept of bioprinting too, various metonymic references are possible, that is, various aspects of the scientific domain could be selected for a discussion of the whole domain, as illustrated in Figure 11.2.

As shown in this figure, those willing to discuss additive biomanufacture have a range of elements to focus on: software, devices, reagents, funding, and so forth. Before

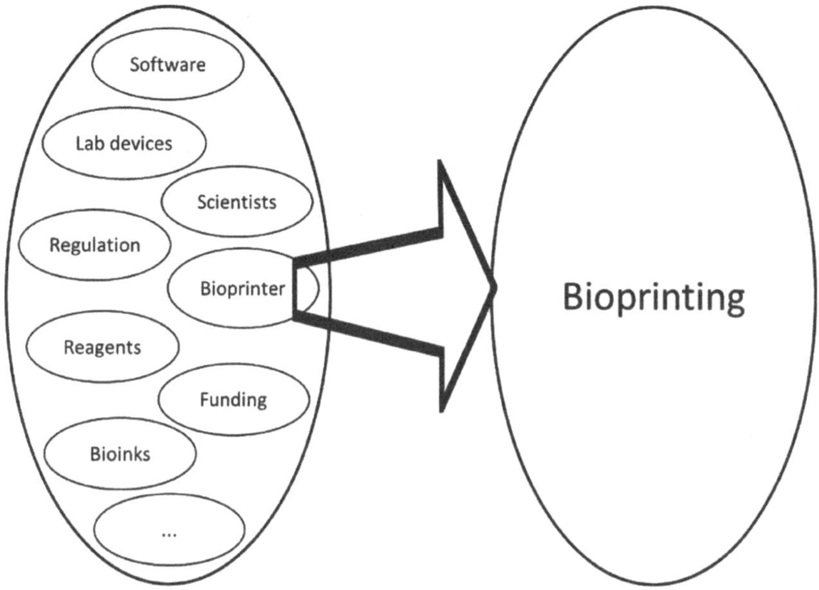

Source: Author.

Figure 11.2 Metonymic mapping of open-source software

those elements, a group of researchers has selected the bioprinter to focus on, thus making a particular metonymic choice: THE SCIENTIFIC INSTRUMENT FOR THE SCIENCE or, more specifically, THE BIOPRINTER FOR BIOPRINTING.

Therefore, the aim of Figure 11.2 is not to present a list of topics that are thematised in this scientific domain. Its aim is to point out that among the various topics that might be discussed by the open-source bioprinting movement, the topic of bioprinters is the one that is metonymically selected to become a reference.

As a result of this choice, all the discussions are made through the topic of bioprinters. This is why the numerous publications of the open-source bioprinting movement – some of which have been reviewed for the preparation of this chapter (Cortez et al., 2022; Darwish et al., 2021; Engberg et al., 2021; Fitzsimmons et al., 2018; Garciamendez-Mijares et al., 2021; Honiball et al., 2021; Ioannidis et al., 2020; Kahl et al., 2019; Koch et al., 2021; Lanaro et al., 2021; McElheny et al., 2017; Reid et al., 2016; Roehm & Madihally, 2018; Schmieden et al., 2018; Wüst et al., 2012) – have, as their main topic of discussion, the features, production, and diffusion of bioprinters.

This open-source movement triggers a political discussion. Secretive, commercial, closed processes are said to generate commercial bioprinters whereas collaborative, open processes are said to generate open-source bioprinters. This approach is concerned with the advancement of commercialisation and the proliferation of bioprinting companies, some of which are gaining multinational reach as explained in previous publications (Bicudo et al., 2021; Choudhury et al., 2018).

Two fundamental characteristics of commercial bioprinters are frequently discussed, and deplored, by this metonymic approach. First, these bioprinting researchers, for the most part based in universities, criticise the cost of commercial bioprinters. It is stressed that these machines have a 'range in cost between $10,000 and >$200,000,' (Darwish et al., 2021, p. 2), a circumstance that 'places them out of reach for many scientists' (Lanaro et al., 2021, p. 2540). Moreover, there is much concern with the situation of 'young research teams especially those teams in the developing countries' (Darwish et al., 2021, p. 2).

In reaction, several scientists have developed some innovative systems, attempting to promote 'low-cost bioprinting' (Honiball et al., 2021, p. 6). For example, Garciamendez-Mijares and colleagues (2021) have designed an affordable system, which for them, is a bioprinter whose construction would range in cost from $50 to $4,000. Other similar examples are proliferating in the bioprinting literature, with reverberations in our interviews, especially those with academic researchers, as well as managers of companies operating in less dynamic countries. For example, an entrepreneur based in Eastern Europe talked about the characteristics of the bioprinters sold by companies now dominating the market, such as Cellink:

> [W]hen we first saw commercial machines, we were like: 'Why so simple? … and why so expensive?' It shouldn't be so expensive because there is no one thing that makes those machines so expensive, and to our belief, people who are buying those machines are overpaying a lot … The bioprinters that are right now on the market … shouldn't cost that much … Well, they earn a lot of money from this business, that's for sure.
>
> *Interviewee 36, bioprinting company, Eastern Europe*

The second feature of commercial bioprinters that is deplored by this metonymic approach is their technical rigidity, that is, the fact that they 'are typically closed-sourced and difficult to modify' (Honiball et al., 2021, p. 2). On the level of basic research, it is frequently necessary to experiment with novel materials, components, parameters, and processes, which is not always possible with commercial bioprinters.

> For example, there are some commercial machines that have only one printhead or two printheads or three printheads, and you need to work with more materials. So the need for working with more or less materials, or with thermoplastic materials, or … with solid materials which become liquid trough UV [ultra-violet light], all of this frequently makes you fail to find a commercial device exactly the way you need.
>
> *Interviewee 10, academic laboratory, UK*

These considerations underpin the emergence of an open-source 'bioprinting research community' (Engberg et al., 2021, p. 2) whose initiatives have multiplied over the last ten years, with a list of ongoing projects being provided by Garciamendez-Mijares and colleagues (2021). Two main features are shared by open-source bioprinters: the publication of their project, making it possible for interested research groups to 'follow the recipe' and build up their own machines; and their technical malleability, making it possible for researchers to use components from several providers. This open-source tactic is gaining force even among small bioprinting companies.

> For us, everything ... is open. You don't depend on our hydrogel kits, you can buy any hydrogel, you don't depend on the syringes that you need to change, because they're disposable. For many bioprinters, different syringes don't fit in, like for Cellink, for example, and also Cellink hydrogels, which are very expensive. With us, everything is open, from software to all inputs ... all the raw materials you need, syringes, needles, everything. You can buy everything in a pharmacy.
>
> *Interviewee 20, bioprinting company, Brazil*

In this example, the metonymic reasoning is applied to companies for the sake of a comparison. In this BIOPRINTER FOR THE COMPANY metonymy, the Cellink bioprinter is described as rigid and expensive whereas the Brazilian bioprinter is framed as an affordable and flexible machine. At the same time, Cellink is metonymically selected to make reference to criticisable commercial strategies whereas the interviewee's company would metonymically make reference to a socially, economically, and scientifically sound open attitude.

The emerging bioprinting community draws on some tactics consolidated by two other open-source communities. On the one hand, the open-source bioprinting community has made extensive use of open-source software, which it also develops with considerable consistency. Elsewhere (Bicudo et al., 2020), we demonstrated that over the last ten years, the number of open-source packages being used in bioprinting has indeed grown more quickly than that of proprietary packages. As declared by Interviewee 34 (academic laboratory, Italy): '[W]e are trying to use only open-source software.' In this metonymic approach, contrary to what was seen for the metaphoric approach, open-source packages are considered reliable products, because of 'the constant updates and improvements that they receive (usually generated by the users themselves), thus, increasing printer capabilities and features' (Garciamendez-Mijares et al., 2021, p. 21).

This kind of claim echoes previous claims from Richard Stallman, one of the pioneers of the free software community, for which software development should be thought of and practised 'in terms of taking a step and realizing that after you've taken a step, other people will take more steps and, together, it will get the job done eventually' (Stallman, 2002a, p. 153). Elsewhere (Bicudo, 2019) we gave several examples of how software development can serve as an anchor for collaboration and communication.

In this way, the open-source bioprinting community has adopted practices that are typical of other open-source software communities. For example, engineering projects for bioprinters, like the one proposed by Lanaro and colleagues (2021), have been shared on GitHub, an online platform widely used in open-source software (Bicudo, 2019).

On the other hand, the bioprinting community has used one of the cornerstones of the do-it-yourself (DIY) (or maker) community: Arduino motherboards (Garciamendez-Mijares et al., 2021; Reid et al., 2016). These motherboards are formed by a group of microchips which must be present in electronic devices in order to transform digital information (such as some bioprinting parameters) into physical outputs (such as the movements of a bioprinter). As we explained elsewhere (Bicudo et al., 2021), the business models of small bioprinting companies have been extensively reliant on Arduino boards.

The DIY movement (Wolf & McQuitty, 2011) had a strong impact on the domain of normal 3D printing. In 2005, Adrian Bowyer, at the University of Bath in England, created RepRap, the first DIY 3D printer, inspiring similar projects in subsequent years (Garciamendez-Mijares et al., 2021; Malone & Lipson, 2007). Reverberations of the DIY movement were seen in several domains, including biomedical research, with the emergence of the so-called DIYbio movement (Landrain et al., 2013). Eventually, the first DIY bioprinter appeared in 2012 with the release of the Standard Inkjet Printer, a project by Owczarczak and colleagues (2012). Thus we are dealing with researchers willing to design fully flexible machines, that is, 'open-source printers with modifiable software and hardware' (Wüst et al., 2012, p. 376).

At this point, it is crucial to point out that the open-source bioprinting community has been formed by professionals based in universities and research institutes, conducting high-level studies supported by major funding agencies and published in peer-reviewed journals. These studies are leading to promising outcomes, as exemplified by one of our interviewees who obtained funding from a government institution to conduct an international collaborative project where an innovative bioprinter has been developed. In this project, they stated, 'we are developing a robotic arm that can be used directly in a surgical room in order to bioprint tissues directly in the human body.'

In the understanding reviewed here, the bioprinter is taken to metonymically represent the whole scientific field. This may gain a lexical manifestation when people use the words *bioprinting* and *bioprinter* interchangeably.

> People are probably afraid of bioprinting because it seems something magic, something automatic. It's another machine, okay? It's just a machine which is able to place, locally, cells.
>
> *Interviewee 32, academic laboratory, Italy*

In this example, the interviewee starts by talking about bioprinting and, in the very next moment, describes it as 'just a machine.' To be sure, this linguistic event – in an interviewee who was interviewed in English but whose native language is not English – may be the outcome of confusion or mispronunciation. However, it arguably also expresses a deep-rooted metonymic understanding by a researcher based in a laboratory with a range of in-house made bioprinters. As this interviewee explained:

> Everything that you see in the lab ... 99% of those printers were built in the lab. Or if they were bought from a producer, they were completely customised with our extruders, our software, and other modifications.

On more profound (non-lexical) cognitive levels, the BIOPRINTER FOR BIOPRINTING metonymy inspires ideological or social concerns. Consequently, this approach goes beyond the technical issues highlighted by the metaphoric approach to assume an almost utopian tone. For example, Honiball and colleagues (2021, p. 2) declare that their project for an open-source bioprinter can 'contribute to the democratization of bioprinting technology and furthermore find application in biomedical education.' In this vein, Interviewee 08 (academic laboratory, UK) explained how he framed bioprinting at the end of the university degree: 'I saw a really powerful technology that could have a real impact and drive the whole healthcare ecosystem and the whole society as we understand it.' In these examples, a sort of metonymic extension occurs whereby bioprinting becomes the part representing the whole scientific field, the whole healthcare system, or even the whole social fabric.

These cognitive extensions are possible because of the referential role played by metonymies, that is, their usefulness in connecting concepts. This has been interpreted as metonymies' capacity to create contexture (Jakobson, 1956) or their capacity to create domains within language (Dirven, 2003). These chains of concepts (such as BIOPRINTER-OPENNESS-COLLABORATION-TRANSPARENCY-SOLIDARITY-DEMOCRACY- and so on) aim to reflect, on the lexical level, the kinds of relations that are sought at the practical level.

This is not to say, however, that the metonymic and metaphoric approaches are always mutually exclusive, as explained below.

11.6 Metaphors, metonymies, and hybrid cases

The differences between metaphor and metonymy, as alternative mappings for human understanding, have been explored before (Barcelona, 2000; Dirven & Pörings, 2003; Jakobson, 1956), but their possible combination has also been stressed. As shown by Dirven (2003), for example, there is a continuum between the metaphoric and the metonymic poles, because some sentences express, at the same time, a metaphor and a metonymy.

In bioprinting, a combination between metaphor and metonymy is possible because companies, whose discourse tends to be in line with the metaphoric reasoning, may also participate in and benefit from open-source projects. For example, Cellink, a successful bioprinting company, recommends that its machines be controlled with Slic3r, an open-source software package.

With such practical and cognitive combinations, hybrid discourses can be generated, as in the following example:

> [W]e like what we see on the 3D printing market, what Ultimaker does ... And Risa Research ... Risa, Czech Republic, Czech manufacturer, very popular 3D printers. They both have great businesses, they earn a lot of money and they both are based on open-source solutions ... they let other companies, other people, use their solutions and change it, manage it, and still maintain very successful businesses. So I think it is a very interesting ... business model.
>
> *Interviewee 36, bioprinting company, Eastern Europe*

On the one hand, this interviewee draws on the formative concepts provided by metaphoric reasoning. The additive manufacturing domain, metaphorically connected to the printing domain, is then framed as precise, technical, and professional, which enables the mobilisation of concepts such as 'market,' 'business models,' and 'solutions.' On the other hand, the flexible nature of products from two companies (Ultimaker and Risa) is metonymically stressed, introducing a preoccupation with 'other people' – that is, other users – who are able to 'change' and 'manage' the technology.

In this way, the cognitive explanation is not Manichean, dichotomous, or dialectical. The metaphoric and metonymic understandings are neither poles in conflict nor players in need of a redemptive synthesis. We can call it a 'complementary' explanation, in the sense intended by Bohr. Indeed, when interpreting metaphors and metonymies, it is possible to repeat Bohr's (1934, p. 56) words: 'We are not dealing with contradictory but with complementary pictures of the phenomena' at stake. Metaphor and metonymy are structured in very different ways, but can coexist in the same sentence (Dirven, 2003). Likewise, a single discourse can be underpinned by both metaphoric and metonymic understandings at the same time. From a political and cognitive point of view, the question is not which reasoning wins out, or how reasonings can mingle together, but how to prevent cognitive imbalances where one reasoning overgrows, suffocating the other one.

Identifying these two approaches, as well as grasping their divisions and combinations, is key to understanding not only the current features of bioprinting but also how cutting-edge scientific domains have been configured. We are dealing with reasonings that have institutional and political entailments, insofar as depending on the stance favoured by social players, they will be likely to support or adopt particular models of technology development, device use, and scientific collaboration. Whether a laboratory is equipped with commercial bioprinters and proprietary software packages or possesses a range of in-house developed machines and algorithms depends not only on issues of funding and institutional networks but also on the (either metaphoric or metonymic) understandings adopted by researchers.

In this way, it is important to clarify that the interpretation proposed by cognitive linguistics – and taken over here – is not causal. It is not simply claimed that a certain understanding causes people to espouse certain political ideologies and advocate for certain governance schemes. Understandings involve practices and experiences, rather than being intellectual conclusions. In this regard, Wittgenstein's admonition is helpful: 'Try not to think of understanding as a "mental process" at all. For that is the expression which confuses you' (Wittgenstein, 1963, p. 61). There is a circularity between people's experiences and trajectories, on the one hand, and people's views, on the other. For those who have explored the scientific and technical aspects of additive biomanufacture, which may include fruitful interactions with companies, the metaphoric understanding tends to be naturally grasped. In their turn, those who have explored economic and equity issues in additive biomanufacturing, which may include engagement with open-source communities, tend to make the metonymic understanding stand out. And, indeed, once people have subscribed to either metaphoric or metonymic views, certain ideologies and projects tend to be defended. In this way, when understanding and practical activity are taken into consideration, it is not possible to say that one causes the other; instead, they emerge together, underpinning each other.

11.7 Final words

This paper has focused on two cognitive stances that various social players – especially researchers – mobilise to make sense of the bioprinting domain. The metaphoric understanding is based on the ADDITIVE BIOMANUFACTURE IS PRINTING metaphor. It takes a specific concept (printing) to specify a complex field (additive biomanufacture), by means of analogies. The outcome is the cognitive constitution of a scientific field, with emphasis on its precise and reproducible capabilities, including an insistence on the need for its professional and/or commercial development.

In their turn, open-source bioprinting groups draw on THE BIOPRINTER FOR BIOPRINTING metonymy. This understanding selects a component part (the bioprinter) to represent the whole domain (additive biomanufacture). The outcome is a cognitive stance that claims for scientific creativity and cooperation, condemning the high prices and technical rigidity of commercial bioprinters as a way to criticise the commercialisation of scientific practice.

According to cognitive linguistics, metaphors and metonymies are not simply figures of speech. They are ways to link concepts together, which is crucial for people to make sense of their experiences. In this sense, metaphors are not used because people would be intent on communicating their views in impressive ways. Rather, metaphors are used because people assimilate a cognitive approach whereby analogies are mobilised to make sense of certain activities – bioprinting, in the case of this paper. We are not dealing with metaphors we select but with 'Metaphors we live by' (Lakoff & Johnson, 1980). Eventually, the metaphor becomes so normalised, strong and effective that bioprinting is framed as 'just technology,' in contrast with the social and collaborative framing proposed by the metonymic approach.

Metaphors and metonymies are seldom used consciously (Dirven & Pörings, 2003; Lakoff & Johnson, 1980). Therefore, the arguments outlined in this chapter, voiced by scientists, entrepreneurs, and regulators, do not always derive from systematic and planned thought. This is not to say that understanding is a highly subjective operation to be unearthed by psychological investigations. If metaphoric and metonymic utterances can be understood by various individuals, this is because metaphoric and metonymic reasonings transcend individual idiosyncrasies. It is this normalised side of understanding that sociology (in the approach proposed here) focuses on.

Metaphors and metonymies have been used in various biomedical domains. Metaphors are useful because it is often hard to conceptualise disciplines of increasing complexity. In gene editing, the GENES ARE LETTERS (OR WORDS) metaphor is proposed; in biomedical engineering, there is the CELLS ARE MECHANICAL PIECES metaphor; and in neuroimaging, brain maps underpin THE BRAIN IS A TERRITORY metaphor. These examples, which can be further studied in the years to come, remind us that: 'Health and illness … are among the experiences that we often talk about through metaphors' (Demjén & Semino, 2016, p. 385).

As for metonymies, examples have also multiplied. Generally, a certain portion of a discipline (such as a device or a product) is selected to represent the whole domain, with a consistent concern with the (either open or proprietary) ways in which that device or product is developed. This cognitive operation can also be targeted in future studies. For example, in cell science there are projects for inexpensive cell processing machines (Schmitt et al., 2019; Walzik et al., 2015), denoting THE CELL PROCESSING DEVICE FOR CELL SCIENCE metonymy. In biomedical laboratories, the maker movement has had considerable impact, with researchers now being able to 3D print their own equipment and tools (Baden et al., 2015), which expresses the LABORATORY EQUIPMENT FOR BIOMEDICINE metonymy. In neuroimaging, many researchers have designed collaborative, open algorithms (Bicudo, 2019), constituting THE ALGORITHM FOR NEUROIMAGING metonymy.

The study of such cognitive bases of society will require both analytical skills and methodological flexibility. As for analytical skills, it is important to assimilate some linguistic concepts pertaining, for example, to the nature of metaphors and metonymies, degrees of metaphoricity and metonymicity, cognitive frames, and the ways in which understandings emerge in discourses. In terms of methods, the use of interviews and document analysis – which is to a large extent familiar to sociologists – can be combined with alternative approaches, such as the analysis of images and videos for the identification of visual metaphors and visual metonymies.

In bioprinting, some strong ideological stances have been elaborated, whereby one tries, for example, to promote '3D bioprinting for everybody' (Wüst et al., 2012, p. 376). In this approach, scientific advancement should foster technical progress but also, and perhaps primarily, social equality and fairness. However, such ideological stances have not reached very high levels of political clarity or generated a campaign against private companies, as has been the case, for example, in the open-source software movement (Ensmenger, 2010; Stallman, 2002b, 2002c; Weber, 2004). This is probably due to the infancy of the bioprinting market where medium-sized companies can still coexist with increasingly globalised corporations (Bicudo et al., 2021). However, as the bioprinting market evolves, with a possible multiplication of mergers and acquisitions, academic researchers may sharpen their metonymic reasoning, as well as their market aversion, at seeing their field of scientific options narrowing down.

In this way, current political debates do not emerge, primarily, as a conflict between alternative metaphors, as claimed in previous analyses (Goatly, 2007; Kövecses, 2010; Lakoff & Johnson, 1980), but as a cognitive *division* between metaphoric and the metonymic understandings. As long as the ongoing models of scientific and market evolution are consolidated, the politics of metaphors and metonymies will continue. In order to refine future research agendas, it is crucial to be aware of, and focus on, these basic sources of human understanding.

Notes

1. https://dictionary.cambridge.org/us/dictionary/english/printing
2. https://www.regenhu.com/bioprinting-applications/#tablet_printing

References

Ahadian, S. & Khademhosseini, A. 2018. A perspective on 3D bioprinting in tissue regeneration. *Bio-Design and Manufacturing*, *1*(3): 157–160.

Baden, T., Chagas, A. M., Gage, G., Marzullo, T., Prieto-Godino, L. L. & Euler, T. 2015. Open labware: 3-D printing your own lab equipment. *PLOS Biology*, *13*(5): 1–12.

Barcelona, A. 2000. *Metaphor and Metonymy at the Crossroads: A Cognitive Perspective*. Berlin: Mouton de Gruyter.

Bartsch, R. 2003. Generating polysemy: Metaphor and metonymy. In Dirven, R. & Pörings, R. (Eds.), *Metaphor and Metonymy in Comparison and Contrast*. Berlin: Mouton de Gruyter, 49–74.

Bicudo, E. 2019. *Neuroimaging, Software, and Communication: The Social Code of Computer Code*. Singapore: Palgrave McMillan.

Bicudo, E. 2023. Cognitive foundations of society: The concept of schemata in cell, gene, and tissue therapies. *Applied Linguistics*, 45(5): 806–828.

Bicudo, E. 2025. *Sociology, cognition, and linguistics: Towards a theory of sociognistics*. Oxon: Routledge.

Bicudo, E., Faulkner, A. & Li, P. 2020. Software, risks, and liabilities: Ongoing and emergent issues in 3D bioprinting. *Journal of Risk Research*, *24*(10): 1319–1334.

Bicudo, E., Faulkner, A. & Li, P. 2021. Sociotechnical alignment in biomedicine: The 3D bioprinting market beyond technology convergence. *Technology in Society*, *66*: 1–12.

Bicudo, E., Morrison, M., Li, P., Faulkner, A., Webster, A., Mourby, M. & Kaye, J. 2022. Patent power in biomedical innovation: Technology governance in biomodifying technologies. *The Journal of World Intellectual Property*, *25*(2): 473–494.

Bohr, N. 1934. *Atomic Theory and the Description of the Nature*. Cambridge: Cambridge University Press.

Choudhury, D., Anand, S. & Naing, M. W. 2018. The arrival of commercial bioprinters: Towards 3D bioprinting revolution! *International Journal of Bioprinting*, *4*(2): 1–20.

Cortez, J. E. P., Sánchez, V. H., Vázquez-Lepe, E., Santiago, G. T., Álvarez, M. M. & Martínez-López, J. I. 2022. Retrofitting of an affordable 3D printer: Towards a material efficient and low-cost bioprinting system. *Procedia CIRP*, *110*: 150–155.

Darwish, L. R., El-Wakad, M. T. & Farag, M. M. 2021. Towards an ultra-affordable three-dimensional bioprinter: A heated inductive-enabled syringe pump extrusion multifunction module for open-source fused deposition modeling three-dimensional printers. *Journal of Manufacturing Science and Engineering*, *143*(12): 1–10.

Demjén, Z. & Semino, E. 2016. Using metaphor in healthcare. In Demjén, Z. & Semino, E. (Eds.), *The Routledge Handbook of Metaphor and Language*. London: Routledge, 385—399.

Dirven, R. 2003. Metonymy and metaphor: Different mental strategies of conceptualisation. In Dirven, R. & Pörings, R. (Eds.), *Metaphor and Metonymy in Comparison and Contrast*. Berlin: Mouton de Gruyter, 75–111.

Dirven, R. & Pörings, R. 2003. *Metonymy and Metaphor: Different Mental Strategies of Conceptualisation*. Berlin: Mouton de Gruyter.

Engberg, A., Stelzl, C., Eriksson, O., O'Callaghan, P. & Kreuger, J. 2021. An open source extrusion bioprinter based on the E3D motion system and tool changer to enable FRESH and multimaterial bioprinting. *Scientific Reports*, *11*(1): 1–11.

Ensmenger, N. 2010. *The Computer Boys Take Over: Computers, Programmers, and the Politics of Technical Expertise*. Cambridge/London: The MIT Press.

Fillmore, C. J. 1985. Frames and the semantics of understanding. *Quaderni di Semantica*, *6*(2): 222–254.

Fitzsimmons, R., Aquilino, M. S., Quigley, J., Chebotarev, O., Tarlan, F. & Simmons, C. A. 2018. Generating vascular channels within hydrogel constructs using an economical open-source 3D bioprinter and thermoreversible gels. *Bioprinting*, *9*: 7–18.

Gao, G., Huang, Y., Schilling, A. F., Hubbell, K. & Cui, X. 2018. Organ bioprinting: Are we there yet? *Advanced Health Care Materials*, *7*(1701018): 1–8.

Garcia-Garcia, L. A. & Rodriguez-Salvador, M. 2018. Uncovering 3D bioprinting research trends: A keyword network mapping analysis. *International Journal of Bioprinting*, *4*(2): 1–8.

Garciamendez-Mijares, C. E., Agrawal, P., Martínez, G. G., Juarez, E. C. & Zhang, Y. S. 2021. State-of-art affordable bioprinters: A guide for the DiY community. *Applied Physics Reviews*, *8*: 1–31.

Goatly, A. 2007. *Washing the Brain: Metaphor and Hidden Ideology*. Amsterdam/Philadelphia: John Benjamins.

Honiball, J. R., Pepper, M. S. & Prinsloo, E. 2021. Step-by-step assembly and testing of a low-cost bioprinting solution for research and educational purposes. *MethodsX*, *8*: 1–9.

Ioannidis, K., Danalatos, R. I., Tsaniras, S. C., Kaplani, K., Lokka, G., Kanellou, A., Papachristou, D. J., Bokias, G., Lygerou, Z. & Taraviras, S. 2020. A custom ultra-low-cost 3D bioprinter supports cell growth and differentiation. *Frontiers in Bioengineering and Biotechnology*, *8*: 1–13.

Jakobson, R. 1956. *Fundamentals of Language*. The Hague: Mouton & Co.

Johnson, M. 1987. *The Body in the Mind: The Bodily Basis of Meaning, Imagination, and Reason*. Chicago: The University of Chicago Press.

Kahl, M., Gertig, M., Hoyer, P., Friedrich, O. & Gilbert, D. F. 2019. Ultra-low-cost 3D bioprinting: Modification and application of an off-the-shelf desktop 3D-printer for biofabrication. *Frontiers in Bioengineering and Biotechnology*, *7*: 1–12.

Knowlton, S. & Tasoglu, S. 2016. A bioprinted liver-on-a-chip for drug screening applications. *Trends in Biotechnology*, *34*(9): 681–682.

Koch, F., Thaden, O., Tröndle, K., Zengerle, R., Zimmermann, S. & Koltay, P. 2021. Open-source hybrid 3D-bioprinter for simultaneous printing of thermoplastics and hydrogels. *HardwareX*, *10*: 1–20.

Kövecses, Z. 2010. *Metaphor: A Practical Introduction*. Oxford: Oxford University Press.

Lakoff, G. 1987. *Women, Fire, and Dangerous Things: What Categories Reveal About the Mind.* Chicago: The University of Chicago Press.

Lakoff, G. & Johnson, M. 1980. *Metaphors We Live By.* Chicago: The University of Chicago Press.

Lakoff, G. & Johnson, M. 1999. *Philosophy in the Flesh: The Embodied Mind and its Challenge to Western Thought.* New York: Basic Books.

Lamastra, C. R. 2009. Software innovativeness: A comparison between proprietary and Free/Open Source solutions offered by Italian SMEs. *R&D Management, 39*(2): 153–169.

Lanaro, M., Luu, A., Lightbody-Gee, A., Hedger, D., Powell, S. K., Holmes, D. W. & Woodruff, M. A. 2021. Systematic design of an advanced open-source 3D bioprinter for extrusion and electrohydrodynamic-based processes. *The International Journal of Advanced Manufacturing Technology, 113*: 2539–2554.

Landrain, T., Meyer, M., Perez, A. M. & Sussan, R. 2013. Do-it-yourself biology: Challenges and promises for an open science and technology movement. *Systems and Synthetic Biology, 7*(3): 115–126.

Ma, X., Liu, J., Zhu, W., Tang, M., Lawrence, N., Yu, C., Gou, M. & Chen, S. 2018. 3D bioprinting of functional tissue models for personalized drug screening and in vitro disease modeling. *Advanced Drug Delivery Reviews, 132*: 235–251.

Maben, A. J. 2016. The CRISPR fantasy: Flaws in current metaphors of gene-modifying technology. *Inquiries Journal, 8*(6): 1–2.

Malone, E. & Lipson, H. 2007. Fab@Home: The personal desktop fabricator kit. *Rapid Prototyping Journal, 13*(4): 245–255.

Mandrycky, C., Wang, Z., Kim, K. & Kim, D.-H. 2016. 3D bioprinting for engineering complex tissues. *Biotechnology Advances, 34*(4): 422–434.

McElheny, C., Hayes, D. & Devireddy, R. 2017. Design and fabrication of a low-cost three-dimensional bioprinter. *Journal of Medical Devices, 11*(4): 0410011–0410019.

Mironov, V., Kasyanov, V., Drake, C. & Markwald, R. R. 2008. Organ printing: Promises and challenges. *Regenerative Medicine, 3*(1): 93–103.

Noor, N., Shapira, A., Edri, R., Gal, I., Wertheim, L. & Dvir, T. 2019. 3D printing of personalized thick and perfusable cardiac patches and hearts. *Advanced Science, 6*(11): 1–10.

O'Keefe, M., Perrault, S., Halpern, J., Ikemoto, L., Yarborough, M. & UC North Bioethics Collaboratory for Life & Health Sciences. 2015. 'Editing' genes: A case study about how language matters in bioethics. *The American Journal of Bioethics, 15*(12): 3–10.

Owczarczak, A. B., Shuford, S. O., Wood, S. T., Deitch, S. & Dean, D. 2012. Creating transient cell membrane pores using a standard inkjet printer. *Journal of Visualized Experiments, 61*: 1–6.

Pragglejaz Group. 2010. MIP: A method for identifying metaphorically used words in discourse. *Metaphor and Symbol, 22*(1): 1–39.

Raymond, E. S. 2001. *The Cathedral & the Bazaar: Musings on Linux and Open Source by an Accidental Revolutionary.* Sebastopol: O'Reilly.

Reid, J. A., Mollica, P. M., Johnson, G. D., Ogle, R. C., Bruno, R. D. & Sachs, P. C. 2016. Accessible bioprinting: Adaptation of a low-cost 3D-printer for precise cell placement and stem cell differentiation. *Biofabrication, 8*(2): 1–12.

Rodríguez-Salvador, M., Rio-Belver, R. M. & Garechana-Anacabe, G. 2017. Scientometric and patentometric analyses to determine the knowledge landscape in innovative technologies: The case of 3D bioprinting. *Plos One, 12*(6): 1–22.

Roehm, K. D. & Madihally, S. V. 2018. Bioprinted chitosan-gelatin thermosensitive hydrogels using an inexpensive 3D printer. *Biofabrication, 10*: 1–14.

Rosch, E. 1978. Principles of categorization. In Rosch, E. & Lloyd, B. B. (Eds.), *Cognition and Categorization.* Hillsdale: Lawrence Erlbaum, 27—48.

Schmieden, D. T., Vázquez, S. J. B., Sangüesa, H., van der Does, M., Idema, T. & Meyer, A. S. 2018. Printing of patterned, engineered E. coli biofilms with a low-cost 3D printer. *ACS Synthetic Biology*, *7*(5): 1328–1337.

Schmitt, M. A., Friedrich, O. & Gilbert, D. F. 2019. Portoporator©: A portable low-cost electroporation device for gene transfer to cultured cells in biotechnology, biomedical research and education. *Biosensors and Bioelectronics*, *131*: 95–103.

Stallman, R. M. 2002a. Copyright and globalization in the age of computer networks. In Gay, J. (Ed.), *Free Software, Free Society: Selected Essays of Richard M. Stallman*. Boston: GNU Press, 133–154.

Stallman, R. M. 2002b. The danger of software patents. In Gay, J. (Ed.), *Free Software, Free Society: Selected Essays of Richard M. Stallman*. Boston: GNU Press, 95–112.

Stallman, R. M. 2002c. Why software should not have owners. In Gay, J. (Ed.), *Free Software, Free Society: Selected Essays of Richard M. Stallman*. Boston: GNU Press, 45–50.

Sun, H., Jia, Y., Dong, H., Dong, D. & Zheng, J. 2020. Combining additive manufacturing with microfluidics: An emerging method for developing novel organs-on-chips. *Current Opinion in Chemical Engineering*, *28*: 1–9.

Sweetser, E. E. 1990. *From Etymology to Pragmatics: Metaphorical and Cultural Aspects of Semantic Structure*. Cambridge: Cambridge University Press.

Walzik, M. P., Vollmar, V., Lachnit, T., Dietz, H., Haug, S., Bachmann, H., Fath, M., Aschenbrenner, D., Mofrad, S. A., Friedrich, O. & Gilbert, D. F. 2015. A portable low-cost long-term live-cell imaging platform for biomedical research and education. *Biosensors and Bioelectronics*, *64*: 639–649.

Weber, S. 2004. *The Success of Open Source*. Cambridge: Harvard University Press.

Wittgenstein, L. 1963. *Philosophische Untersuchungen / Philosophical Investigations*. Oxford: Basil Blackwell.

Wolf, M. & McQuitty, S. 2011. Understanding the do-it-yourself consumer: DIY motivations and outcomes. *AMS Review*, *1*: 154–170.

Wüst, S., Godla, M., Schwilch, P. & Müller, R. 2012. 3D bioprinting for everybody: Application of low-cost 3D printers in tissue engineering. *Journal of Tissue Engineering and Regenerative Medicine*, *6*: 376.

Yun, Y. E., Jung, Y. J., Choi, Y. J., Choi, J. S. & Cho, Y. W. 2019. Artificial skin models for animal-free testing. *Journal of Pharmaceutical Investigation*, *48*: 215–223.

12 Medical travel for AMR treatment

Trang Do and Andrea Whittaker

12.1 Introduction

Antimicrobial resistant (AMR) infections are a global health problem. They became the leading cause of mortality in 2019 with 4.95 million deaths associated with bacterial AMR worldwide (Murray et al., 2022), with forecasts that AMR could claim 10 million lives every year by 2050 (O'Neill, 2016). Statistics on AMR morbidity are largely missing, however, if predictions of the increasing incidences of AMR infections are correct (OECD, 2018), the burden of living with these infections will continue to grow. Yet, there is little known about living with such infections and how people affected by AMR manage or seek treatments. In this chapter, we describe the findings from a study of the therapeutic journeys experienced by a small sample of people with complex AMR infections. In doing so, the chapter considers new research directions for studying AMR in a context where the number of cases of AMR infections increases globally, creating the imperative to understand the 'chronic lives' of patients and their resorts to care.

AMR is not a singular phenomenon but describes the characteristics of various pathogens which have become less susceptible to biomedical treatment such as antibiotics and antifungals. AMR describes the changes to microbes' responses to antimicrobial drugs that enable them to limit the activity of the drugs, become less permeable to antimicrobials, or actively eject drugs (Centers for Disease Control, 2021; World Health Organization, 2021). AMR occurs through exposure to antimicrobials and selective pressures favouring resistant microbes. In addition, microbes may transfer resistance traits in their DNA to other microbes they come into contact with. The emergence and spread of drug-resistant pathogens poses a significant threat to modern medicine by making it harder to treat infections and perform critical medical procedures. It also impacts animal and plant health, reduces farm productivity, and threatens food security, leading to higher healthcare costs and economic burdens globally (World Health Organization, 2021).

Medical travel has emerged as a global phenomenon with profound implications for the patient experience and the health systems in both sending and receiving countries (Whittaker et al., 2010). As the world becomes more interconnected, the dynamics of medical travel have evolved, presenting both opportunities and challenges for healthcare providers, policymakers, and the patients themselves. International medical travel (IMT) – temporary movements by patients across national borders to seek medical treatments – has become a normalised option for patients seeking treatments and care in many parts of the world. The travellers are from diverse socio-economic backgrounds, their travels are differently funded, and they may travel by air, overland, individually, or in groups. To date, most research involving travel and AMR is about the risk of gaining resistant infections while travelling. Medical travel to foreign hospitals in particular is considered to put patients at high risk of contracting novel resistant infections due to higher distributions of AMR infections in some countries, iatrogenic infections during surgical procedures, or because of the possible misuse of antibiotics and poor stewardship by professionals. However, in this chapter we describe the travel by patients with AMR infections to seek care in foreign settings for non-orthodox treatments. This care-seeking experience is poorly known in the current body of literature on medical travel or the lived experience of AMR. We aim to address this gap by focusing on international medical travel for AMR, as we anticipate this practice will continue to grow, given that most conventional treatment for AMR infections is complex, costly, and in many cases may not be effective.

In this chapter, we begin with a review of conceptualisations surrounding medical travel that once caused substantial debate in academic and public literature. The chapter then goes on to provide prominent conceptual and theoretical frameworks that guide the work in this field. We then present main findings in the existing literature in relation to what has motivated medical travellers to seek care overseas and influenced their choice of destinations. Subsequently, the chapter turns to describing the situation of phage therapy – the use of viral bacteriophages or viruses that attack bacteria, which has recently regained its popularity to treat infections as an alternative to antibiotics in managing AMR but has received scant attention in the social sciences. We then present two cases of patients who had travelled overseas to obtain phage therapy from our qualitative study that explored the lived experiences of AMR. By examining existing scholarly literature supplemented by our empirical work, we aim to provide a broad understanding of the trends, implications, and future trajectories of medical travel. As the demand for alternative treatment in the context of the rise of AMR, a nuanced examination of this phenomenon becomes valuable to inform decision-making, policy development, and the delivery of patient-centred care.

12.2 Medical travel

Much of the burgeoning popular media on 'medical tourism' promotes an image of people from the Global North travelling to foreign destinations to receive fertility treatment, dental treatment, or life-transforming cosmetic surgery (Jones, 2008; Lunt et al., 2016; Lunt and Carrera, 2010). It is often envisaged as patients from high-income backgrounds who can afford high-end, costly healthcare services overseas (Lunt et al., 2016), however, the reality is that many people travel to access various forms of care and may have gone into debt in order to afford their treatment. Scholars have criticised the term 'medical tourism' (sometimes 'health tourism' (Goodrich, 1993) is used interchangeably), arguing that it inadequately encapsulates the realities of seeking healthcare services outside one's home coun and implies adventure, joy, and pleasure (Cham et al., 2021; Connell, 2015, 2016; Inhorn and Patrizio, 2009; Ormond, 2015; Whittaker, 2008). The use of the term 'tourism' has met with harsh critiques from the academic community and individuals travelling for medical services outside of their home countries out of desperate need for treatment (Inhorn, 2015), who may view the language as insensitive and even offensive to their suffering as their experiences are stressful and far from being pleasant in nature (Inhorn and Patrizio, 2009).

Social scientists have suggested alternative terminology that better covers the complexity and dynamics of this global phenomenon and the diverse stakeholders involved in this practice, such as 'transnational or international medical travel' (Kangas, 2010; Turner, 2013), 'transnational therapeutic travel' (Ormond and Lunt, 2020), or 'therapeutic mobility' (Franchina et al., 2022). Frenz (2019) has adopted the term 'movements for healthcare' to reflect the practice of international border crossings or mobility within a nation-state to seek medical treatment. They argue that the use of 'healthcare' instead of 'medical' allows for broader inclusion of biomedical, but also alternative care that is sought by many people when travelling overseas. Some scholars adopt terms that are more politically charged (Ormond and Lunt, 2020) such as 'medical migration' to emphasise the importance of social interactions, cultural inflections, and nuanced understanding of motivations surrounding cross-border care (Chee and Whittaker, 2020). Others have argued for using 'medical refugees' or 'medical exiles' when describing those 'forced' to travel from their home countries where certain reproductive procedures are illegal, inaccessible due to the expense, or unavailable (Inhorn, 2012; Matorras, 2005).

In this chapter, our preference is to opt for the term 'international medical travel' to acknowledge that not all journeys for medical treatment across borders involve tourism-related activities (Turner, 2013). This neutral, more generic term allows us to understand the complex nature of the movement and capture the diversity of intentions and stakeholders involved in this practice, as well as the social and structural context within which the international travel occurs.

A substantial body of scholarly work on medical travel now exists (Hanefeld et al., 2013, 2014; Ormond and Lunt, 2020; Smith and Jenner, 2000; Whittaker, 2015; Whittaker et al., 2019). This work finds that people seeking medical treatments, procedures, or surgeries outside their home countries are largely driven by a wish to pursue medical treatments that are unavailable or of poor quality in their home countries rather than to access more affordable services (Frenz, 2019; Whittaker et al., 2017). For example, patients from neighbouring countries travel to South Africa to obtain basic medical care that is not offered in their own countries (Crush and Chikanda, 2015) ranging from basic to specialised procedures such as abortion (Crush et al., 2015), reconstructive surgery, chemotherapy (Ahwireng-Obeng and van Loggerenberg, 2011), fertility treatment (Moll et al., 2022), drug rehabilitation, and transplants (Crush et al., 2012; Scheper-Hughes, 2011). Seeking high-quality healthcare has also been shown to be the greatest motivation explaining the flow of patients within Southeast Asia (Whittaker and Chee, 2015), sometimes due to mistrust of the health services and professionals in their home coun (Whittaker et al., 2017).

Patients also travel to access services that may be restricted in their home countries. This is the case in assisted reproduction (Inhorn, 2015; Inhorn and Gürtin, 2011; Whittaker et al., 2019). Access to third party donor materials is an important reason to cross borders, such as the case of French women crossing the border to Belgium for assisted reproduction to evade the laws prohibiting treatment with donor sperm in France (Van Hoof et al., 2015); Europeans travelling to Spain for ready access to donated ova (Bergmann, 2011; Closas, 2021); or people travelling for social sex selection or surrogacy (Everingham and Whittaker, 2023; König, 2023; Pande, 2014; Whittaker et al., 2019). Other studies have documented the travel by patients for experimental treatments such as stem cell therapies in China, motivated by hope of a cure (Brophy, 2017; Petersen et al., 2017). In summary, existing research in the social sciences has illustrated that medical travel is primarily driven by the pursuit of high-quality treatments, for instance, specialised procedures, assisted reproduction, and experimental treatments, which are unavailable or restricted in patients' home countries, rather than cost considerations. Their findings emphasise the need for attending to the personal, socio-economic, and political factors influencing patient decisions to seek medical care abroad and the nuances of their experiences during and after treatment.

12.3 Phage therapy

The AMR crisis has revitalised interest in using bacteriophages as an alternative approach (Kutter et al., 2015; Luong et al., 2020; Saha and Mukherjee, 2019; Suh Gina et al., 2022). Phages, made up of protein or proteolipidic capsids containing fragments of nucleic acids, are the most represented biological entity on Earth (Brives and Pourraz, 2020). Phage therapies involve the use of viral bacteriophages that attack bacteria to treat infections as an alternative to the use of antibiotics. Specific bacteriophages act on the target bacteria to destroy it through a process called 'lysis.' In clinical settings, phages can be tailored specifically for a patient's infection (personalised or custom approach), or treatment can utilise commercial phage preparations, which come with pre-defined phage compositions. They can also be prepared by small biotech and academic institutions for individual patients on compassionate use (Patey et al., 2018).

The use of bacteriophages or phages – viruses that infect bacteria – dates back to nearly a century ago when Felix d'Herelle, a French-Canadian microbiologist, successfully isolated the first bacteriophage in 1917 and then used an oral phage preparation to treat bacterial dysentery in 1919 (Kutateladze and Adamia, 2008). After its discovery, phage therapy was used extensively across the world, particularly in former Soviet Union countries. Clinics in Georgia, for instance, began administering phage therapy for various bacterial infections, among which the Eliava Institute of Bacteriophages, Microbiology, and Virology in Tbilisi, Georgia, has been a pioneer in phage research and production since its establishment in the 1920s (Álvarez et al., 2020; Sacher and Zheng, 2021). The Eliava Institute has become a popular destination for international patients travelling in search of a more effective treatment for managing antibiotic resistant infections, including informants interviewed in our study.

In Western countries, however, phage application was abandoned after the Second World War (Kakasis and Panitsa, 2019; Kutateladze and Adamia, 2008). This was partly due to the inadequate understanding of phage biology and varied results of its efficacy (Kutateladze and Adamia, 2008), but mainly on account of the discovery and introduction of antibiotics, which acted as a kind of powerful epistemological infrastructure inhibiting the development of phage therapy (Brives and Pourraz, 2020). Although it has been a respected therapy option in France and many Eastern European and post-Soviet countries, there is a paucity of data with which to judge its effectiveness. Much of the reporting on success with phage therapy is through uncontrolled case reports (Suh Gina et al., 2022) and the few randomised, placebo-controlled, double-blind clinical trials show no significant advantage of readily available standard phage preparations over placebos (Leitner et al., 2021; Suh Gina et al., 2022). However, it has been noted that the production of a rigorous trial is difficult given the personalised nature of the treatment for each specific infection, the difficulty in recruiting a patient population with the same resistant infections, the lack of funding and interest from pharmaceutical companies, and regulatory barriers (Álvarez et al., 2020).

Many countries have now reconsidered bacteriophages as a viable alternative to antibiotics to treat infections. In Belgium, for example, a recent study found that external requests for phage therapy received at a Brussels-based military hospital increased remarkably to 260 over the 2016–2018 period, with 151 requests recorded alone in 2017 (Djebara et al., 2019). Apart from the Eliava Institute in Tbilisi mentioned above, only a few places in the world offer bacteriophage treatment. These include Queen Astrid Military Hospital, Belgium; Hospices Civils de Lyon, France; Phage Therapy Unit, Poland; Center for Innovative Phage Applications and Therapeutics, California, US (Álvarez et al., 2020; Sacher and Zheng, 2021). Outside of those countries, phage therapy has not yet been approved as a medicine and can only be administered for compassionate use (Sacher and Zheng, 2021; Suh Gina et al., 2022). Compassionate use denotes the use of medicines that are unauthorised or only available in other countries for patients suffering from a disease who have exhausted standard therapy (Helsinki Declaration of the World Medical Association, 2014). Regulations of compassionate drug use vary across countries. For instance, in Australia where our study was based, drugs that are not included in the Australian Register of Therapeutic Goods (unregistered drugs) can be obtained through the Special Access Scheme, the Authorised Prescriber Scheme, or by personal importation, and are considered experimental (Donovan, 2017). The Therapeutic Goods Administration has allowed the administration of phage therapy to patients on compassionate grounds (Fabijan et al., 2019).

Under those circumstances, initiating the process of administering the use of phage therapy requires the consent of both the treating physician and the patient diagnosed with a multidrug-resistant bacterial infection, or their guardian (McCallin et al., 2019). Obtaining approval is often an arduous process for physicians, as they may be required to explain the therapy to an institutional review board and national health authority, as well as safety evaluation and oversight for their patients when phage is administered (McCallin et al., 2019; Sacher and Zheng, 2021). Finding sources of phages poses an additional challenge for physicians because they cannot use the same method as ordering approved medicines (Sacher and Zheng, 2021). Therefore, patients often face significant barriers to access compassionate phage therapy in countries where phage is not approved for clinical use, which prompts them to look for alternative options elsewhere. As yet, there have been few studies of medical travel for phage therapy.

12.4 A qualitative study on AMR survivorship

To address the gap in medical travel literature, we report on the quest for phage therapy using data collected from a qualitative study capturing the social burden of AMR. We present the care-seeking experiences of patients who had travelled overseas to Georgia to undergo phage treatment and others who had ordered phage via post. Within this study, we conducted semi-structured interviews with nine 'survivors' and six caregivers across 2021/22, including seven men and eight women. We described the procedure for collecting data and the participant background in a previous publication (Whittaker et al., 2023).

12.4.1 Case study 1: Sandra

Sandra (37 years old), who lived in Germany at the time of our study, had suffered with copious malodorous nasal discharge from her left nostril despite continuous use of antibiotics and multiple surgical procedures since the age of 15. When really severe, the infection affected her eyesight and gave her headaches and constant dark green discharge. From a South African background, she had ear-nose-throat (ENT) surgery in 2003 in South Africa. With the problems continuing, for the last 15 years prior to our interview she has taken antibiotics (Ciprofloxacin/Levofloxacin) in a low dose. She moved to Germany for work, and in late 2019 and early 2020 her condition was getting worse. Sandra recalled the situation at that time:

> Come January, February 2020 obviously I'm super stressed with the situation that's happening with the pandemic. The nose situation has literally reached a level of the most heightened it has ever been. So just to give you an explanation, I'm blowing my nose literally – no exaggeration, ten times per hour … And in the April of 2020 we are locked down, and I'm in a new coun. I have no support … I want to see an ENT, but then I'm like no, I just need to wait, because we have a pandemic.

Because of the persistent infections, Sandra experienced significant difficulty in her social life during the pandemic:

> So it's a bit of a different situation than being in the office where I would constantly be blowing my nose. But I had been doing this before. It's really not great. I mean people look at you weird. Now we're in a pandemic they look at you even if you're breathing, because you

> have COVID ... But imagine going out and having lunch with your friends. Imagine having a conversation here, and I'm like: 'Hold on I need to blow my nose.' It just makes you feel like – I'm like, why me?

It was not until June that year that Sandra could have an appointment with an ENT specialist in Frankfurt who tested her and diagnosed her as having resistant *Pseudomonas aeruginosa* and *Enterobacter cloacae* infections. They explained that she had been previously given the wrong class of antibiotics to treat a nasal infection and that because of the vast years of antibiotic misuse the *P. aeruginosa* strain was now resistant to most antibiotics.

Her journey to seek phage therapy first started with a recommendation from an ENT specialist following a month-long hospitalisation and several surgical procedures, which could only manage *Enterobacter cloacae* and were ineffective against nasal *Pseudomonas aeruginosa* infection. Sandra remembered feeling confused and disappointed with the lack of information about phage therapy from the ENT specialist:

> And she explained to me: 'Unfortunately you cannot be on Meropenem [a strong antibiotic used to treat serious bacterial infections which is often given intravenously] again ... your next step is phage.' And I'm like: 'What is phage?' And then she gave me a brief explanation. And she said: 'You can do it at a Belgium hospital. This procedure is going to *fix* it.' And then she's like: 'You'd need to Google, because it's not provided in Germany, because the German healthcare does not pay for this.' A little in my mind did I know that it's not approved by FDA.

After that conversation, Sandra's anxiety grew as she was unable to find reliable, up-to-date information about phage therapy on the internet:

> [W]hen I started my research, using my best friend Google, I was very disappointed, because the amount of information on the internet is few and far between. I was getting cases of people that had the same issue as me in the year 1987 ... There was no information. Absolutely nothing.

She recollected visiting the website of the hospital in Belgium which the ENT specialist mentioned but was dissuaded because she could not access the information in English:

> And when I was doing my research in Belgium the hospital only speaks – I think it's French and Dutch. When I opened their website, it was in French or Dutch. I was like, forget it, I can't go through this.

Sandra believed her experience could have been improved if she had access to some peer support throughout this process. She expressed her opinion in favour of 'find[ing] someone who has pseudomonas,' while admitting the difficulty of locating any community with a common condition and mutual experience:

> But I wish there was like a forum where people can talk one-on-one and share their experience … I want a proper medical forum where I can say, here's my information, here's what I have. If somebody has a similar as to what I have, let's and get in touch, and – and see what we've been through. But I can't find anything like this.

In a situation of frustration, Sandra accidentally read some news articles about phage experiments conducted in the US and Australia and contacted some of the scientists mentioned in those articles. To her surprise, one of them responded to her and provided her with the information about the Eliava Institute in Tbilisi, Georgia. With that piece of information from a researcher affiliated with a prestigious academic institution, she researched the Eliava Institute on the internet and was impressed by what she found on their website, as she told us in the interview:

> [E]verything was on their website. It's clean, it's clear, it's crisp. You know what's going to happen to you before you get there. It's very detailed.

Being able to find the information and communicate with the clinic staff in English motivated Sandra to pursue the therapy there. She remembered her first encounter with the Eliava Institute:

> They have an amazing marketing department, speaking in English. You just reach out to them, they correspond in English.

However, the travel to Georgia did not commence seamlessly, due to the requirements related to phage susceptibility testing prior to treatment, along with COVID-19 restrictions across Europe. In our interview, Sandra recalled being anxious for lacking control over the sample sent to the Georgian clinic:

> I sent my sample on the 3rd of November. Again, because of the pandemic, it only reached them on the 16th of December. I was like, in my mind, the sample is not going to survive. It is going to be dead. They are going to come up with nothing. I have just wasted [money] – because you pay to send it, you pay to test it.

Speaking highly of her experience overseas, Sandra often used words such as 'phenomenal' or 'absolutely amazing' to recognise the professional care she had received at the Eliava Institute. For example, Sandra complimented the efficient communication with the medical staff and the organisation of service offered by the clinic there:

> I had two young doctors who are obviously in their fifth or sixth year, speaking in English, adding me to the WhatsApp, explaining to me the process. I then met an older doctor who was an ENT [specialist]. I then met another coordinator. The process of them, and how they treated me, and just every patient, made this experience absolutely amazing. So I had to start with the treatment that I received from them. And just the whole – they were so with it, like WhatsApping, I could call them. It's just like real time.

In addition, Sandra made a remark about hospitable service from the non-medical staff during her stay, describing it like a 'royal treatment:'

> [T]hey do everything for you. They were even recommending tours that I should do … Apart from being there to fix obviously a medical situation, they also throw you into the culture, and let you experience a bit of the coun.

During her fortnight in Tbilisi, she was given two bottles containing standard phage treatment which she took every morning and evening by drinking them with saline water. She also used a nebuliser to inhale phage twice a day and was advised not to drink anything else 30 minutes before or after taking the phage. During her time there, she was also sent out for several tests and a scan. The two-week-long treatment generated positive outcomes for Sandra. Nasal discharge decreased substantially following the hospital-based treatment in Georgia. Sandra continued with self-administered phage treatment after returning to her coun of residence to maintain its effectiveness in controlling the *Pseudomonas* infection. Each batch of treatment is 60 days' duration (with 3 rounds of 20 days each and two intervals of 2 weeks in between). She continued to receive her second batch of treatment while in Germany and administered it herself, and at the time of the interview was going to continue with a third batch. Upon her return to Germany, she recognised her condition was better controlled although not eliminated. Her most recent test had suggested that the *Pseudomonas* was at a minimal level.

While having a positive experience with the Georgian clinic and successful treatment, Sandra's trip overseas inevitably involved a stressful part, as she was travelling alone to an unfamiliar former Soviet coun. Out-of-pocket expenses were another issue for Sandra, like for most people travelling overseas to seek medical treatment. While public healthcare is free in her coun of residence, the phage therapy-seeking process in Georgia cost Sandra approximately €6,000 (or US$6,560), including all medical costs, air tickets, accommodation, and meals. When receiving phage delivered to Germany, each time Sandra paid about €500 (US$547) for the phage, plus €100 (US$109) for the shipping fee. Because phage treatment is not approved in Germany, she cannot claim those expenses for tax deduction as those applied for other medical services incurred in Germany.

12.4.2 Case study 2: Albert

Albert, a 63-year-old Australian man, was diagnosed with bacterial prostatitis which started with an infection in his prostate in 2016, five years prior to our interview. At that time, he started to experience a range of symptoms and dysfunctions, such as headache, frequent urination, and what he described in the interview as hot 'peeing,' which caused significant disruptions to his professional and personal lives. Albert was prescribed several types of antibiotics, but all the medications failed to contain his infection. His infectious disease specialist then sent him out for numerous additional tests, including a cystoscopy, which suggested a Methicillin-resistant *Staphylococcus* infection.

In 2017 he watched a television programme about using phage therapy in which the Eliava Institute was mentioned. He learned about the long history and success of using phage to treat infections in Europe:

> [T]hey get all sorts of Europeans go there as well. Dutch, Germans, they all go there. And the East Europeans love it because it's a more simple and cheaper process than standard antibiotics that pretty much don't work much.

Albert was not concerned about the effectiveness of phage therapy, despite it not being a standard treatment approved in Australia. He explained to us:

> I didn't see any risk that was detrimental, because a lot of people are using it. A lot of East Europeans and Georgians, they're commonly using it – phages to treat other conditions besides what I had. They're more simple treatments than we use [in Australia].

Similarly to Sandra, Albert contacted the Eliava Institute directly and booked an appointment with them without the facilitation of any intermediaries and started to send his sperm sample overseas for initial examination. However, unlike Sandra's experience, Albert's travel to Georgia in 2018 was lengthier and more arduous, as it involved a 21-hour flight from Melbourne, Australia to Tbilisi. In addition, his communication with the treating doctor was facilitated by a translator that the Eliava Institute provided, as the physician 'didn't know much English, but enough to get by.' Despite this, Albert spoke positively about his experience in Georgia and was satisfied with the doctors and treatment he received there:

> I was happy with it. And they said, 'you're *cured*, you're finished.' They said they couldn't find any infection.

After returning from Georgia, Albert 'felt 100% better.' Unfortunately, the infection came back around four weeks later, demanding him to continue to use phage imported from Georgia. Monitoring phage therapy at home appeared problematic and caused him a lot of distress, despite the help of his partner, who was a nurse. He brought back phage that required daily injection. Albert described the difficult situation when they could not administer the injected dose correctly:

> Yeah, I followed the treatment for a while, but I didn't follow it up as well as I should, because I couldn't handle the needles in the urethra, the syringes ... My partner is a nurse, but it was just too stressful, especially when we got the volumes wrong ... Too hard, too painful for me.

Albert attempted to seek consultations and help from medical specialists in Australia. However, both specialists he reached out to responded in an unsupportive manner:

> I just wanted to talk to him [the first specialist] about it, and he says, that was your business going over there, all I can suggest is other antibiotics, that was it. And I went and saw the

> infectious disease expert, and he said 'Oh you need to have the operation.' So, I haven't seen them in two years.

In Albert's opinion, their reluctance was because he had received an unorthodox therapy provided by an overseas medical facility. His remark draws attention to the disruption in the continuity of care when patients like Albert return to their home countries after receiving treatment in a foreign coun:

> It's crossing their medical line. They're not going to get involved with it because it's not an official treatment in Australia.

12.4.3 Travelling Phages

Other patients in our sample had not travelled to receive phage therapies, but instead phages travelled to them. Currently, the alternative to patients travelling overseas for phage therapies is to purchase the phages directly. For example, a man who has bronchiectasis knew about phage therapy after reading reports and scientific journal articles and books on the subject and contacted a scientist after seeing him present on television about his research on bacterial phages. He had his infectious disease specialist assist him in receiving a phage sample specific for the pathogen he carried, which was delivered to Australia in a phial and administered by his specialist or GP. The procedure would cost him about AU$4,000 (~ US$2,705) out of pocket. In our interview, he described himself as an experiment and believed that if his case was successful, it would also help other people with bronchiectasis. Similarly, a woman patient (who has a *Pseudomonas* infection in the bone behind her ear) read about phage therapy on the internet after her nine-year-old grandson watched a YouTube programme about phages. She contacted a microbiologist and an infectious disease specialist about phage therapy and was advised that her treating specialist would have to apply to the Therapeutic Goods Administration for approval if she wished to phage therapy in Australia. She was not considering travelling to Europe, so intended to pursue this option.

12.5 Considerations for future research

A contribution of this chapter is to describe international medical travel for phage therapy and the movement of phages across borders to treat chronic AMR infections. We provide a glimpse of the experience of patients travelling overseas to seek phage therapy through several cases collected as part of a recent qualitative study exploring the social burden of living with AMR. In doing so, we address a knowledge gap in the current body of scholarship on medical travel and the lived experience of AMR. In this concluding section, we highlight the common themes found in the patient cases presented in this chapter and recommend several areas for future research to focus on.

Travel for all kinds of healthcare has become part of people's repertoire of potential options for healthcare when access is unavailable, restricted, of poor quality, or unaffordable in their home country. Travel for phages in particular is occurring among highly vulnerable patients. As the two case studies of Sandra and Albert suggest, patients reported difficulty in obtaining reliable and comprehensible information prior to and throughout their journeys of seeking phage therapy, which remains an unorthodox treatment in most Western countries. For both patients, they relied heavily on the internet to research phage and the potential place of care. The internet played a vital role in shaping the travel experience overseas and contributing to the continuity of care. Travellers turned to the websites of the clinics they wished to receive phage from as the primary source of treatment information. Informants used emails to source expert knowledge from scientists across the world when communication with their local care team about phage was challenging. Emails and internet-based instant messaging (such as WhatsApp) were also common means of communication with the clinic in their medical travel destination prior to one's arrival to arrange for pre-treatment sample testing and receive necessary information at the time of treatment. Online communication continued beyond the hospital-based treatment when patients required the use of phage upon returning to their coun of residence.

Patients were often left on their own to make the decision to travel overseas to obtain phage with minimal involvement of a medical team in their home coun. Their travelling accounts point to the urgent need for greater access to information on phage therapy for patients and clinicians to help them better navigate through the options available for managing antibiotic resistant infections. As living, dynamic, evolving, and specific entities, phages do not easily fit into regulatory categorisation, norms, and dominant models of drug development (Brives and Pourraz, 2020). It is very difficult to design standard double-blinded placebo-controlled trials for phage therapy, given the complexity of infections, the fact that many patients have other medical conditions which have contributed to their AMR infections, and the variation in the phage treatments given to control them. Generally, case reports have been the favoured means of reporting on effectiveness. This has hampered the development and legitimacy of the treatment. Further research into the effectiveness of phage therapies and viable models of phage production and scalability would greatly facilitate the dissemination of knowledge of phages and their potential as an alternative to treatments with antimicrobials.

Findings from the existing literature often note the intermediary role of a third party, usually facilitation companies, in influencing the decision-making, the choice of the treatment destination, and the experience of medical travel, for instance, in terms of selecting providers, facilitating provider-patient communication, or assisting with the logistics of their trips (Hunter, 2020; Whittaker, 2018). In our study, we only interviewed one man who used a medical tourism company to arrange his medical travel after experiencing mistrust with conventional biomedical treatment and the medical team in his home coun. The patient had travelled to China and India for non-orthodox treatment before going to Georgia to obtain phage therapy – a mark of his desperation and frustration to find a treatment after repeated courses of antibiotics had offered little relief to his chronic infections and his frustration with the therapies offered to him. China is among the few places in the world treating chronic prostate infections with antibiotic injections into the urethra. It is a destination associated with experimental treatments in 'grey areas' between approved clinical practices and unauthorised experimentation (Sleeboom-Faulkner, 2016) and has come under criticism in the science media (Cyranoski, 2012), attracting the moniker of the 'Wild East' (Chen, 2009; Song, 2011). In that specific case, the medical tourism company helped the patient resolve a conflict with the foreign hospital where he received treatment, which involved an additional charge of a multiple-thousands-dollar bill. Utilising the service of any facilitating party was however not observed for most of the patient cases we interviewed who travelled overseas to receive phage therapy. While this may mitigate the risks of being exploited by the facilitators (Hartmann, 2019; Whittaker, 2018), patients are left to privately deal with the intricacies of international travel, from coping with language barriers to navigating throughout a foreign health system they are unfamiliar with. Compounding with the unwillingness of the doctors in their coun of residence to discuss options such as phage therapies, the heavy reliance on the internet for seeking information, this lack of assistance from a facilitating third party leaves patients vulnerable to potentially harmful or exploitative practices and with few legal protections should they fall subject to malpractice.

Both case studies highlight the need to attend to the monitoring of phage when patients returned to their home coun, which often became frustrating and interfered with the effectiveness of their treatment overseas and the continuity of care. The current scholarship has captured the risks to medical travellers, highlighting the fragmented care they experience post-treatment (Chen and Wilson, 2013; Kundury et al., 2024). When complications result from a treatment that is not widely recognised in mainstream care such as phage therapy, patients are often constrained when seeking post-travel care due to the unavailability of expertise and resources to attend to their issues within the current health sector. Patients like Albert met with resistance from local medical specialists when handling follow-up care, which may deter patients from seeking timely help and render the post-travel care a personal struggle hidden to the health system in their home coun.

Access to therapies across borders is only an option for those with the financial resources and physical health to travel. Our sample includes other patients whose conditions did not permit them to travel for treatments. Many of those with severe AMR infections are not in a position to undertake journeys for therapies. While alternative treatments like phage therapy remain available only for compassionate use, the demand for cross-border treatment is likely to rise. As the AMR crisis heightens globally, there will be a growing demand for a range of treatments for AMR, including not only new therapies, but old therapies used in new ways such as travelling phages. The question of equity of access to care and treatment and inequalities (Brives and Pourraz, 2020) needs examination – it should not depend upon one's income or ability to travel.

The distress and social burden of AMR infections are growing. The stories of these patients travelling to engage in phage therapies underline not only the suffering caused by these infections but also the determination of patients as agents in seeking treatments, often at considerable personal expense. More research is needed into the social and psychological burdens of AMR infections and the 'chronic living' (Wahlberg et al., 2021) of AMR 'survivors' and their pursuits for treatment. From a public health perspective, further research with larger samples is needed to address the needs and options for those living with chronic AMR infections that prove intractable to standard treatments, particularly as the numbers of people with AMR infections grow. In addition, in-depth analyses of the travelling experience to different treatment destinations and accounts of patients receiving compassionate phage therapy are critical to inform patient decision-making and strategies to mitigate medical travel-related risks. Knowledge from such studies is especially valuable to health policymakers, insurance regulators, and the medical community of the sending countries who are concerned with the delivery of patient-centred care in the fight against AMR.

One of the major challenges we faced when conducting the study on the lived experience of AMR was recruiting due to the lack of a community of people who self-identified as suffering from AMR. As a result, this sample represents a small purposive sample of people who recognise themselves as having AMR infections. We only interviewed one man who actively engaged with fellow patients while pursuing treatment overseas and positioned himself as a pioneer and patient advocate. The majority of patients had a similar experience to Sandra in one of the two cases illustrated in this chapter, who pointed to the perceived lack of social support and the need to connect with peers suffering similar medical conditions. Unlike conditions such as cancer or HIV, which are linked with strong patient advocacy and community action (Rabinow, 2010; Petersen et al., 2019), there are few AMR patient advocacy initiatives globally (IDSA, 2022; Narrative, 2023). It is difficult for people suffering from AMR infections to constitute a 'biosocial' group (Rabinow, 2010) whose collective identity is formed around aspects of their biological status. People living with chronic AMR infections experience a wide range of infections affecting various parts of their bodies, making it difficult for them to identify as a single biosocial group with a single common condition. This lack of a unified social identity hinders the formation of a cohesive survivor community and limits the development of effective support programmes and policies. Consequently, there is a critical need for social science researchers to explore patient activism and identity formation in the context of AMR. In addition, understanding how individuals with chronic AMR infections develop a shared identity can identify areas for strengthening community bonds and support networks for the AMR survivor community. By focusing on these areas, future research in the social sciences can contribute to the development of a supportive and empowered community for those affected by AMR, ultimately improving their health outcomes and quality of life.

12.6 Ethics approval

Ethical clearance was sought through the Monash University Human Research Ethics Committee (Project ID: 29413). All participants provided written informed consent to participate in the study. All names used in this chapter are pseudonyms.

References

Ahwireng-Obeng, F. and van Loggerenberg, C. (2011) 'Africa's middle class women bring entrepreneurial opportunities in breast care medical tourism to South Africa', *The International Journal of Health Planning and Management*, *26*(1), 39–55.

Álvarez, A., Fernández, L., Iglesias, B., Rodríguez, J., Rodríguez, A. and García, P. (2020) 'Phage therapy: Unexpected drawbacks to reach hospitals', *Future Virology*, *14*(12), 779–782.

Bergmann, S. (2011) 'Reproductive agency and projects: Germans searching for egg donation in Spain and the Czech Republic', *Reproductive Biomedicine Online*, *23*(5), 600–608.

Brives, C. and Pourraz, J. (2020) 'Phage therapy as a potential solution in the fight against AMR: Obstacles and possible futures', *Palgrave Communications*, *6*(1), 1–11.

Brophy, J. (2017) 'Navigating the "grey areas": Australian medical travellers in China's stem cell bionetwork', *Asia Pacific Viewpoint*, *58*(2), 216–227.

Centers for Disease Control (2021) *How Antimicrobial Resistance Happens*. https://www.cdc.gov/antimicrobial-resistance/about/?CDC_AAref_Val=https://www.cdc.gov/drugresistance/about/how-resistance-happens.html

Cham, T.-H., Lim, Y.-M., Sia, B.-C., Cheah, J.-H. and Ting, H. (2021) 'Medical tourism destination image and its relationship with the intention to revisit: A study of Chinese medical tourists in Malaysia', *Journal of China Tourism Research*, *17*(2), 163–191.

Chee, H. L. and Whittaker, A. (2020) 'Moralities in international medical travel: Moral logics in the narratives of Indonesian patients and locally-based facilitators in Malaysia', *Journal of Ethnic and Migration Studies*, *46*(20), 4264–4281.

Chen, H. (2009) 'Stem cell governance in China: From bench to bedside?', *New Genetics and Society*, *28*(3), 267–282.

Chen, L. H. and Wilson, M. E. (2013) 'The globalization of healthcare: Implications of medical tourism for the infectious disease clinician', *Clinical Infectious Diseases*, *57*(12), 1752–1759.

Closas, A. M. (2021) *Taming Egg Donors: The Production of the Egg Donation Bioeconomy in Spain*. PhD, Monash University, Melbourne.

Connell, J. (2015) 'From medical tourism to transnational health care? An epilogue for the future', *Social Science & Medicine*, *124*, 398–401.

Connell, J. (2016) 'Reducing the scale? From global images to border crossings in medical tourism', *Global Networks*, *16*(4), 531–550.

Crush, J. and Chikanda, A. (2015) 'South–South medical tourism and the quest for health in Southern Africa', *Social Science & Medicine*, *124*, 313–320.

Crush, J., Chikanda, A. and Maswikwa, B. (2012) 'Patients without borders: Medical tourism and medical migration in Southern Africa', *The Southern African Migration Programme*, Migration Policy Series No. 57.

Crush, J., Chikanda, A., Sanders, D. and Maswikwa, B. (2015) 'The rise of medical tourism to South Africa'. In Lunt, N., Horsfall, D. and Hanefeld, J. (Eds.), *Handbook on Medical Tourism and Patient Mobility*. Edward Elgar Publishing, 323—331.

Cyranoski, D. (2012) 'China's stem-cell rules go unheeded: Health minis's attempt at regulation has had little effect', *Nature*, *484*(7393), 149–151.

Djebara, S., Maussen, C., De Vos, D., Merabishvili, M., Damanet, B., Pang, K. W., De Leenheer, P., Strachinaru, I., Soentjens, P. and Pirnay, J.-P. (2019) 'Processing phage therapy requests in a Brussels military hospital: Lessons identified', *Viruses*, *11*(3), 265.

Donovan, P. (2017) 'Access to unregistered drugs in Australia', *Aust. Prescr.*, *40*(5), 194–196.

Everingham, S. G. and Whittaker, A. (2023) 'Trends in engagement in surrogacy by nationality 2018–2020: A survey of surrogacy agencies', *Global Reproductive Health*, *8*(1), e64.

Fabijan, A. P., Lin, R. C. Y., Ho, J., Maddocks, S., Iredell, J. R., Westmead Bacteriophage Therapy Team (2019) 'Safety and tolerability of bacteriophage therapy in severe Staphylococcus aureus infection', *bioRxiv*, p. 619999.

Franchina, L., Sarradon-Eck, A., Arnault, Y., Le Corroller, A.-G., Zunic, P. and Marino, P. (2022) 'Lived experience of State-sponsored intra-national overseas therapeutic mobility for stem cell transplantation', *Social Science & Medicine, 301*, 114957.

Frenz, M. (2019) 'Introduction: Medical tourism or movement for healthcare? Reflections on (inter-)national cross-border mobility', *Global Public Health, 14*(3), 321–325.

Goodrich, J. N. (1993) 'Socialist Cuba: A study of health tourism', *Journal of Travel Research, 32*(1), 36–41.

Hanefeld, J., Smith, R., Horsfall, D. and Lunt, N. (2014) 'What do we know about medical tourism? A review of the literature with discussion of its implications for the UK National Health Service as an example of a public health care system', *Journal of Travel Medicine, 21*(6), 410–417.

Hanefeld, J. D., Horsfall, D. P., Lunt, N. P. and Smith, R. P. (2013) 'Medical tourism—cure or malaise for the National Health Service: A mixed methods study', *The Lancet (British Edition), 382*(S3), S40.

Hartmann, S. (2019) 'Mobilising patients towards transnational healthcare markets–insights into the mobilising work of medical travel facilitators in Delhi', *Mobilities, 14*(1), 71–86.

Helsinki Declaration of the World Medical Association (2014) 'Ethical principles of medical research involving human subjects', *Pol Merkur Lekarski, 36*(215), 298.

Hunter, B. M. (2020) 'Going for brokerage: Strategies and strains in commercial healthcare facilitation', *Globalization and Health, 16*(1), 49.

IDSA (2022) *Patient Stories: The Faces of Antimicrobial Resistance*. https://amr.solutions/2017/03/22/idsas-faces-of-antimicrobial-resistance-faor-report/

Inhorn, M. C. (2012) 'Reproductive exile in global Dubai: South Asian stories', *Cultural Politics, 8*(2), 283–306.

Inhorn, M. C. (2015) *Cosmopolitan Conceptions: IVF Sojourns in Global Dubai*. Duke University Press.

Inhorn, M. C. and Gürtin, Z. B. (2011) 'Cross-border reproductive care: A future research agenda', *Reproductive Biomedicine Online, 23*(5), 665–676.

Inhorn, M. C. and Patrizio, P. (2009) 'Rethinking reproductive "tourism" as reproductive "exile"', *Fertility and Sterility, 92*(3), 904–906.

Jones, M. R. (2008) *Skintight: An Anatomy of Cosmetic Surgery*. Berg Publishers.

Kakasis, A. and Panitsa, G. (2019) 'Bacteriophage therapy as an alternative treatment for human infections. A comprehensive review', *International Journal of Antimicrobial Agents, 53*(1), 16–21.

Kangas, B. (2010) 'Traveling for medical care in a global world', *Medical Anthropology, 29*(4), 344–362.

König, A. (2023) 'Reproductive entanglements in times of war: Transnational gestational surrogacy in Ukraine and beyond', *Medical Anthropology*, 1–14.

Kundury, K. K., Shylaja, K. C. and Namitha (2024) 'Concerns and considerations in medical tourism: An overview', in Chaudhary, B., Bhatia, D., Patel, M., Singh, S. and Sharma, S. (Eds.), *Medical Tourism in Developing Countries: A Contemporary Approach*. Springer Nature Singapore, 35–51.

Kutateladze, M. and Adamia, R. (2008) 'Phage therapy experience at the Eliava Institute', *Médecine et Maladies Infectieuses, 38*(8), 426–430.

Kutter, E. M., Kuhl, S. J. and Abedon, S. T. (2015) 'Re-establishing a place for phage therapy in western medicine', *Future Microbiol, 10*(5), 685–688.

Leitner, L., Ujmajuridze, A., Chanishvili, N., Goderdzishvili, M., Chkonia, I., Rigvava, S., Chkhotua, A., Changashvili, G., McCallin, S. and Schneider, M. P. (2021) 'Intravesical bacteriophages for treating urinary tract infections in patients undergoing transurethral resection of the prostate: A randomised, placebo-controlled, double-blind clinical trial', *The Lancet Infectious Diseases*, *21*(3), 427–436.

Lunt, N. and Carrera, P. (2010) 'Medical tourism: Assessing the evidence on treatment abroad', *Maturitas*, *66*(1), 27–32.

Lunt, N., Horsfall, D. and Hanefeld, J. (2016) 'Medical tourism: A snapshot of evidence on treatment abroad', *Maturitas*, *88*, 37–44.

Luong, T., Salabarria, A.-C. and Roach, D. R. (2020) 'Phage therapy in the resistance era: Where do we stand and where are we going?', *Clin. Ther.*, *42*(9), 1659–1680.

Matorras, R. (2005) 'Reproductive exile versus reproductive tourism', *Hum. Reprod.*, *20*(12), 3571; author reply 3571–3572.

McCallin, S., Sacher, J. C., Zheng, J. and Chan, B. K. (2019) 'Current state of compassionate phage therapy', *Viruses*, *11*(4), 343.

Moll, T., Gerrits, T., Hammarberg, K., Manderson, L. and Whittaker, A. (2022) 'Reproductive travel to, from and within sub-Saharan Africa: A scoping review', *Reproductive Biomedicine & Society Online*, *14*, 271–288.

Murray, C. J., Ikuta, K. S., Sharara, F., Swetschinski, L., Aguilar, G. R., Gray, A., Han, C., Bisignano, C., Rao, P. and Wool, E. (2022) 'Global burden of bacterial antimicrobial resistance in 2019: A systematic analysis', *The Lancet*, *399*(10325), 629–655.

Narrative, A. (2023) *The AMR Narrative – Voices Together for Antimicrobial Resistance*. https://amrnarrative.org/.

OECD (2018) *Stemming the Superbug Tide: Just a Few Dollars More*. OECD Paris.

O'Neill, J. (2016) 'Tackling drug-resistant infections globally: Final report and recommendations'. https://amr-review.org/sites/default/files/160518_Final%20paper_with%20cover.pdf

Ormond, M. (2015) 'Solidarity by demand? Exit and voice in international medical travel–the case of Indonesia', *Social Science & Medicine*, *124*, 305–312.

Ormond, M. and Lunt, N. (2020) 'Transnational medical travel: Patient mobility, shifting health system entitlements and attachments', *Journal of Ethnic and Migration Studies*, *46*(20), 4179–4192.

Pande, A. (2014) *Wombs in Labor: Transnational Commercial Surrogacy in India*. Columbia University Press.

Patey, O., McCallin, S., Mazure, H., Liddle, M., Smithyman, A. and Dublanchet, A. (2018) 'Clinical indications and compassionate use of phage therapy: Personal experience and literature review with a focus on osteoarticular infections', *Viruses*, *11*(1), 18.

Petersen, A., Munsie, M., Tanner, C., MacGregor, C. and Brophy, J. (2017) *Stem Cell Tourism and the Political Economy of Hope*. Springer.

Petersen, A., Schermuly, A. C. and Anderson, A. (2019) 'The shifting politics of patient activism: From bio-sociality to bio-digital citizenship', *Health*, *23*(4), 478–494.

Rabinow, P. (2010) 'Artificiality and enlightenment: From sociobiology to biosociality', *Politix*, *2*, 21–46.

Sacher, J. C. and Zheng, J. (2021) 'Phage therapy collaboration and compassionate use', *Bacteriophages: Biology, Technology, Therapy*, 1069–1098.

Saha, D. and Mukherjee, R. (2019) 'Ameliorating the antimicrobial resistance crisis: Phage therapy', *IUBMB Life*, *71*(7), 781–790.

Scheper-Hughes, N. (2011) 'Mr Tati's holiday and João's safari. Seeing the world through transplant tourism', *Body & Society*, *17*(2–3), 55–92.

Sleeboom-Faulkner, M. E. (2016) 'The large grey area between "bona fide" and "rogue" stem cell interventions—Ethical acceptability and the need to include local variability', *Technological Forecasting and Social Change*, *109*, 76–86.

Smith, C. and Jenner, P. (2000) 'Health tourism in Europe', *Travel & Tourism Analyst*, *1*, 41–59.

Song, P. (2011) 'The proliferation of stem cell therapies in post-Mao China: Problematizing ethical regulation', *New Genetics and Society*, *30*(2), 141–153.

Suh, G. A., Lodise, T. P., Tamma, P. D., Knisely, J. M., Alexander, J., Aslam, S., Barton, K. D., Bizzell, E., Totten, K. M. C., Campbell, J. L., Chan, B. K., Cunningham, S. A., Goodman, K. E., Greenwood-Quaintance, K. E., Harris, A. D., Hesse, S., Maresso, A., Nussenblatt, V., Pride, D., Rybak, M. J., Sund, Z., van Duin, D., Van Tyne, D. and Patel, R. (2022) 'Considerations for the use of phage therapy in clinical practice', *Antimicrobial Agents and Chemotherapy*, *66*(3), e02071-21.

Turner, L. (2013) 'Transnational medical travel: Ethical dimensions of global healthcare', *Cambridge Quarterly of Healthcare Ethics*, *22*(2), 170–180.

Van Hoof, W., Pennings, G. and De Sutter, P. (2015) 'Cross-border reproductive care for law evasion: A qualitative study into the experiences and moral perspectives of French women who go to Belgium for treatment with donor sperm', *Social Science & Medicine*, *124*, 391–397.

Wahlberg, A., Jieun, M., Dokumaci, A., Kingod, N., Svensson, M. and Heinsen, L. (2021) Chronic living: Ethnographic explorations of daily lives swayed by (multiple) medical conditions. *Somatosphere*. https://somatosphere.com/2021/chronic-living.html/

Whittaker, A. (2008) 'Pleasure and pain: Medical travel in Asia', *Global Public Health*, *3*(3), 271–290.

Whittaker, A. (2015) 'The implications of medical travel upon equity in lower and middle income countries', in Hanefeld, J., Lunt, N. and Horsfall, D. (Eds.), *Handbook on Medical Tourism and Patient Mobility*. Edward Elgar Publishing, 112—122.

Whittaker, A. (2018) *International Surrogacy as Disruptive Indus in Southeast Asia*. Rutgers University Press.

Whittaker, A. and Chee, H. L. (2015) 'Perceptions of an "international hospital" in Thailand by medical travel patients: Cross-cultural tensions in a transnational space', *Social Science & Medicine*, *124*, 290–297.

Whittaker, A., Chee, H. L. and Por, H. H. (2017) 'Regional circuits of international medical travel: Prescriptions of trust, cultural affinity and history', *Asia Pacific Viewpoint*, *58*(2), 136–147.

Whittaker, A., Do, T. T., Davis, M. D. M. and Barr, J. (2023) 'AMR survivors? Chronic living with antimicrobial resistant infections', *Global Public Health*, *18*(1), 2217445.

Whittaker, A., Inhorn, M. C. and Shenfield, F. (2019) 'Globalised quests for assisted conception: Reproductive travel for infertility and involuntary childlessness', *Global Public Health*, *14*(12), 1669–1688.

Whittaker, A., Manderson, L. and Cartwright, E. (2010) 'Patients without borders: Understanding medical travel', *Medical Anthropology*, *29*(4), 336–343.

World Health Organization (2023) 'Antimicrobial resistance'. https://www.who.int/news-room/fact-sheets/detail/antimicrobial-resistance

13 A psychedelic research agenda? The quest for therapeutic and legal legitimacy

Muireann Quigley and Matt Hayler

13.1 Introduction

We are demonstrably in the middle of a mental health crisis. In the European Union (EU), for instance, a recent Eurobarometer survey estimated that 21 million people, or 4.5% of European citizens, are affected by depressive disorders alone (European Council, 2024). The cost of mental ill health to the UK economy has been estimated to be £118 billion per year, or 5% of GDP. Meanwhile, for the EU, this is estimated to be in the region of €600 billion, or more than 4% of GDP (European Council, 2024). Although these figures are likely to be significant underestimates of the true costs, they do give a sense of the vast scale of real human suffering. Yet, despite this, and the arguably questionable efficacy of existing treatments (Penn & Tracy, 2012), very few new drug therapies for mental health disorders get approved. For instance, in 2024 the European Medicines Agency (EMA) recommended 114 new medicines for approval for human use (EMA, 2025a, p. 1). In 2023, this number was 77 (EMA, 2024a, p. 1). However, in 2024, only three of these were listed in the psychiatric medicines category (one antipsychotic for treating schizophrenia and two for ADHD) (EMA, 2024a, p. 6). The previous year none were for treating mental health disorders of any variety. This is compared, for example, to 28 and 25 new drugs, respectively, for a variety of cancers in these years (EMA, 2024a, p. 3; EMA, 2025a, p. 3). This is despite the prevalence of depressive mental ill health, for instance, being roughly similar to that of cancer (around 5% of European citizens have had a cancer diagnosis in their lifetimes) (EU Science Hub, 2024).

Against this background, so-called psychedelics – such as psilocybin, lysergic acid diethylamide (LSD), N,N-dimethyltryptamine (DMT), and 3,4-methylenedioxymethamphetamine (MDMA/midomafetamine) – offer new and potentially highly efficacious treatments for conditions that are widespread, debilitating, difficult to treat, and surrounded by stigma. Following their near-blanket ban from the 1970s to the early 2000s, there has been an escalating resurgence of interest in, research on, and use of psychedelics to treat a range of psychological disorders. These include depression, anxiety, obsessive-compulsive disorder, eating disorders, substance abuse, and post-traumatic stress disorder (PTSD) (Yao *et al.*, 2024). Clinical studies on these substances – for example, the use of psilocybin for the treatment of major depressive disorder and treatment-resistant depression, and the use of MDMA-assisted therapy (MDMA-AT) for PTSD – are showing some promising results regarding both immediate symptomatic relief and long-term improvements to quality of life (Carhart-Harris *et al.*, 2016; Mitchell *et al.*, 2023). In light of this research, there has been increasing pressure from some quarters to (facilitate research in order to) make these substances available for therapeutic use (Neill, 2024; Bliss, 2025). Indeed, if substances such as psilocybin and MDMA can be shown to help even a fraction of those affected, they would represent a revolution in care. However, nothing, as they say, is that simple.

The principal reason for this is that in many jurisdictions around the world, including European countries, psychedelics (including psilocybin and MDMA) are so-called 'Schedule 1' substances under national drugs laws.[1] This means that, according to the law, they are considered to have no therapeutic value and to pose a high public health risk. As Schedule 1 substances, they are subject to the highest level of restrictions under national regimes, generally meaning that their use, possession, and sale are illegal. Consequently, for a psychedelic substance to be legally prescribed, dispensed, and used, it would require not only medicines authorisation by the relevant medicines regulators, but also rescheduling under national drugs control laws. Until recently, both things seemed unlikely. Yet, within a relatively short time span, we have moved from a situation where this was considered by many researchers and legislators to be functionally impossible, to one where, if the hype in some circles was to be believed, the path to new and better psychedelic futures was all but assured.

In recent years, psilocybin, MDMA, and LSD have all been granted 'breakthrough therapy' designation by the US Food and Drug Administration (FDA) and so-called Innovation Passports (as part of their Innovative Licensing and Access Pathway) by the UK's Medicines and Healthcare products Regulatory Agency (MHRA). Further, in 2023, although not approved for use by their medicines regulator, the Therapeutic Goods Administration (TGA), Australia rescheduled both psilocybin and MDMA and made them available for therapeutic use (with a prescription from a specialist psychiatrist) (TGA, 2023). On the back of all of this, and following a series of apparently successful clinical trials, it had been widely expected that in 2024 the FDA would approve a New Drug Application (NDA) from Lykos Therapeutics for an MDMA/midomafetamine-assisted therapy (MDMA-AT) for the treatment of PTSD (Reardon, 2023). However, following a meeting of the Psychopharmacologic Drugs Advisory Committee (AdCom) (an independent advisory panel to the FDA) in June 2024, the FDA rejected the application, leaving unresolved questions about if, when, and how this might now become possible.

In this chapter, we examine the quest for psychedelic therapeutic and legal legitimacy that is currently playing out in Europe and elsewhere. We begin by looking at what psychedelics are, the therapeutic promissory which has developed in relation to these substances, and how they differ from standard drug treatments for their target disorders. We will see that they are qualitatively different from other sorts of drugs that are ordinarily used to treat mental health conditions in clinical medicine; something which stems from both the psychotherapeutic or psychological-assistance component of these therapies, as well as the distinctive pharmacological modes of action and effects of the substances themselves. Noting that these substances are set against a socio-cultural and academic backdrop of over 50 years of prohibition, we then examine the ongoing quest for legitimacy in this area. On this, we demonstrate how psychedelics' legal status as Schedule 1 substances represents a significant impediment to this quest, not only to their clinical use, but also in terms of generating the evidence necessary to support such use. Given this, in the final section, we examine some of the hurdles which need to be surmounted if the psychedelic promissory is to move beyond hype and be proven to be safe, effective, and ethical.

13.2 The psychedelic therapeutic promissory

The term psychedelics includes a wide range of psychoactive substances that can be broadly divided into the so-called 'classical' and 'non-classical' psychedelics. The classical psychedelics – or serotonergic psychedelics – consist of substances such as: psilocybin, which is found in magic mushrooms; LSD, a synthetic substance first discovered and produced by Albert Hofmann in 1943; N,N-dimethyltryptamine (DMT), the active ingredient in ayahuasca, a brew used in the Amazon basin for at least 3,000 years; and mescaline, from the San Pedro or peyote cactus, used by Native Americans as part of indigenous religious ceremonies. Meanwhile, the 'non-classical' psychedelics include substances such as: ketamine, which is already licensed around the world for certain uses, including as a sedative, anaesthetic, and painkiller; and MDMA, also known more commonly as molly or ecstasy (particularly when in pill form). Whilst all of these (and more) have potential clinical applications, in this chapter, we focus mainly on psilocybin and MDMA. We do this because these have garnered the most mainstream attention, have long histories of recreational usage, represent examples from the two broad categories described, and have been the targets of the most research and promise in therapeutic settings. They also represent test cases where their relative success or failure in clinical application may well shape how other compounds are received, both clinically and by regulatory bodies.

The modes of action and the effects of psychedelics are of a qualitatively different ilk to standard pharmaceuticals used within the clinical sphere because they induce states of altered mood and consciousness. Significantly, for some, these modes of altered subjectivity are thought to be part of how these substances work (Yaden and Griffiths, 2021). Whilst both classical and non-classical psychedelics significantly alter mood, perception, and cognition, classical psychedelics such as psilocybin and ayahuasca also induce powerful hallucinations as part of their mode of action. The non-classical psychedelics such as MDMA do not (except at very high doses and for some users) have hallucinogenic effects. The different substances have distinct modes of action, and there are a variety of theories about how they bring about their therapeutic effects (McCulloch *et al.*, 2022). Users of both classes of these substances, including participants in clinical trials, describe a multitude of experiences distinct to psychedelics. Depending on the substance, these can include vivid visual hallucinations; feelings of the self or ego dissolving away; states of greater 'openness' and 'connection' (to fellow humans, non-human animals, and to environments); spiritual awakenings; insights into trauma; the capacity to communicate difficult experiences; being jolted out of negative and ruminatory thought loops; and viewing the world in a different way (Belser *et al.*, 2017; Holze *et al.*, 2020).

Whilst these psychedelic experiences are often positive, it is not uncommon for users to experience difficulties. Research by Evans and colleagues, for example, indicates a range of issues – social, perceptual, cognitive, emotional, existential, and ontological – which may be challenging following a psychedelic experience. They also document how those who have used psychedelics can experience subsequent problems of self-perception, somatic and behavioural difficulties, and how they can, for some, trigger psychotic episodes (Evans *et al.*, 2023). Capturing these challenging experiences, then, is crucial to ensuring a balanced evaluation of psychedelics' effects. The positives, and seemingly low rate of negative incidents, of psychedelic-assisted therapies might well justify the risk for any one individual (as with the justification of side effects of any number of commonly used pharmaceuticals, including anti-depressants). Nevertheless, better awareness of psychedelics' most deleterious effects, their true frequency, and common risk factors is necessary, not least so that patients can be adequately informed should these substances become more widely available for therapeutic use.

The clinical use of psychedelics also stands apart from other therapeutics in two significant ways. First, they are not pill-a-day type therapies. In contrast to standard medication for depression, for instance, those being treated with psilocybin will take maybe two to three doses spaced a few weeks apart. Whilst this could be repeated in the future, perhaps in 6 to 12 months if the patient experiences a regression with regard to their symptoms, this is far from a pill-a-day therapy. Second, and perhaps even more significantly, the psychedelic will typically be administered as part of a psychotherapeutic encounter involving a talking therapy (typically a bespoke, non-directive approach) that is modified by a drug for one or two sessions. As we will explain shortly, these are variously (and varyingly) understood as 'psychedelic-*assisted*' or 'psychedelic-*supported*' therapies. Thus, psychedelic therapies are not simply a different class of pharmaceutical; they are hybrid therapeutic encounters.

Whilst the psychedelic-assisted or -supported encounter can vary significantly, a semi-standardised treatment model is starting to emerge where attention is paid to the total 'set, setting, and support system' of the encounter (MAPS, 2017, p. 6). This model consists of four stages: assessment, preparation, the psychedelic experience, and integration. First, the patient is assessed to ensure that they are suitable for the therapy; in particular, that there are no contraindications, such as a history of psychosis. Second, they are actively prepared for what they will experience. Third, they are provided with a safe environment in which to immerse themselves and experience the psychedelic therapy (Roseman, Nutt, & Carhart-Harris, 2018). Fourth, they are supported beyond the immediate psychedelic experience to ensure that they can process and integrate 'insights' from what can be an intense process. As we will see in more detail in section four, and despite this emerging model, concerns about the exact nature and role of the psychotherapeutic component of psychedelic-assisted or -supported therapies loomed large during the FDA AdCom discussion and likely played a significant role in the eventual rejection by the FDA of Lykos Therapeutics' application for the approval of MDMA-AT.

Nevertheless, whether principally led by the effects of the compounds themselves or their combination with the psychotherapeutic settings in which they are administered, the results from clinical studies of both classical and non-classical psychedelics indicate that these substances could become positioned as supplements to, alternatives to, or even replacements for existing pharmacological and psychotherapeutic interventions (e.g. Carhart-Harris *et al.*, 2016; Wighton, 2016; Mithoefer *et al.*, 2018; Bogenschutz *et al.*, 2022). If this promise holds, deepens, or reveals further avenues for treatment in larger studies, then the therapeutic potential of these substances cannot be overstated, particularly in light of the mental health crisis noted in the introduction.

13.3 The (ongoing) quest for psychedelic legitimacy?

Arguably, the principal impediment to both the clinical use of, and indeed the generation of clinical evidence regarding, psychedelics is their legal status. As mentioned, they are listed in the UN Convention on Psychotropic Substances as 'Schedule 1' drugs. The Convention was drafted explicitly to address concerns regarding 'the public health and social problems resulting from the abuse of certain psychotropic substances' and to acknowledge that 'rigorous measures are necessary to restrict the use of such substances to legitimate purposes' (United Nations, 1971, p. 1). The most 'rigorous' measures in this respect – that possession, use, sale, and supply of these substances are illegal – are reserved for Schedule 1 drugs. Being listed as Schedule 1, in the terms of the Convention, means that they were (and indeed still are until they are rescheduled) considered to have little, or typically no, therapeutic benefits and to carry serious public health risks, whatever that might be taken to mean (United Nations, 1971, p. 17). The impact of the inclusion of these substances in the Convention cannot be overstated. It is a hugely influential international treaty with 185 state signatories, including the US, UK, and all EU member states (United Nations, 1971). Moreover, many countries' national drugs control laws mirror the provisions of the Convention (Rolfe & Lancaster, 2024), meaning that, in the eyes of the law, they are considered to have no medicinal value.

Interestingly, up until the 1960s and 1970s, when the convergence of reactionary politics and social conservatism meant that these substances were de facto banned, psychedelics had been reasonably commonly used by psychiatrists and psychotherapists to treat a variety of conditions. We do not lay out this history here, which is in any case well documented elsewhere (Langlitz, 2013; Pollen, 2018), but note that, as a result of intentional political will, psychedelics became constructed and reconfigured as a kind of pharmaceutical bogeyman within mainstream consciousness. Moreover, this lack of legitimacy was then reinforced by the introduction of the UN scheduling and the mirroring of this by national drugs control laws. Apart from the more obvious consequences for individuals (in terms of the criminalisation of and lack of access to these substances for recreational use), the scheduling of psychedelic substances has meant that their research and medical use has been subject to an almost complete ban. In the UK, for instance, as Schedule 1 drugs, doctors cannot prescribe psychedelics such as psilocybin and MDMA. Meanwhile, although it is not impossible in principle to do research on psychedelics, political, legal, and socio-cultural factors have combined to make it extremely difficult. Again, in the UK, a domestic licence from the Home Office is required to conduct research using these substances, along with an import licence if the drugs are not available domestically (Bunn & Naulls, 2023). Once the relevant licences are obtained, these also come with numerous restrictive requirements; for instance, licensing and compliance site visits will be mandated (Home Office, 2019), along with the need to have extensive and specific security arrangements in place for the storage and movement of the drugs (Home Office, 2022). This makes even basic research costly and time-consuming, which, particularly when accompanied by social and disciplinary stigma, is enough to prevent most researchers from carrying out such research (Howard *et al.*, 2021; Nutt, 2023).

Having said all of this, and despite the manifold hurdles imposed, by the mid-2000s and into the 2010s the so-called 'psychedelic renaissance' was well underway with a plethora of studies on psilocybin and MDMA in particular (Griffiths *et al.*, 2006; Griffiths *et al.*, 2008; Carhart-Harris *et al.*, 2012). Thus, the tide began to turn, at first slowly, and then, recently, very rapidly with the emergence of an increasingly convincing body of evidence relating to psychedelic substances for a range of disorders (Tupper *et al.*, 2015). The Multidisciplinary Association for Psychedelics Studies (MAPS) Public Benefit Corporation, a spinout of MAPS later rebranded to Lykos Therapeutics, submitted the first application for 'breakthrough therapy' status for MDMA-AT for PTSD, with the FDA assessing and granting the request in 2017 (MAPS, 2017). Following this, breakthrough designation has been granted to four other sponsors: in 2018 to Compass Pathways (a UK-based company) for the use of psilocybin for treatment-resistant depression (Compass Pathways, 2018); in 2019, to a US-based non-profit, the Usona Institute, for developing a treatment for major depressive disorder using psilocybin (BusinessWire, 2019); and in March 2024 to Mind Medicine for the use of LSD in generalised anxiety disorder and to Cybin for psilocybin for major depressive disorder (Cybin, 2024; MindMed, 2024). Additionally, for MDMA and psilocybin respectively, in 2022 MAPS and Compass Pathways were both given so-called Innovation Passports by the UK's MHRA (MAPS, 2022; Compass Pathways, 2022).

Given the Schedule 1 status of these compounds, we should not underestimate the significance of all of this. Substances granted FDA breakthrough designation, and those on the MHRA's Innovative Licencing and Access Pathway (ALAP), benefit from being able to access a range of extra and dedicated support. These authorisations represent watershed moments in the history of psychedelics and a move towards mainstream acceptance that hadn't been conceivable in at least half a century. The move from counterculture and the fringes of research back into mainstream consciousness was also, seemingly, further solidified in 2023. Although they have not been approved by the TGA, Australia's medicines regulator, both psilocybin and MDMA were nevertheless rescheduled, thus making them available, in practice, for therapeutic use in Australia by specialist prescribers (Therapeutic Goods Administration, 2023). Interestingly, absent from much of the reporting around this is the fact that this change was the result of intensive lobbying by the mental health interest group Mind Medicine Australia (Ministry of Health, Welfare and Sport (The Netherlands), 2024, pp. 190–192) and that the final decision from the TGA in favour of rescheduling was preceded by three negative interim decisions (Mind Medicine Australia, n.d.). Nevertheless, subsequent to this, much of the reporting around Lykos' application for MDMA-AT for PTSD suggested that regulatory approval was a foregone conclusion (Psychedelic Alpha, 2023), with the probability of authorisation and rescheduling of other substances, and in other jurisdictions, predicted to increase thereafter (Reardon, 2023). However, as noted earlier, in August 2024, and following the AdCom discussion in June that year (Hardman, 2024), the FDA rejected Lykos' application. In so doing, and as we will see in more detail in the next section, the quest for psychedelic legitimacy has arguably shifted from the political and socio-cultural battlegrounds which characterised previous decades to more evidential and methodological disputes which need to be resolved if psychedelic medicine is to move forward.

13.4 Towards better psychedelic futures? Hope not hype

For those who fought the earlier battles in search of psychedelic legitimacy, the FDA decision came as both a bitter blow and an unwelcome setback (Price, 2024). However, by attending to some of the various challenges brought into focus by the mainstreaming of the therapeutic use of psychedelics, there is now an opportunity to move towards better and more solid psychedelic futures. In this final section, therefore, we take a closer look at some of these challenges – legal and regulatory, methodological, ethical, and practical – and at what needs to happen in order to address them. Whilst there is not space to deal with all of these in detail, we offer an overview of some of the most pressing areas, indicating what we believe to be the most significant current and future research topics and directions in this area.

13.4.1 Evidence and Ethics in Psychedelics Trials

Although prior to the FDA AdCom panel meeting there had been widespread belief amongst activists and advocates that Lykos Therapeutics' application for MDMA-AT would be approved, in the run-up to the meeting there were indications that approval might not be as smooth a process as had come to be assumed. A draft report by the Institute for Clinical and Economic Review (ICER), published just a couple of months before the AdCom meeting, set out a litany of methodological and ethical concerns regarding Lykos' proposed therapy (Mustafa *et al.*, 2024). Moreover, the FDA briefing document, which preceded the AdCom meeting, mirrored these concerns which then dominated discussion on the day. Key amongst these were: (1) concerns about the experimental design and validity of the data, in particular issues of functional unblinding, expectation bias, and selection bias; (2) the exact contribution of the psychotherapeutic component to the overall treatment effect; (3) a failure to adequately record and capture the treatment's negative sequelae; and (4) ethical concerns about both the conduct of the trials and even trial therapists (FDA, 2024; Mustafa *et al.*, 2024).

Functional unblinding refers to the fact that, due to the psychopharmacological effects of a drug (in this case MDMA), it is effectively impossible to blind participants as to whether they are in the active or placebo arm of a trial. Expectation bias occurs when a person's prior expectations or beliefs about the treatment affect the results. In this specific case, some trial participants may have held strong beliefs regarding the efficacy of MDMA-AT (FDA, 2024). On this, the ICER report noted that participants' 'feelings around psychedelics lead the community to engage with them more like a religious movement than like pharmaceutical products' (Mustafa *et al.*, 2024). Any expectation bias here is likely related to a pronounced selection bias in the recruitment of trial participants: 'the participants in the trials, including therapists and some number of the patients, came from a community with strong prior beliefs about the value of psychedelics for management of serious mental health conditions' (Mustafa *et al.*, 2024, p. 8). Given these potential biases, there were concerns about how this affected the validity of the data from the trials. Moreover, concerns over selection bias also fed into those regarding the safety of MDMA-AT. The fact that 40% of Lykos' clinical trial participants had previously taken MDMA may have made the safety data seem better than it otherwise would have been (Hardman, 2024).

In addition to these issues, there were significant questions raised about the role of the psychotherapeutic component in the overall therapy, and whether and how the effect of this could be disentangled from the pharmacological effects of the MDMA itself (FDA, 2024, pp. 38–39; Hardman, 2024). Comments in this respect ranged from statements about how the regulation of psychotherapies does not fall within the FDA's remit to concerns about the fact that no comparison had been made with existing psychotherapeutic modalities (Hardman, 2024). In essence, the fact that the psychotherapeutic component in both active and placebo arms was MAPS/Lykos' own bespoke therapy means that the efficacy of MDMA-AT had not been compared to existing gold standard treatments for PTSD (Mustafa *et al.*, 2024). The AdCom discussion also contained allegations of pressure to report good outcomes in order to bolster the results of the trial, and that negative outcomes were downplayed (or potentially even suppressed) (Mustafa *et al.*, 2024). Meanwhile, the ICER report contained a troubling allegation of sexual misconduct by therapists during Lykos' Phase II trial (Mustafa *et al.*, 2024, p. 8).

The failure of Lykos to secure FDA approval for MDMA-AT could be viewed as a particularly concrete instantiation of what Yaden and colleagues have dubbed the 'bursting of the psychedelic hype bubble' (Yaden, Potash, & Griffiths, 2021, p. 943). The hype bubble, as Noorani and colleagues describe it, 'had created sector-wide investment volatility and premature enthusiasm about clinical trial outcomes, alongside concern about methodological rigour' (Noorani *et al.*, 2023). Further, they note that '[t] he number of registered clinical trials has exploded, raising concerns about poorly designed, underpowered trials, the use of questionable research practices, and a lack of transparency' (Noorani *et al.*, 2023). Against this backdrop, the FDA decision could be viewed as a much-needed course correction, offering an opportunity to redress the balance away from exaggerated claims and overhyped expectations towards more realistic, evidence-based, attainable, and ethical psychedelic futures. Exactly how this should be done, however, especially to the satisfaction of the regulators, is one of the pressing challenges for researchers in this area.

13.4.2 Regulating Psychedelics as Medicines

The FDA decision notwithstanding, in numerous respects we are still headed towards more permissive law and policy regarding the therapeutic use of psychedelics. Albeit as a result of lobbying, and not universally welcomed (Rossell *et al.*, 2023, p. 935), we have already seen that Australia is leading the way in this respect. Concurrently, several states in the US and Canada have relaxed, or are in the process of relaxing, their approach to psychedelics (Psychedelic Alpha, 2024a, 2024b). In the UK and mainland Europe, appetite for change regarding these substances, and indeed the practicalities of moving them from research into clinical application, seems to be gathering pace, with increased engagement on a number of fronts. There has been an increase in activism from a variety of groups regarding the therapeutic use of psychedelics (Francis, 2023; Bliss, 2025). These include long(er)-standing organisations such as Psychedelics Europe (an association of private, NGO, and academic researchers) and Drug Science (a committee of scientists, academic researchers, and policy makers), but also the establishment of new interest groups such as the Psychedelic Access and Research European Alliance (PAREA, a non-profit that brings together academia with private research, patient organisations, and medical associations) (Hawrot, 2022). In the UK, there has been an increasingly open approach to questions regarding the use of psychedelics for therapeutic purposes during Parliamentary debates (Price, 2023; Rough, Garratt, & Sutherland, 2023). This has been accompanied by a series of POSTbriefs on different aspects of psychedelics from the Parliamentary Office of Science and Technology (POST) (Bunn & Naulls, 2023).

Further, at the end of 2023, the UK Government's Advisory Council on the Misuse of Drugs (ACMD) published its advice on barriers to research on Schedule 1 controlled drugs, advising that, for certain purposes, Schedule 1 drugs be treated *as if* they were on Schedule 2 (ACMD, 2023). This was followed in 2025 by the announcement of a pilot to exempt universities and hospitals 'from the need to apply for a Home Office domestic licence and instead to operate in accordance with the requirements of Schedule 2 Controlled Drugs' (Home Office, 2025). Also in 2025, following a lengthy public consultation period, the EMA's Guideline on the clinical investigation of medicinal products in the treatment of depression came into effect. This included a section on psychedelics (EMA, 2025b). Additionally, during the consultation period, in early 2024, the EMA hosted a multi-stakeholder workshop on psychedelics (EMA, 2024b). Amongst other things, the workshop participants discussed different regulatory perspectives, as well as methodological, safety, and implementation challenges and considerations. Around the same time, the State Commission on MDMA (a government commission) in the Netherlands published a report (hereafter, Dutch Report) which recommended that efforts be made to make MDMA-AT available (albeit the report does not recommend rescheduling at the moment). Nevertheless, whilst all of this speaks to the increasing legitimation of psychedelics, significant barriers remain; many of which are a result of the current legal and regulatory landscapes. The primary issue here is the restrictive scheduling of these substances.

Because current scheduling affects the ability of researchers to generate the kind of evidence necessary to satisfy the various medicines regulators (discussed in the previous section), if we are to move forward and build a more solid evidence base regarding therapeutic use, then addressing the scheduling of psychedelics is likely to be necessary sooner rather than later. Part of the problem, as noted in the ACMD's report, is the time and cost implications associated with the controlled drugs licensing process and permissions for Schedule 1 drugs (ACMD, 2023, pp. 7–9). Moving these drugs down one schedule to Schedule 2 would significantly reduce these, and so previously there have been calls for the wholesale rescheduling of these substances (Royal Pharmaceutical Society, n.d.; Hawkes, 2018; Howard *et al.*, 2021). However, whilst rescheduling might, on the face of it, look like the simpler and more expedient option, the scheduling of controlled drugs is not just about use in the research context. The schedule in which a drug is placed also dictates whether it can be prescribed, dispensed, bought and sold, and legally possessed. Given this, although calls for psychedelics to be rescheduled are understandable, to do so now might be to put the clinical cart before the research horse in terms of regulatory reform. This is because, as section 13.4.1 demonstrated in the context of MDMA-AT, there are still evidential, methodological, and indeed ethical challenges which need to be addressed regarding the clinical use of psychedelics.

It is perhaps for this reason that the ACMD's preferred approach consists of options that involve, for instance, exempting research in universities and hospitals, or that which is conducted as part of clinical trials, from the need for a domestic licence, and allowing research in these contexts to operate in accordance with the less onerous requirements of Schedule 2 drugs (ACMD, 2023). Broadly, such an approach seems sensible since, as set out in section 13.4.1, one of the principal sticking points currently is the need for more and better evidence regarding the therapeutic benefits of these substances (whether this comes as integrally bundled with a psychotherapeutic component or not). However, there are two things to note here. First, although, as already noted, and acting on the ACMD report, a limited pilot to treat Schedule 1 controlled drugs as if they are on Schedule 2 has been announced by the UK Government, the exact shape and scope of this was not publicly available at the time of writing. Whilst this is undoubtedly a crucial first step for more and better evidence generation (Neill, 2024), the likely success and impact of the pilot will lie in the detail. Second, in the longer term, if and when evidence is produced to the satisfaction of the regulators, and they approve the first psychedelics as medicines, scheduling beyond the research context would need to be revisited. This is because, as we have already noted, a drug's scheduling affects who can legally possess it, use it, prescribe it, and so on. Therefore, once, for example, psilocybin or MDMA has been approved by a regulator, then in order for it to be able to be used in practice, it would need to be moved out of Schedule 1. In the UK, one solution would be for psychedelics with medicines approvals to join other commonly prescribed controlled drugs on Schedule 2: for example, diamorphine/heroin. However, even this may prove less straightforward than it arguably ought to be.

Post-Brexit, whilst drugs control, such as a drug's scheduling, is a UK-wide matter, medicines authorisations are not. Pursuant to the Northern Ireland Protocol, the MHRA is responsible for medicines authorisations in Great Britain (England, Scotland, and Wales), whilst Northern Ireland continues to fall under the purview of the EU's EMA. Thus, we may end up in a situation of regulatory divergence between the different UK jurisdictions (as is already occurring in other areas such as medical devices regulation (Quigley *et al.*, 2023)). The situation in mainland Europe is even more complicated. Medicines authorisation is a centralised process, meaning that once the EMA approves a medicine, that substance is automatically approved for use as a medicine in each EU member state. However, drugs control is not 'harmonised' across EU member states. As such, each member state may have to reschedule newly approved psychedelics nationally, something which would likely lead to delays and be subject to a range of political and socio-cultural factors which might either help or hinder the process in each country.

13.4.3 Psychedelics in (Clinical) Practice

Before we finish, it is important to acknowledge that even if the evidential and ethical challenges outlined are addressed to the satisfaction of various medicines regulators, and even if psychedelics are approved for therapeutic use and the particular substances rescheduled to permit their prescription, practical barriers to their more widespread use would nevertheless remain. These range from a lack of availability domestically of pharmaceutical grade versions of these substances, to a lack of infrastructure for importing and distributing them, to the fact that, even if moved to Schedule 2, a stringent set of requirements would need to be met for would-be importers, manufacturers, prescribers, and other actors. This is something aptly demonstrated by the example of cannabis-based products for medicinal use (CBPMs). These were moved from Schedule 1 to Schedule 2 in 2018. Yet, despite this, they have not gained widespread clinical use. There are a range of reasons for this, but key amongst them are the continuing licensing requirements (see, e.g., MHRA, 2020), as well as the continued framing and treatment of these products as 'contested objects' by various professional bodies and regulators (Case, 2021). It is likely that the more widespread clinical use of psychedelics could encounter similar issues. Unlike CBPMs which remain unlicensed, it may be that these issues could be at least partially mitigated if and when psychedelic substances, such as psilocybin and/or MDMA, gain medicines authorisations. However, even this may not be the panacea that some may hope for.

As outlined in section 13.2, at least in the short term, psychedelic-assisted therapies are more time and resource intensive than standard 'pill-a-day' therapies. This is especially the case within the increasingly standardised four-phase model which includes psychotherapist-led assessment, preparation, and later integration phases, as well as the monitored psychedelic experience itself. As such, there will be significant cost, infrastructure, and resource issues in rolling out psychedelic-assisted therapies at scale. In the UK, for example, there are already exceedingly long waiting times for people to be able to access talking therapies within the National Health Service (NHS). This situation would almost certainly be exacerbated with the introduction of a drug therapy which also has a psychotherapeutic component, particularly if rapid, high efficacy, and low risk results for common mental health conditions become widely publicised. Demand for experienced psychiatrists, psychotherapists, and prescribing clinicians, all working in tandem, would likely also reinforce regional differences in care.

Psychedelic-assisted therapies could also not simply be rolled out within existing infrastructures. As we have explored above, they are not the same as standard clinical psychological therapies, such as pill-a-day approaches or Cognitive Behavioural Therapy (CBT). Those acting in supportive therapeutic roles before, during, and after psychedelic experiences will need specific training (Phelps & Henry, 2022), not least because existing therapeutic training is not up to the task of preparing therapists for the levels of power imbalance that can be experienced working with a highly dependent client in a psychedelic state (Caporuscio & Kind, 2024). Such training would require thousands of therapists' will/motivation (something which may be significantly shaped by psychedelics' social history and changing place in the mainstream), time (at least multiple weeks, but typically months), money (in the thousands-of-pounds per therapist or funded by government), and expertise (knowledge sharing being vital to the rapid, informed, and ethical growth of psychedelic therapy pedagogy).

Whilst organisations, such as MAPS and Fluence in the US, and Clerkenwell Health and PsyEdu in the UK, have created and started deploying such training (Fluence, n.d.; PsyEdu, n.d.;MAPS, 2023; Clerkenwell Health, 2024), arguably the type and form that any psychotherapeutic component ought to take is not yet supported by a convincing evidence base (something that was one of the issues for the FDA when assessing Lykos' application). As yet, although there are emerging sets of practices, there is not an established body of learning and resources for psychedelic therapy that comes anywhere close to being comparable with that which exists for more standard psychotherapeutic modalities available privately or through the NHS. As a recent British Association for Counselling and Psychotherapy (BACP) article asks, 'are the counselling and psychotherapy professions in a position to react quickly enough to get on board' if there is a sudden regulatory change (Jackson, 2023)? We would suggest that, currently, they are not. Indeed, the question of the kinds of expertise therapists might require goes beyond theory. There is a live debate as to whether or not first-hand, subjective experience of these substances by those administering the therapy is necessary (or indeed ought to be mandatory in experiential training). Psychedelic experiences, and the work involved in processing them, can be profound, yet theoretically shareable. And whilst therapists with lived psychedelic experiences might better understand their patients and, thus, be better equipped to build the trust vital to therapeutic encounters, commentators are divided on whether lived psychedelic experience is necessary (Dames *et al.*, 2024; Emmerich & Humphries, 2024).

In short, whilst medicines regulation is a significant piece of the psychedelic puzzle, psychotherapy's own regulatory bodies, such as the BACP and the UK Council for Psychotherapy, will also need to prepare and act if the psychedelic promissory is to include psychedelic-assisted therapies, with all that they might offer.

13.5 Conclusion

Despite the recent setback (in the eyes of some) in the US with the FDA rejection of Lykos Therapeutics' NDA, an ever-growing set of promissory visions, futures, and, indeed, economies still surround psychedelics. Moreover, the psychedelic promissory and attendant imaginaries are not only actively reshaping the social and legal landscapes in which these substances sit (Schwarz-Plaschg, 2022), but potentially 'the nature of the interventions themselves' (Noorani, Bedi, & Muthukumaraswamy, 2023, p. 5892). This is evident from the increased (and increasingly successful) lobbying of organisations such as Mind Medicine Australia and PAREA in the EU. It is also evident from the shifting legal and regulatory contexts, such as the rescheduling of psilocybin and MDMA in Australia and their decriminalisation and licensing in certain US states. As we have seen throughout this chapter, the challenges in relation to this mainstreaming of the therapeutic use of psychedelics are manifold. They range from issues of evidence and ethics, which currently threaten to derail the psychedelic therapeutic promissory, and the (arguably overhyped) expectations surrounding this, to the practicalities of navigating misaligned medicines regulation and national drugs control systems.

Given this, there are a number of issues – scientific/methodological/clinical, socio-legal, political, institutional, and policy-related – which need to be explored further and addressed if the psychedelic promissory is to be realised and turned into a desirable reality in Europe. Future research agendas, then, must at least in part be interdisciplinary, ensuring that researchers are communicating insights and enabling new knowledge that could not be achieved in disciplinary silos. We suggest that the most pressing areas include: (1) better establishing efficacy (and particularly in light of whether and how these substances assist/are assisted by psychotherapeutic support); (2) dealing with trial issues such as functional unblinding; (3) understanding the implications of rescheduling, and exploring alternatives to support psychedelic research; (4) establishing patterns of need and desire in both publics and practitioners; and (5) identifying bottlenecks and un-/under-examined issues – infrastructural, practical, ethical – specific to psychedelics ahead of any potential rollout consequent upon regulatory regime change. Psychedelics hold the potential to mitigate one of the great public health issues of our time, but progress will stall, in Europe and elsewhere, without prioritising the careful and un-hyped exploration and resolution of these issues.

Acknowledgements

We would like to thank Helena da Costa, Alana Farrell, and Matt Jordan for their research assistance on work that contributed to this piece. We would also like to thank Tehseen Noorani, Christoph Bublitz, Josh Hardman, and Louise Hatherall for helpful discussion and comments. All errors remain our own. Work on this piece was supported by the University of Birmingham's College Research Fund and through the University's Institute of Advanced Studies funded 'Psychedelics and Regulatory Decision-making' project.

Note

1. Note that some countries number their schedules differently; for example, in Australia Schedule 9 is the equivalent of Schedule 1. However, for ease, we refer to these as Schedule 1 substances throughout.

References

ACMD (2023) *ACMD Consideration of Barriers to Research Part 2: Schedule 1 Controlled Drugs*, 22 December, pp. 1–25. https://assets.publishing.service.gov.uk/media/65857643ed3c3400od3bfdc5/221223-_Barriers_to_Research_II_Report__final_.pdf

Belser, A. B. *et al.* (2017) 'Patient experiences of psilocybin-assisted psychotherapy: An interpretative phenomenological analysis', *Journal of Humanistic Psychology*, *57*(4): 354–388.

Bliss, C. (2025) 'PsychedeliCare launches first European citizens' initiative demanding political action on psychedelic-assisted therapies', *Psychedelic Alpha*, 14 January. https://psychedelicalpha.com/news/psychedelicare-launches-first-european-citizens-initiative-demanding-political-action-on-psychedelic-assisted-therapies

Bogenschutz, M. P. *et al.* (2022) 'Percentage of heavy drinking days following psilocybin-assisted psychotherapy vs placebo in the treatment of adult patients with alcohol use disorder: A randomized clinical trial', *JAMA Psychiatry*, *79*(10): 953–962.

Bunn, S. & Naulls, S. (2023) 'Psychedelic drugs to treat depression', Rapid response POSTbrief, 7 August. https://doi.org/10.58248/RR09

Caporuscio, C. & Kind, A. (2024) 'Therapist, trip sitter or guide? A second-person perspective on psychedelic-assisted psychotherapy', in R. Lovering (Ed.), *The Palgrave Handbook of Philosophy and Psychoactive Drug Use*. Cham, Switzerland: Palgrave Macmillan, 513–530.

Carhart-Harris, R. L. *et al.* (2012) 'Neural correlates of the psychedelic state as determined by fMRI studies with psilocybin', *Proceedings of the National Academy of Sciences of the United States of America*, *109*(6): 2138–2143.

Carhart-Harris, R. L. *et al.* (2016) 'Psilocybin with psychological support for treatment-resistant depression: An open-label feasibility study', *The Lancet Psychiatry*, *3*(7): 619–627.

Case, P. (2021) 'Medicinal cannabis prescribing: A study of boundary work and medico-legal risk', *Modern Law Review*, *84*(6): 1189–1226.

Clerkenwell Health (2024) 'Clerkenwell Health launches new therapist free training programme to remove bottlenecks in the psychedelic industry', 10 May [press release]. https://www.clerkenwellhealth.com/blog/psychedelic-therapist-training

Compass Pathways (2018) 'COMPASS pathways received FDA breakthrough therapy designation for psilocybin therapy for treatment-resistant depression', 23 October [press release]. https://ir.compasspathways.com/News--Events-/news/news-details/2018/COMPASS-Pathways-receives-FDA-Breakthrough-Therapy-designation-for-psilocybin-therapy-for-treatment-resistant-depression/default.aspx

Compass Pathways (2022) 'Annual review 2022', p. 4. https://compasspathways.com/wp-content/uploads/2023/03/Compass-Pathway-Annual-Review-2022.pdf

Cybin (2024) 'Cybin receives FDA breakthrough therapy designation for its novel psychedelic molecular CYB003 and announces positive four-month durability data in major depressive disorder', 13 March [press release]. https://ir.cybin.com/investors/news/news-details/2024/Cybin-Receives-FDA-Breakthrough-Therapy-Designation-for-its-Novel-Psychedelic-Molecule-CYB003-and-Announces-Positive-Four-Month-Durability-Data-in-Major-Depressive-Disorder/default.aspx

Dames, S. *et al.* (2024) 'Psychedelic-assisted therapy training: An argument in support of firsthand experience of nonordinary states of consciousness in the development of competence', *Psychedelic Medicine*, *2*(3): 130–137.

EMA (2024a) *Human Medicines Highlights 2023*, 16 January.https://www.ema.europa.eu/en/documents/other/human-medicines-highlights-2023_en.pdf

EMA (2024b) 'EMA multi-stakeholder workshop on psychedelics – Workshop report', 16–17 April. https://www.ema.europa.eu/en/documents/report/report-ema-multi-stakeholder-workshop-psychedelics_en.pdf

EMA (2025a) *Human Medicines in 2024*, 16 January. https://www.ema.europa.eu/en/documents/report/human-medicines-2024_en.pdf

EMA (2025b) *Draft Guideline on the Clinical Investigation of Medicinal Products in the Treatment of Depression, EMA/CHMP/185423/2010*, Revision 3 (20 January 2025).

Emmerich, N. & Humphries, B. (2024) 'Is the requirement for first-person experience of psychedelic drugs a justified component of a psychedelic therapist's training?', *Cambridge Quarterly of Healthcare Ethics*, *33*(4): 548–557.

EU Science Hub (2024) *Cancer Burden: 1 in 20 Europeans Has Faced a Cancer Diagnosis in their Lifetime*. Belgium: Joint Research Centre, 31 January. https://joint-research-centre.ec.europa.eu/jrc-news-and-updates/cancer-burden-1-20-europeans-has-faced-cancer-diagnosis-their-lifetime-2024-01-31_en

European Council (2024) *Mental Health*. Last updated: 23 April. https://www.consilium.europa.eu/en/policies/mental-health/#state

Evans, J. *et al.* (2023) 'Extended difficulties following the use of psychedelic drugs: A mixed methods study', *PloS One*, *18*(10): e0293349.

FDA (2024) 'Briefing document: Psychopharmacologic drugs advisory committee meeting', 4 June. https://www.fda.gov/media/178984/download

Fluence (n.d.) 'Psychedelic therapy education'. https://www.fluencetraining.com/

Francis, S. (2023) 'Relax rules on research into illegal drugs, say advisers', *BBC*, 22 December. https://www.bbc.co.uk/news/uk-politics-67801919

Griffiths, R. R. *et al.* (2006) 'Psilocybin can occasion mystical-type experiences having substantial and sustained personal meaning and spiritual significance', *Psychopharmacology*, *187*(3): 268–292.

Griffiths, R. *et al.* (2008) 'Mystical-type experiences occasioned by psilocybin mediate the attribution of personal meaning and spiritual significance 14 months later', *Journal of Psychopharmacology*, *22*(6): 621–632.

Hardman, J. (2024) 'Live coverage: FDA advisory committee reviews MDMA-assisted therapy for PTSD', *Psychedelic Alpha*, 4 June. https://psychedelicalpha.com/news/live-coverage-fda-advisory-committee-reviews-mdma-assisted-therapy-for-ptsd

Hawkes, N. (2018) 'Cannabis based drugs should be rescheduled to make research and prescribing easier, says Chief Medical Officer', *BMJ (Clinical Research Ed.)*, *362*, 5 July.

Hawrot, T. (2022) Interviewed by *VJ Neurology*. Austria: European Academy of Neurology Congress 2022 (26 June). https://www.vjneurology.com/video/_jameqlulpi-parea-psychedelic-assisted-therapies-in-europe/

Holze, F. *et al.* (2020) 'Distinct acute effects of LSD, MDMA, and D-amphetamine in healthy subjects', *Neuropsychopharmacology*, 45: 462–471.

Home Office, UK (2019) *Controlled Drugs: Domestic Licences* (online). https://www.gov.uk/guidance/controlled-drugs-domestic-licences

Home Office, UK (2022) *Security Guidance for All Existing or Prospective Home Office Controlled Drug Licensees and/or Precursor Chemical Licensees or Registrants* (online). https://assets.publishing.service.gov.uk/media/63a1b6c8e90e075874d91825/Security_Guidance_for_all_Businesses_and_Other_Organisations_v1.5_Nov_2022.pdf

Howard, A. *et al.* (2021) 'Schedule 1 barriers to research in the UK: An in-depth qualitative analysis', *Drug Science, Policy and Law*, *7*.

Jackson, C. (2023) 'The big issue: Is working with psychedelics the future of therapy?', *Therapy Today*, *34*(6). https://www.bacp.co.uk/bacp-journals/therapy-today/2023/july-august-2023/the-big-issue/

Langlitz, N. (2013) *Neuropsychedelia*. California: University of California Press.

MAPS (2017) 'FDA grants breakthrough therapy designation for MDMA-assisted therapy for PTSD, agrees on special protocol assessment for phase 3 trials', 26 August (press release). https://maps.org/news/media/press-release-fda-grants-breakthrough-therapy-designation-for-mdma-assisted-psychotherapy-for-ptsd-agrees-on-special-protocol-assessment-for-phase-3-trials/

MAPS (2022) 'MAPS is granted innovation passport in United Kingdom for MDMA as an adjunct to therapy for PTSD', 25 January (press release). https://maps.org/2022/01/25/maps-is-granted-innovation-passport-in-united-kingdom-for-mdma-as-an-adjunct-to-therapy-for-ptsd/

MAPS (2023) 'MDMA therapy training program update', 18 January (press release). https://maps.org/2023/01/18/mdma-therapy-training-program-update-january-2023/

McCulloch, D. E.-W. *et al.* (2022) 'Psychedelic resting-state neuroimaging: A review and perspective on balancing replication and novel analyses', *Neuroscience and Biobehavioral Reviews*, *138*: 104689.

MHRA (2020) *The Supply, Manufacture, Importation and Distribution of Unlicenced Cannabis-Based Products for Medicinal Use in Human 'Specials'*. https://assets.publishing.service.gov.uk/media/5e58eefb86650c53a363f77c/Cannabis_Guidance__unlicensed_CBPMs__updated_2020.pdf

MindMed (2024) 'MindMed received FDA breakthrough therapy designation and announces positive 12-week durability data from phase 2B study of MM120 for generalized anxiety disorder', 7 March (press release). https://ir.mindmed.co/news-events/press-releases/detail/137/mindmed-receives-fda-breakthrough-therapy-designation-and-announces-positive-12-week-durability-data-from-phase-2b-study-of-mm120-for-generalized-anxiety-disorder

Mind Medicine Australia (n.d.) 'TGA rescheduling'. https://mindmedicineaustralia.org.au/tga/

Ministry of Health, Welfare and Sport (The Netherlands) (2024) 'MDMA /// beyond ecstasy', *Report of the State Commission on MDMA*. https://www.government.nl/documents/reports/2024/05/31/mdma-beyond-ecstasy

Mitchell, J. M. *et al.* (2023) 'MDMA-assisted therapy for moderate to severe PTSD: A randomized, placebo-controlled phase 3 trial', *Nature Medicine*, *29*(10): 2473–2480.

Mithoefer, M. C. *et al.* (2018) '3,4-Methylenedioxymethamphetamine (MDMA)-assisted psychotherapy for post-traumatic stress disorder in military veterans, firefighters, and police officers: A randomised, double-blind, dose-response, phase 2 clinical trial', *Lancet Psychiatry*, 5(6): 486–497.

Mustafa, R. A. *et al.* (2024) *3,4-Methylenedioxymethamphetamine Assisted Psychotherapy for Post-Traumatic Stress Disorder: Effectiveness and Value. Draft Evidence Report.* Institute for Clinical and Economic Review, 26 March. https://icer.org/wp-content/uploads/2024/03/PTSD_Draft-Report_For-Publication_03262024.pdf

Neill, J. (2024) 'It is high time the U.K. changes psychedelics laws', *The Regulatory Review*, 22 April. https://www.theregreview.org/2024/04/22/neil-it-is-high-time-the-u-k-changes-psychedelics-laws/

Noorani, T. *et al.* (2023) 'A perspective from the "reimagining psychedelic trials" working group – psychedelic alpha', *Psychedelic Alpha*, 2 February. https://psychedelicalpha.com/news/a-perspective-from-the-reimagining-psychedelic-trials-working-group

Noorani, T., Bedi, G. & Muthukumaraswamy, S. (2023) 'Dark loops: Contagion effects, consistency and chemosocial matrices in psychedelic-assisted therapy trials', *Psychological Medicine*, 53(13): 5892–5901.

Nutt, D. (2023) *Psychedelics: The Revolutionary Drugs that Could Change Your Life – A Guide from the Expert.* London: Yellow Kite.

Penn, E. & Tracy, D. K. (2012) 'The drugs don't work? Antidepressants and the current and future pharmacological management of depression', *Therapeutic Advances in Psychopharmacology*, 2(5): 179–188.

Phelps, J. & Henry, J. (2022) 'Foundation for training psychedelic therapists', *Current Topics in Behavioural Neurosciences*, *56*: 93–109.

Pollen, M. (2018) *How to Change Your Mind: The New Science of Psychedelics*. London: Allen Lane.

Price, S. (2023) 'UK advisory body issues rapid response on psychedelic research', *Psychedelic Health*, 24 August. https://psychedelichealth.co.uk/2023/08/24/uk-advisory-body-rapid-response-on-psychedelic-research/

Price, S. (2024) 'What's next for MDMA therapy following FDA rejection?', *Psychedelic Health*, 21 August. https://psychedelichealth.co.uk/2024/08/21/whats-next-for-mdma-therapy-following-fda-rejection/

Psychedelic Alpha (2023) 'Second phase 3 study of MDMA-assisted therapy reports positive results, paving way for new drug application', 14 September. https://psychedelicalpha.com/news/second-phase-3-study-of-mdma-assisted-therapy-reports-positive-results-paving-way-for-new-drug-application

Psychedelic Alpha (2024a) 'Mapping psychedelic drug policy reform in the United States', 14 March. https://psychedelicalpha.com/data/psychedelic-laws

Psychedelic Alpha (2024b) 'Worldwide psychedelic laws tracker'. https://psychedelicalpha.com/data/worldwide-psychedelic-laws

PsyEdu (n.d.) 'Professional certificate in psychedelic practice'. https://www.psyedu.co.uk/professional-certificate-in-psychedelic-practice

Quigley, M. *et al.* (2023) 'The shape of medical devices regulation in the United Kingdom? Brexit and beyond', *Law, Technology and Humans*, 5(2): 21–42.

Reardon, S. (2023) 'US could soon approve MDMA therapy – Opening an era of psychedelic medicine', *Nature*, 19 April. https://www.nature.com/articles/d41586-023-01296-3

Rolfe, E. & Lancaster, H. (2024) 'Psychedelic medicines 2024', *Mackrell Solicitors* (last updated 21 November). https://practiceguides.chambers.com/practice-guides/comparison/1322/14777/23117-23123-23126

Roseman, L., Nutt, D. & Carhart-Harris, R. (2018) 'Quality of acute psychedelic experience predicts therapeutic efficacy of psilocybin for treatment-resistant depression', *Frontiers in Pharmacology*, 8(974).

Rossell, S. L. *et al.* (2023) 'Why didn't the TGA consult with Australian researchers and clinicians with experience in psilocybin-assisted psychotherapy for treatment-resistant major depressive disorder?', *Australian & New Zealand Journal of Psychiatry*, *57*(7): 935–936.

Rough, E., Garratt, K. & Sutherland, N. (2023) 'Debate On Access to Psilocybin Treatments', Commons Library Debate Pack No CDP 2023/0108, House of Commons Library, 18 May.

Royal Pharmaceutical Society (n.d.) 'Rescheduling of Cannabis for Medical Use'. https://www.rpharms.com/recognition/all-our-campaigns/policy-a-z/rescheduling-of-cannabis-for-medical-use

Schwarz-Plaschg, C. (2022) 'Socio-psychedelic imaginaries: Envisioning and building legal psychedelic worlds in the United States', *European Journal of Futures Research*, *10*(10): 1–16.

Therapeutic Goods Administration (2023) 'Re-scheduling of psilocybin and MDMA in the poisons standard: Questions and answers', *Australian Government: Department of Health and Aged Care*, 3 February. https://www.tga.gov.au/news/media-releases/change-classification-psilocybin-and-mdma-enable-prescribing-authorised-psychiatrists

Tupper, K. W. *et al.* (2015) 'Psychedelic medicine: A re-emerging therapeutic paradigm', *CMAJ: Canadian Medical Association Journal = Journal de l'Association Medicale Canadienne*, *187*(14): 1054–1059.

United Nations (1971) *Convention on Psychotropic Substances, 1971*. No. 14956.

Usona Institute (2019) 'FDA grants breakthrough therapy designation to Usona Institute's psilocybin program for major depressive disorder', 22 November. https://www.usonainstitute.org/updates/fda-grants-breakthrough-therapy-designation-to-usona-institutes-psilocybin-program-for-major-depressive-disorder

Wighton, K. (2016) 'Magic mushroom compound tested for treatment-resistant depression', *Imperial College Press*, 17 May. https://www.imperial.ac.uk/news/172407/magic-mushroom-compound-tested-treatment-resistant-depression/

Yaden, D. B. & Griffiths, R. R. (2021) 'The subjective effects of psychedelics are necessary for their therapeutic efficacy', *ACS Pharmacology & Translational Science*, *4*(2): 568–572

Yaden, D. B., Potash, J. B. & Griffiths, R. R. (2022) 'Preparing for the bursting of the psychedelic hype bubble', *JAMA Psychiatry*, *79*(10): 943–944.

Yao, Y. *et al.* (2024) 'Efficacy and safety of psychedelics for the treatment of mental disorders: A systematic review and meta-analysis', *Psychiatry Research*, *335*: 115886.

Index